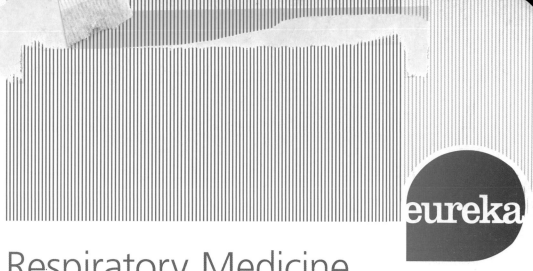

Respiratory Medicine

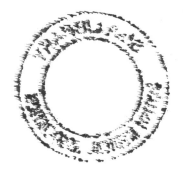

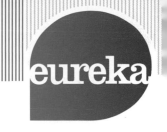

Respiratory Medicine

Laura-Jane Smith MBBChir MRCP
FHEA
Honorary Clinical Lecturer in Medical
Education
UCL Medical School
Respiratory and Medical Registrar
North East London
London, UK

Jennifer Quint MRCP PhD MSc
Senior Lecturer in Epidemiology
London School of Hygiene & Tropical
Medicine
Honorary Consultant in Thoracic
Medicine
University College Hospital
London, UK

Jeremy S Brown MBBS MRCP DPhil
Professor of Respiratory Infection
UCL Medical School
Honorary Consultant
University College Hospital
London, UK

Series Editors

Janine Henderson MRCPsych
MClinEd
MB BS Programme Director
Hull York Medical School
York, UK

David Oliveira PhD FRCP
Professor of Renal Medicine
St George's, University of London
London, UK

Stephen Parker BSc MS DipMedEd
FRCS
Consultant Breast and General
Paediatric Surgeon
St Mary's Hospital
Newport, UK

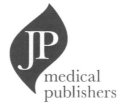

JP
medical
publishers

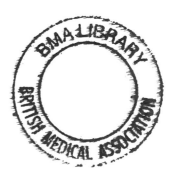

London · Philadelphia · New Delhi · Panama City

© 2015 JP Medical Ltd.

Published by JP Medical Ltd, 83 Victoria Street, London, SW1H 0HW, UK

Tel: +44 (0)20 3170 8910   Fax: +44 (0)20 3008 6180

Email: info@jpmedpub.com   Web: www.jpmedpub.com

ISBN: 978-1-907816-72-7

British Library Cataloguing in Publication Data
A catalogue record for this book is available from the British Library

Library of Congress Cataloging in Publication Data
A catalog record for this book is available from the Library of Congress

Publisher:	Richard Furn
Development Editors:	Thomas Fletcher, Paul Mayhew, Alison Whitehouse
Editorial Assistant:	Sophie Woolven
Copy Editor:	Kim Howell
Graphic narratives:	James Pollitt
Cover design:	Forbes Design
Page design:	Designers Collective

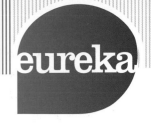

Series Editors' Foreword

Today's medical students need to know a great deal to be effective as tomorrow's doctors. This knowledge includes core science and clinical skills, from understanding biochemical pathways to communicating with patients. Modern medical school curricula integrate this teaching, emphasising how learning in one area can support and reinforce another. At the same time students must acquire sound clinical reasoning skills, working with complex information to understand each individual's unique medical problems.

The *Eureka* series is designed to cover all aspects of today's medical curricula and reinforce this integrated approach. Each book can be used from first year through to qualification. Core biomedical principles are introduced but given relevant clinical context: the authors have always asked themselves, 'why does the aspiring clinician need to know this'?

Each clinical title in the series is grounded in the relevant core science, which is introduced at the start of each book. Each core science title integrates and emphasises clinical relevance throughout. Medical and surgical approaches are included to provide a complete and integrated view of the patient management options available to the clinician. Clinical insights highlight key facts and principles drawn from medical practice. Cases featuring unique graphic narratives are presented with clear explanations that show how experienced clinicians think, enabling students to develop their own clinical reasoning and decision making. Clinical SBAs help with exam revision while Starter Questions are a unique learning tool designed to stimulate interest in the subject.

Having biomedical principles and clinical applications together in one book will make their connections more explicit and easier to remember. Alongside repeated exposure to patients and practice of clinical and communication skills, we hope *Eureka* will equip medical students for a lifetime of successful clinical practice.

Janine Henderson, David Oliveira, Stephen Parker

About the Series Editors

Janine Henderson is the MB BS undergraduate Programme Director at Hull York Medical School (HYMS). After medical school at the University of Oxford and clinical training in psychiatry, she combined her work as a consultant psychiatrist with postgraduate teaching roles, moving to the new Hull York Medical School in 2004. She has a particular interest in modern educational methods, curriculum design and clinical reasoning.

David Oliveira is Professor of Renal Medicine at St George's, University of London (SGUL), where he served as the MBBS Course Director between 2007 and 2013. Having trained at Cambridge University and the Westminster Hospital he obtained a PhD in cellular immunology and worked as a renal physician before being appointed as Foundation Chair of Renal Medicine at SGUL.

Stephen Parker is a Consultant Breast & General Paediatric Surgeon at St Mary's Hospital, Isle of Wight. He trained at St George's, University of London, and after service in the Royal Navy was appointed as Consultant Surgeon at University Hospital Coventry. He has a particular interest in e-learning and the use of multimedia platforms in medical education.

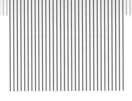
Preface

Respiratory diseases are both common and varied, and include chronic inflammatory conditions, malignancy and infectious diseases. A sound understanding of the common respiratory diseases is essential for all clinicians.

Eureka Respiratory Medicine provides the key skills to succeed in treating respiratory conditions: the ability to take a good history, interpret examination findings, integrate investigation results and apply these to the management of patients.

The book is structured to make it easy to find information in practice and during revision, and is highly illustrated to aid understanding of key concepts. Chapter 1 provides the core respiratory anatomy, physiology and immunology that are essential for an understanding of respiratory disorders. Chapter 2 outlines the clinical approach to patients, i.e. how to make sense of symptoms and signs, and the range of investigations and management options available to the clinician. The subsequent chapters describe the important respiratory diseases. Each chapter is introduced by one or more detailed cases that show how patients present, how clinicians think through the diagnosis and how they decide which investigations to perform. Chapter 11 gives concise information on respiratory emergencies and Chapter 12 explores important but often overlooked aspects of caring for patients with respiratory disease. Finally, a chapter of SBA questions with detailed answers is provided to aid revision.

We hope *Eureka Respiratory Medicine* provides students with all of the tools they require to become successful clinicians in the future.

Laura-Jane Smith, Jennifer Quint, Jeremy Brown
April 2015

About the Authors

Laura-Jane Smith is a Respiratory Registrar and Honorary Clinical Lecturer in Medical Education at University College London. She has been involved in clinical teaching throughout her career and pursued this interest further by taking a year out of training as a teaching fellow to complete a Postgraduate Certificate in Medical Education.

Jennifer Quint is a Senior Lecturer in Epidemiology at the London School of Hygiene and Tropical Medicine and a Consultant in Thoracic Medicine at University College London Hospital. She has extensive experience in teaching undergraduates and postgraduates and is a Fellow of the Higher Education Academy.

Jeremy Brown is a Consultant in Respiratory Medicine with 25 years' experience of teaching medical students, for the past 12 years at the University College of London Medical School. As well as lecturing and examining finals, he holds a weekly bedside teaching session which emphasises the importance of clinical skills.

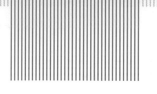

Contents

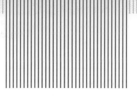

Glossary

A–a	alveolar–arterial
A1AT	α_1-antitrypsin
ABG	arterial blood gas
ABPA	allergic bronchopulmonary aspergillosis
AC	adenylyl cyclase
ACE	angiotensin-converting enzyme
ACh	acetylcholine
ACTH	adrenocorticotropic hormone
ANCA	anti–neutrophil cytoplasmic antibody
BALT	bronchus-associated lymphoid tissue
BCG	bacille Calmette–Guérin
cAMP	cyclic AMP
Ca_{O_2}	oxygen-carrying capacity of arterial blood
CAP	community-acquired pneumonia
CFA	cryptogenic fibrosing alveolitis
CFTR	cystic fibrosis transmembrane conductance regulator
CMV	cytomegalovirus
COPD	chronic obstructive pulmonary disease
CPAP	continuous positive airway pressure
CPE	complicated parapneumonic effusion
CT	computerised tomography
CTPA	computerised tomography pulmonary angiography
Cv_{O_2}	oxygen-carrying capacity of venous blood
D_{O_2}	oxygen delivery to tissues
DPLD	diffuse parenchymal lung disease
2,3-DPG	2,3-diphosphglycerate
DVLA	Driver and Vehicle Licensing Agency
EBUS	endobronchial ultrasound
ECG	electrocardiogram
EGFR	epidermal growth factor receptor
EPGA	eosinophilic granulomatosis with polyangiitis

ERV	expiratory reserve volume
ESR	erythrocyte sedimentation rate
EUS	endoscopic ultrasound
FDG	fluorodeoxyglucose
FEV_1	forced expiratory volume (in 1 s)
Fi_{O_2}	fractional concentration of oxygen in inspired air
FRC	functional residual capacity
FVC	forced vital capacity
GOLD	Global Initiative for Chronic Obstructive Lung Disease
GP	general practitioner
GPA	granulomatosis with polyangiitis
G_s	G protein
HAP	hospital-acquired pneumonia
HP	hypersensitivity pneumonitis
HSCT	haematopoietic stem cell transplant
IC	inspiratory capacity
ICS	inhaled corticosteroid
Ig	immunoglobulin
IL	interleukin
ILD	interstitial lung disease
INR	international normalised ratio
IPF	idiopathic pulmonary fibrosis
IRV	inspiratory reserve volume
K_{CO}	transfer coefficient of the lung for carbon monoxide
LABA	long-acting β_2 agonist
LAMA	long-acting muscarinic anticholinergic
LDH	lactate dehydrogenase
LLL	left lower lobe
LMWH	low-molecular-weight heparin
LUL	left upper lobe
MRC	Medical Research Council
MRI	magnetic resonance imaging

mRNA	messenger RNA	SABA	short-acting β_2 agonist
MRSA	methicillin-resistant *Staphylococcus aureus*	SAMA	short-acting muscarinic antagonist
		Sao_2	arterial oxygen saturation
NSCLC	non-small-cell lung cancer	SCLC	small-cell lung cancer
NSIP	non-specific interstitial pneumonia	SIADH	syndrome of inappropriate antidiuretic hormone hypersecretion
NTM	non-tuberculous mycobacteria		
		Svo_2	venous oxygen saturation
$PA–ao_2$	alveolar–arterial oxygen partial pressure gradient		
		TBNA	transbronchial needle aspiration
$Paco_2$	alveolar partial pressure of carbon dioxide	Th	T helper
		TLC	total lung capacity
$Paco_2$	arterial partial pressure of carbon dioxide	T_{LCO}	transfer factor of the lung for carbon monoxide
PAMP	pathogen-associated molecular pattern	TNF	tumour necrosis factor
Pao_2	alveolar partial pressure of oxygen	TNM	tumour size, nodal involvement and metastases
Pao_2	arterial partial pressure of oxygen		
PB	barometric pressure	UIP	usual interstitial pneumonia
PEF	peak expiratory flow	URTI	upper respiratory tract infection
PEFR	peak expiratory flow rate		
PET	positron emission tomography	V_A	alveolar volume
PKA	protein kinase A	VAP	ventilator-acquired pneumonia
Po_2	partial pressure of oxygen	VATS	video-assisted thoracoscopic surgery
PS	performance status	VC	vital capacity
Pvo_2	venous partial pressure of oxygen	V_{gas}	gas transfer through a membrane
		VO_2	oxygen consumption
R	respiratory quotient	VQ	ventilation–perfusion
RLL	right lower lobe	VQ scan	ventilation–perfusion scan
RML	right medium lobe	VT	tidal volume
RUL	right upper lobe		
RV	residual volume	WHO	World Health Organization

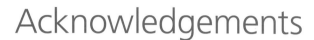

Acknowledgements

Thanks to the following medical students for their help reviewing chapters: Jessica Dunlop, Aliza Imam, Roxanne McVittie, Daniel Roberts and Joseph Suich.

Figures 2.1, 2.3, 2.4 and 2.14 are copyright of Sam Scott-Hunter and are reproduced from: Tunstall R, Shah N. *Pocket Tutor Surface Anatomy*. London: JP Medical, 2012.

Figures 2.22, 2.23, 2.24d, 2.25, 2.26, 2.27, 2.28a c -d, 2.31, 3.2, 6.1, 7.1, 7.4, 7.5, 7.11, 8.6, 8.12, 8.15, 8.17 and 9.3 are reproduced from: Darby M, et al. *Pocket Tutor Chest X-Ray Interpretation*. London: JP Medical, 2012.

Figure 10.3 is reproduced from James S, Nelson K. *Pocket Tutor ECG Interpretation*. London: JP Medical, 2011.

Figures 2.20 and 8.4 are reproduced from: Behera D. *Textbook of Pulmonary Medicine, 2e, Vol 1*. Delhi: Jaypee Brothers Medical Publishers, 2010.

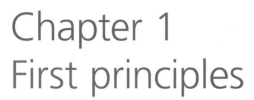

Chapter 1
First principles

Overview of the respiratory system

Starter questions

Answers to the following questions are on page 57.

1. Does the respiratory system have a role in more than breathing?
2. Do humans have an efficient respiratory system?

The respiratory system comprises the nose, the mouth, the pharynx, the larynx, the trachea and the bronchial tree and alveoli (**Figure 1.1**). The system also includes the pleurae (the two membranes covering the whole of the lungs) and the muscles and bones of the chest wall and diaphragm.

Roles of the respiratory system

The main role of the respiratory system is to supply the blood with oxygen. Oxygenated blood is then distributed throughout the body by the circulatory system (the heart and blood vessels). Oxygen is essential for the generation of energy for cellular processes.

The respiratory system also excretes carbon dioxide, which is a waste product of cellular reactions. Carbon dioxide diffuses from cells into the blood, which is then transported to the lungs by the circulatory system. Failure to excrete carbon dioxide from the lungs would result in an increased amount of carbon dioxide in the body. The increased carbon dioxide would, in turn, increase the amount of acid in the body and have other toxic effects.

More severe respiratory conditions prevent the supply of oxygen to the blood, result in failure to excrete carbon dioxide, or both. The consequences are life-threatening.

The respiratory system also regulates temperature, defends against pathogens and creates the sounds that allow us to talk.

Structure and function of the respiratory system

Oxygen uptake by the lungs begins with inhalation of air through the mouth or nose.

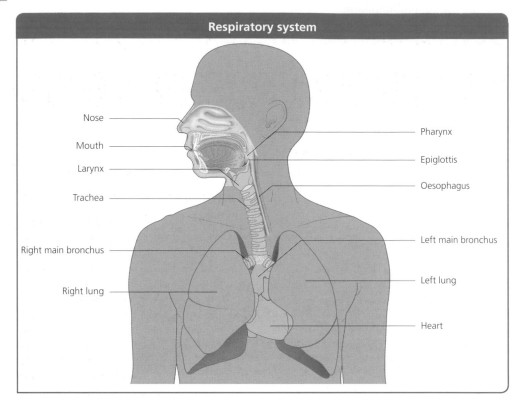

Figure 1.1 Structure of the respiratory system.

This process uses the muscle power of the diaphragm and chest wall. From the mouth or nose, inhaled air flows through the pharynx and larynx. The air travels into the lungs through the bronchial tree (**Figure 1.2**).

The bronchial tree starts with the trachea, which splits into two smaller tubes: the right main bronchus and the left main bronchus. The right and left main bronchi supply air to their respective lungs. Both main bronchi divide further into smaller and smaller tubes. These tubes eventually supply air to small air sacs called alveoli.

Oxygen in the air diffuses into the blood carried by capillaries (small blood vessels) surrounding the alveoli. At the same time, carbon dioxide passes from the blood in the capillaries to the alveoli. The carbon dioxide is then removed from the body during expiration. This process expels air from the lungs, following the same path as inhalation but in reverse.

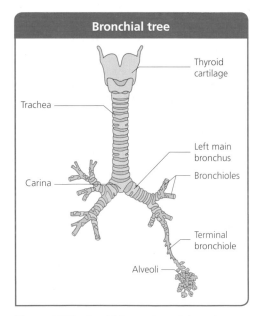

Figure 1.2 The brochial tree. As each bronchus divides into smaller bronchioles, less and less cartilage surrounds the airway.

Development of the respiratory system

Starter questions

Answers to the following questions are on page 57.

3. Do fetuses breathe in the womb?

4. Can babies survive if their respiratory system does not develop normally?

The development of the respiratory system is complicated and mostly happens in utero and postnatally, although the respiratory system continues to develop into adolescence.

Fetal development

The respiratory system develops from the midsection of the foregut, just anterior to the pharynx, in the 4th week of gestation (about 22 days after implantation) (**Figure 1.3**). First, a laryngeotracheal groove forms on the ventral side of the foregut. The groove deepens to become a pouch called the respiratory diverticulum. The diverticulum separates from the oesophagus, then splits into a right and a left bronchial bud around day 26.

Over the next 2 weeks, secondary bronchi are produced by further branching. By week 5, asymmetrical branching has occurred and the lung lobes have formed. By week 6, the main divisions of the bronchial tree are in place.

The distal end of the respiratory diverticulum develops into the tracheal bud. This structure gives rise to the trachea.

All cells derive from one of the three embryonic germ cell layers: the endoderm (inner layer), the mesoderm (middle layer) or the ectoderm (outer layer). The respiratory diverticulum is lined by endoderm. Therefore all the respiratory epithelium and the glands of the trachea, bronchi and alveoli are endodermal in origin. Supporting structures, such as cartilage, blood vessels, muscles and connective tissue, derive from the mesoderm surrounding the respiratory diverticulum. The mesoderm regulates the way in which branching occurs; mesoderm around the trachea inhibits branching, and mesoderm around the bronchi stimulates it.

The further development of the respiratory system is divided into three stages: the glandular period, the canalicular period and the terminal saccular period. Development is

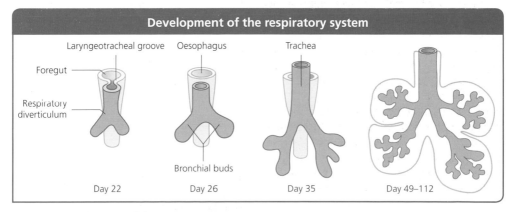

Development of the respiratory system

Laryngeotracheal groove   Oesophagus   Trachea

Foregut

Respiratory diverticulum

Bronchial buds

Day 22   Day 26   Day 35   Day 49–112

Figure 1.3 Development of the respiratory system.

regulated by several factors. These factors and their functions are shown in **Table 1.1**.

Glandular period

In the glandular period (weeks 7–16), all the major lung elements develop. The bronchial tree repeatedly branches to the level of the terminal bronchioles. The glandular period is so-called because the terminal bronchioles resemble small clusters of gland cells called glandular acini.

Canalicular period

In the canalicular period (weeks 16–26), the bronchioles, alveolar ducts (connecting the bronchioles to the sacs containing the alveoli) and primitive alveoli develop. The lung tissue becomes very vascular and capillaries develop.

Terminal saccular period

In the terminal saccular period, weeks 26–40, more alveoli develop and mature. Alveolar cells differentiate into type 1 and type 2 pneumocytes.

- Type 1 pneumocytes predominate and are the specialised cells responsible for gas exchange.
- Type 2 pneumocytes secrete the pulmonary surfactant that decreases the surface tension of the mucoid lining of the alveoli.

Also in this period, the epithelium thins as it develops and surfactant secretion begins. Capillaries continue to develop around the alveoli.

> **Surfactant reduces the effort needed to expand the lungs by** decreasing surface tension and increasing pulmonary compliance (expansion in response to transmural pressure). Because surfactant secretion does not start until weeks 26–40 some premature babies develop infant respiratory distress syndrome.

Development of pleural cavities and diaphragm

The major body cavities originate from spaces in the lateral plate mesoderm and the cardiogenic mesoderm. The two spaces fuse to form a horseshoe-shaped cavity. Part of this becomes the pericardial cavity; the other part becomes the peritoneal and pleural cavities. As the lungs develop, pleural sacs form around them. The diaphragm develops from the septum transversum, pleuroperitoneal membranes, dorsal mesentery of the oesophagus and body cavity walls.

The fetus aspirates fluid into the lungs throughout development. This fluid contains surfactant, mucus and amniotic fluid. At birth, the fluid is rapidly reabsorbed into blood and lymph vessels.

Regulatory factors for respiratory system development		
Factor	Produced by	Role
Fibroblast growth factor-10	Mesoderm	Stimulates lung bud outgrowth
Hox genes	Lung buds	Expression of different Hox genes specifies regions of the respiratory system
Sonic hedgehog	Endoderm	Inhibits fibroblast growth factor-10 and stimulates bone morphogenic protein-4
N-Myc	Mesoderm	Stimulates branching
Fibronectin	Mesoderm	Stabilises branching
Syndecan	Mesoderm	Stabilises epithelia
Epimorphin	Mesoderm	Organises and arranges epithelium

Table 1.1 Factors regulating development of the respiratory system

Postnatal development

The lungs of a newborn baby contain about 30 million alveoli. Alveoli multiply rapidly in the first 2–3 years of life. Little multiplication occurs subsequently, and an adult's lungs contain about 500 million.

The number of alveoli plateaus in early childhood. However, their size and surface area increase into adolescence.

> **The lungs provide a huge surface area for gas exchange.** They contain 2400 km of airways, about the distance from London to Istanbul. The surface area of the 500 million alveoli within is around 100 m², the same surface area as a tennis court.

Anatomy of the respiratory tract

Starter questions

Answers to the following questions are on page 57–58.

5. Why is the nose important for breathing?
6. Why do we need bronchioles and alveoli?
7. Why are the lungs of an athlete bigger than those of a non-athlete?

The whole airway extends from the nostrils and lips to the alveoli in the lungs. At the level of the vocal cords, the respiratory tract splits into the upper airway and the lower airway. Any part of this system can be affected by respiratory disease.

Upper airway

The upper airway comprises the nose and nasal cavity, the mouth and oral cavity, and the pharynx and larynx. Its overall function is to provide a passage for air to be inhaled and exhaled.

Nose

The nose:

- moistens, warms and filters air
- provides the sense of smell

The external part of the nose consists mostly of cartilage but also of bone (frontal, nasal and maxillary) (**Figure 1.4**). Bones form part of the nasal bridge superiorly. This part of the nose is covered by skin and muscle, and is lined by a mucous membrane and coarse hairs. It contains sweat glands and sebaceous glands.

The nasal airway extends from the nostrils (anterior nares) on the face to the choanae (posterior nares) at the pharynx. Two nasal vestibules lead to a common nasal cavity.

The nasal cavity extends from the vestibule horizontally and is lined by ciliated columnar epithelium. It has an arched ceiling that extends upwards to the olfactory area. This region is made of olfactory epithelium over the cribriform plate, and is supported by nasal, frontal, ethmoid and sphenoid bones.

The medial wall of the nose, the nasal septum, separates the two nasal cavities. The septum is formed by the ethmoid bone and the vomer. The inferior aspect of the nose comprises the palatine process of the maxilla, the palatine bone and the soft palate. The lateral wall of the nasal cavity consists of maxillary and ethmoid bones.

Anatomy of the nose

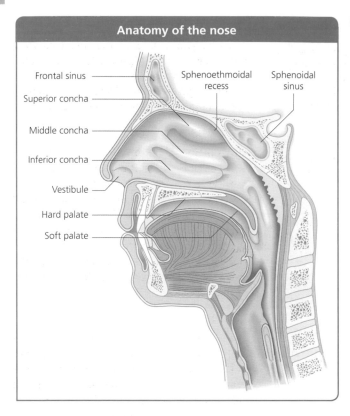

Frontal sinus

Superior concha

Middle concha

Inferior concha

Vestibule

Hard palate

Soft palate

Sphenoethmoidal recess

Sphenoidal sinus

Figure 1.4 Anatomy of the nose.

Inflammation of the nasal passages (rhinitis) or sinuses (sinusitis) result in airflow obstruction, excess mucus secretion and sinus pain. It is caused by infectious, allergic or non-allergic conditions that are frequently associated with lung disease, e.g. allergic rhinitis (one component of hay fever) is associated with asthma, and viral rhinitis with acute bronchitis.

Three bony folds (the superior, middle and inferior turbinates) run horizontally and increase the surface area of the nose.

- The nasolacrimal duct runs into the inferior meatus below the inferior nasal cavity
- The frontal, anterior, ethmoidal and maxillary sinuses drain into the middle meatus
- The posterior ethmoidal sinus drains into the superior meatus

The sinuses are lined by mucus-secreting respiratory epithelium.

The sphenoethmoidal recess is a small area of the nose that sits above the superior turbinates in front of the sphenoid bone. The sphenoidal air sinus opens into this area.

Blood supply

The nose is supplied by the ophthalmic, maxillary and facial arteries. Venous drainage is to the facial vein and pterygoid venous plexus.

Nerve supply

The olfactory mucosa is supplied by the olfactory (first cranial) nerve. Olfactory nerve fibres arise from olfactory cells in the olfactory mucous membrane. The fibres reach the olfactory bulbs through the cribiform plate.

The rest of the nasal cavity is supplied by the first and second divisions of the trigeminal nerve. The anterior part of the nose is supplied by the anterior ethmoidal nerve and the posterior part from the pterygopaltine ganglion.

> Anosmia, lack of the sense of smell, has numerous causes, which affect any part of the pathway from the olfactory mucosa to the brain. Congenital causes include primary ciliary dyskinesia. Acquired causes include nasal polyps, snorting cocaine, tumours (e.g. suprasellar meningioma), trauma to the cribriform plate, inflammation (e.g. granulomatosis with polyangiitis) and brain lesions (e.g. cerebrovascular accident).

Lymphatics

The lymphatics of the vestibules drain into the submandibular nodes. The rest of the lymphatic drainage of the nose is to the upper deep cervical nodes.

> Cancer cells and the inflammatory response to infection spread along the route of local lymph drainage. Therefore knowing the lymphatic drainage for a particular organ is important for identifying potential sites of lymphadenopathy caused by metastases and infection.

Histology

Excluding the vestibules, the nasal cavity is lined by mucous membrane. The olfactory mucous membrane covers the upper part of the superior turbinates and sphenoethmoidal recess. It also lines the roof of the nasal septum. This area contains olfactory neurone and is therefore essential for sensing smell.

The lower part of the nasal cavity is lined by respiratory mucous membrane. The role of the respiratory mucous membrane is to warm, moisten and clean inspired air. The air is warmed by a plexus of veins in the submucous connective tissue. Moisture comes from mucus secreted by glands and goblet cells. The sticky surface of the mucous membrane helps remove dust from the air. The ciliary action of the columnar ciliated epithelia on the surface moves the mucus backwards towards the pharynx, where it is swallowed.

Pharynx

The pharynx is behind the nasal cavities, mouth and larynx (**Figure 1.5**). It has a musculomembranous wall, except anteriorly, where the posterior nasal apertures, opening of the mouth and inlet of the larynx sit.

Nasopharynx

This portion of the pharynx is between the nasal cavities and soft palate. The nasopharynx has a roof and a floor, as well as anterior, posterior and lateral walls. The sphenoid and occipital bones support the roof. The floor is formed by the soft palate, the anterior wall by the posterior nasal apertures, and the posterior wall by the anterior arch of the atlas. The lateral walls contain the opening of the auditory tubes.

Oropharynx

The oropharynx extends from behind the mouth to the soft palate and upper border of the oesophagus. Its roof is formed by the underside of the soft palate and pharyngeal isthmus. The floor is formed by the posterior third of the tongue and the space between the tongue and the epiglottis.

■ The anterior wall opens into the mouth through the oropharyngeal isthmus.

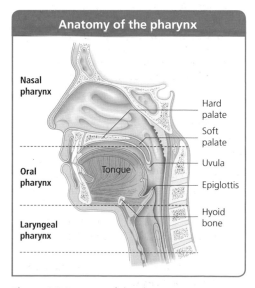

Anatomy of the pharynx

Nasal pharynx

Hard palate

Soft palate

Oral pharynx

Tongue

Uvula

Epiglottis

Hyoid bone

Laryngeal pharynx

Figure 1.5 Anatomy of the pharynx.

- The posterior wall is supported by the 2nd and 3rd cervical vertebrae.
- The lateral walls have palatoglossal and palatopharyngeal arches, folds of mucous membrane covering the palatoglossus muscle.

> **Snoring is the coarse sound produced by vibration of the soft palate and other tissue in the upper airway.** It results from partial blockage of airflow in the nose, oropharynx or base of the tongue. This blockage can have serious physiological consequences in a disease called obstructive sleep apnoea.

Hypopharynx

The hypopharynx sits behind the opening of the larynx and posterior laryngeal surface. It runs from the upper border of the epiglottis to the lower border of cricoid cartilage. The anterior wall is formed by the inlet and posterior surface of the larynx. The posterior wall is supported by the 3rd to 6th vertebrae, and the lateral wall by the thyroid cartilage and thyrohyoid membrane.

Blood supply

Arterial supply to the pharynx is from branches of the ascending pharyngeal, ascending palatine, facial, maxillary and lingual arteries. Veins drain into the pharyngeal venous plexus, which drains into the internal jugular vein.

Nerve supply

Nerve supply is from the pharyngeal plexus. The plexus consists of branches of glossopharyngeal, vagus and sympathetic nerves.

Lymphatics

The tonsils sit in the roof of the pharynx. Lymph vessels drain into deep cervical, retropharyngeal or paratracheal nodes.

Histology

The pharyngeal wall has three layers: a mucous membrane, a fibrous layer and a muscle layer.

- The first layer, the mucous membrane, is continuous with the mouth, nasal cavities and larynx. It is also continuous with the tympanic cavity, through the auditory tubes. The upper part of the membrane is lined by ciliated columnar epithelium, and the lower part with stratified squamous epithelium.
- The middle layer of the pharyngeal wall is a fibrous layer. It is thick at the top, where it connects with the base of the skull, and continuous with the submucosa of the oesophagus.
- The third layer is a muscle layer. It consists of the superior, middle and inferior constrictor muscles, as well as the stylopharyngeus and salpingopharyngeus muscles.

Larynx

The larynx is:

- a conduit for the passage of air
- a sphincter that closes during swallowing to prevent food from entering the respiratory tract
- the organ of phonation (including speech).

The larynx is also essential for effective coughing and for Valsalva's manoeuvre.

The larynx sits between the trachea and the pharynx (**Figure 1.6**). It is anterior to the oesophagus, at the level of the 3rd to 6th cervical vertebrae, and extends from the epiglottis to the cricoid cartilage.

The thyrohyoid membrane suspends the larynx from the hyoid bone. This membrane is made of three single cartilages (thyroid, epiglottic and cricoid) and three paired cartilages (arytenoid, corniculate and cuneiform), combined with ligaments, membranes and muscles.

The main body of the larynx is formed by the thyroid cartilage (Adam's apple). The Adam's apple is connected superiorly to the thyrohyoid membrane. It is formed by two laminae that join anteriorly at the midline. The posterior aspects of the laminae have superior and inferior horns. These horns articulate inferiorly with the cricoid cartilage.

Anatomy of the larynx

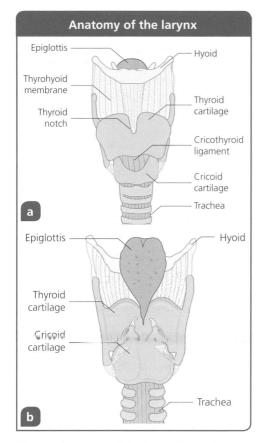

Figure 1.6 Anatomy of the larynx. (a) Anterior view. (b) Posterior view.

The epiglottic cartilage arises from the posterior surface of the thyroid cartilage. During breathing, the leaf shaped epiglottis remains in an upward position, allowing air to pass into the trachea. During swallowing, the epiglottis projects superiorly to cover the laryngeal inlet, diverting food to the oesophagus and away from the trachea. Thus the epiglottis prevents aspiration of food.

The male larynx and female larynx are similar in size during childhood. However, at puberty the male larynx enlarges significantly, reaching an average size in men of 45 mm long and 35 mm in diameter. The average size of the larynx in women is 35 mm by 25 mm.

The cricoid cartilage forms the only complete ring around the larynx, providing it with a rigid structure. Posteriorly, the cricoid cartilage is connected to the trachea by the cricotracheal ligament. Superiorly, it is connected to the thyroid and arytenoid cartilages by the cricothyroid membrane.

The arytenoid cartilages are two pyramidal structures that articulate with the posterior border of the cricoid. Their anterior projections are the vocal processes, which form the posterior attachment for the vocal cords.

The corniculate and cuneiform cartilages are small protrusions above the arytenoid cartilages.

Vocal cords

These are attached to the vocal processes posteriorly and the back of the thyroid cartilage anteriorly (**Figure 1.7**).

The vocal cords are tensed by the cricothyroid muscle, which pulls the arytenoid cartilages posteriorly. Conversely, the thyroarytenoid muscle relaxes the cords.

The posterior cricoarytenoid muscle externally rotates the arytenoid cartilages to induce vocal cord abduction. In contrast, the lateral and interarytenoid muscles cause adduction by internal rotation.

Figure 1.7 Coronal view of the vocal cords.

Anatomy of the vocal cord

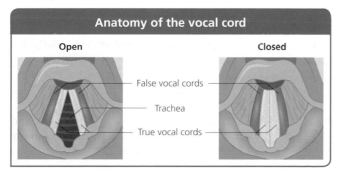

Blood supply

The superior and inferior laryngeal arteries derive from the superior and inferior thyroid arteries, respectively. Venous drainage occurs into the internal jugular and brachiocephalic veins through the superior and inferior thyroid veins.

Nerve supply

The vagus nerve innervates the larynx through the superior and recurrent laryngeal nerves. Sensory supply is provided by the internal branch of the superior laryngeal nerve above the vocal cords, and the recurrent laryngeal nerve below.

The external branch of the superior laryngeal nerve provides motor supply to the cricothyroid muscle. All other intrinsic muscles are innervated by the recurrent laryngeal nerve.

> **Paralysis of the left vocal cord is occasionally a sign of lung cancer.** The left recurrent laryngeal nerve has an unusual course, running through the mediastinum and around the left main bronchus before reaching the larynx. Therefore it can be paralysed by left-sided hilar tumours or enlarged lymph nodes.

Lymphatics

The lower and upper deep cervical lymph nodes receive lymphatic drainage from below and above the vocal cords, respectively.

Histology

Above the vocal cords, the larynx is lined by stratified squamous non-keratinised epithelium. Below the vocal cords, it is lined by ciliated columnar pseudostratified epithelium containing numerous goblet cells (**Figure 1.8**).

Trachea

The trachea (**Figure 1.2**) is a mobile tube that is both cartilaginous and membranous. It starts at the lower border of the cricoid cartilages of the larynx. It then runs inferiorly along the midline of the neck. The trachea ends by

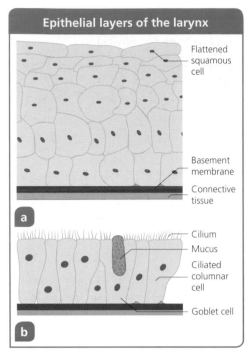

Epithelial layers of the larynx

Flattened squamous cell

Basement membrane

Connective tissue

a

Cilium
Mucus
Ciliated columnar cell

Goblet cell

b

Figure 1.8 Epithelial layers of the larynx. (a) Non-keratinised stratified squamous epithelium. (b) Ciliated columnar pseudostratified epithelium.

dividing into the two main bronchi in the thorax at the level of the 4th and 5th thoracic vertebrae.

The trachea is flattened posteriorly, so it is D-shaped in cross-section. It is about 11 cm long and 2–2.5 cm in diameter.

In the neck, skin, fascia, isthmus of the thyroid, inferior thyroid veins, jugular arch, sternothyroid muscles and sternohyoid muscles run in front of the trachea. The right and left recurrent laryngeal nerves, oesophagus and vertebrae run behind it. Lateral to the trachea are lobes of the thyroid gland and carotid sheath. In the thorax, the manubrium sterni, thymus, left innominate vein, aortic arch, innominate and left common carotid arteries, and deep cardiac plexus sit in front of the trachea.

In the thorax, the trachea sits in the superior mediastinum. On the right side, the trachea is in contact with the pleura, right vagus nerve and innominate artery. On the left side, it is in contact with the left recurrent nerve, aortic arch, and left common carotid and subclavian veins.

The trachea runs just in front of the oesophagus. Oesophageal tumours can erode into the trachea to cause oesophagotracheal fistulas. Tracheal tumours sometimes block the oesophagus to cause dysphagia (difficulty swallowing).

Blood supply

In the neck, the inferior thyroid arteries supply the trachea. In the chest, it is supplied by the bronchial arteries. The bronchial arteries form anastomotic networks with branches of the inferior thyroid artery.

Nerve supply

The trachea is innervated by the vagus nerve, recurrent laryngeal nerves and sympathetic trunks. Sympathetic fibres from sympathetic trunks supply smooth muscle and blood vessels.

Lymphatics

In the neck, lymphatic vessels drain into pretracheal and paratracheal lymph nodes. In the chest, drainage is into tracheobronchial lymph nodes. Paratracheal lymph nodes drain into the thoracic and mediastinal thoracic ducts.

Histology

The trachea is lined by a mucous membrane that is continuous with the larynx and bronchi. The membrane consists of a basement membrane and a stratified epithelium. The top layer is made of ciliated columnar epithelium. Below the basement membrane are elastic fibres and a submucosal layer containing connective tissue, blood vessels, mucous glands and nerves.

Lower airway

The lower airway comprises the trachea, bronchi, bronchioles and alveoli. Its main function is gas exchange.

Lungs

The lungs sit on either side of the mediastinum and fill most of the thorax. These two conical organs are separated by the heart, great vessels and other mediastinal structures. They comprise the bronchial tree and alveoli, and are covered by a thin membrane, the visceral pleura.

The lungs are soft, sponge-like and elastic. In children, they are pink. However, they darken with age because of the accumulation of inhaled dust particles.

To accommodate the heart, the left lung is about 10% smaller than the right lung. An oblique fissure divides the left lung into upper and lower lobes. An oblique and a horizontal fissure divide the right lung into upper, middle and lower lobes. Each lobe is further subdivided into segments (**Figure 1.9**).

Each lobe is supplied by a separate lobar bronchus. Each bronchus subdivides into segmental bronchi. Each segmental bronchus is part of a bronchopulmonary segment, which has its own segmental artery, lymph nodes and nerves.

In situs inversus, the major organs in the thorax and abdomen are on the opposite side to normal. When the heart is on the right (dextrocardia), the left lung has three lobes and the right lung has two. This congenital condition usually has no adverse effects for the patient. However, it can confuse physicians during clinical examinations. Situs inversus sometimes coexists with ciliary dysfunction. In such cases, it is associated with bronchiectasis and called Kartagener's syndrome.

The mediastinal (medial) surface of each lung contains a hilum. This is where bronchi, lymphatic vessels, nerves and pulmonary blood vessels enter and leave the lung. These structures are held in place by connective tissue and pleura.

Bronchial tree

The trachea branches into the right and left main bronchi; these are the primary bronchi (**Figure 1.2**). The division point is called the carina. The right bronchus is shorter, more vertical and wider than the left.

The walls of the primary bronchi contain

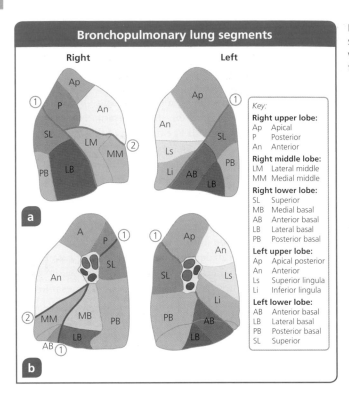

Figure 1.9 Bronchopulmonary segments of the lung. (a) Lateral view. (b) Medial view. (1) Oblique fissures. (2) Horizontal fissure.

incomplete cartilaginous rings, like the trachea, and divide into secondary bronchi as they enter the lungs. Cartilage is present until the small bronchi. The right main bronchus divides into superior, middle and inferior lobar bronchi. The left divides into superior and inferior lobar divisions, corresponding to the lung lobar divisions.

Secondary bronchi branch into tertiary bronchi. These bronchi, in turn, branch into bronchioles. Further branching eventually produces terminal bronchioles. From the trachea to the terminal bronchioles there are about 25 orders of branching. The bronchi and bronchioles originating from the branching of the trachea make up the bronchial tree.

Blood supply

Blood is supplied to the bronchial tree by bronchial arteries. The bronchial arteries arise from the descending aorta (**Table 1.2**). The bronchial veins drain into the azygous and hemiazygous veins (**Table 1.3**).

Nerve supply

The bronchial tree is innervated by the pulmonary plexus, which is formed by branches of the vagus and sympathetic trunk (**Table 1.4**).

The release of adrenaline (epinephrine) and noradrenaline (norepinephrine) relaxes smooth muscle in the bronchioles, which dilates the airway. Parasympathetic mediators have the opposite effect.

> **The right main bronchus is wider and more vertical than the left.** This arrangement means that inhaled foreign bodies are more likely to enter the right main bronchus.

Lymphatics

Drainage is into the superficial and deep plexuses. These groups of lymphatic capillaries converge to form large lymphatic vessels and drain into bronchial lymph nodes.

Arteries supplying the thoracic cavity			
Artery	Source(s)	Branch(es)	Regions supplied
Bronchial artery	Left: descending thoracic aorta Right: 3rd right posterior intercostal artery	Right bronchial artery (occasionally)	Lower trachea Bronchial tree Visceral pleura Lung lymphatics
Pulmonary artery	Right ventricle	Right and left pulmonary arteries Further division into superior lobar (upper lobes) and inferior lobar (lower lobes and middle lobe) arteries	Alveoli and lung interstitium

Table 1.2 Arteries supplying the thoracic cavity

Veins draining the thoracic cavity			
Veins	Tributaries	Drains into	Regions drained
Right and left bronchial veins	Lobar veins	Azygous and hemiazygous pulmonary veins	Proximal and distal bronchial tree
Right and left upper and lower pulmonary veins	Lobar veins	Left atrium	Alveoli and interstitium

Table 1.3 Veins draining the thoracic cavity

Nerves supplying the thoracic cavity				
Nerve(s)	Source	Branches	Motor innervation	Sensory innervation
Phrenic nerve	Ventral rami C3–C5 (cervical plexus)	No named branches	Respiratory skeletal muscle Diaphragm	Diaphragmatic, mediastinal and costal pleura and pericardium
Pulmonary plexus	Autonomic plexus formed by vagus nerve and sympathetic trunk	No named branches	Parasympathetic: bronchial tree smooth muscle and glands Sympathetic: lung vasculature and smooth muscle	None
Vagus nerve	Medulla	Auricular nerve Pharyngeal nerve Superior and recurrent laryngeal nerves Cardiac nerves (multiple) Pulmonary, cardiac and oesophageal plexuses Anterior and posterior vagal trunks	Larynx Pharynx Palate Bronchial smooth muscle Respiratory tree mucous glands Upper gut Heart	Skin of external auditory meatus Epiglottis Viscera of head, neck, thorax and proximal gut

Table 1.4 Nerves supplying the thoracic cavity

Histology

The bronchial tree is lined by pseudostratified ciliated columnar epithelium (**Figure 1.8b**). Bronchioles also contain some non-ciliated columnar cells called club (Clara) cells. Club cells produce surfactant protein and can also act as stem cells. Stem cells have the potential to develop into various types of epithelial cell (**Figure 1.8**).

Alveoli and interstitium

The terminal bronchioles at the end of the bronchial tree open into small cavities in the lung parenchyma. These cavities are the alveoli (**Figure 1.10**).

Each terminal bronchiole supplies several alveoli, which are lined by respiratory epithelium. Alveoli are closely associated with an extensive network of capillaries, which cover about 70% of their surface.

Each lung of an adult human contains about 500 million alveoli. These provide a massive surface area for gas exchange: about $75\,m^2$ in an adult.

Blood supply

The lungs have a dual circulation.

- The bronchial circulation supplies oxygenated blood for metabolic activity by the bronchial tree, lymphatics, visceral pleura and pulmonary vessels
- The pulmonary circulation (**Figure 1.11**) is a low-pressure system. It supplies the alveoli and interstitium with deoxygenated blood for oxygenation

The pulmonary artery arises from the right ventricle. It then divides into right and left pulmonary arteries, which follow the right and left main bronchi, respectively, to enter the lung at the hilum.

As the pulmonary arteries follow the bronchi, they divide further in the same pattern as the bronchial tree. At the terminal bronchioles, pulmonary arterioles supply the capillary plexus, which covers the alveoli, with deoxygenated blood.

Oxygen diffuses from the alveoli into the blood. Carbon dioxide diffuses from the blood into the alveoli.

Oxygenated blood from the alveolar capillaries drains into pulmonary venules. The venules merge to form pulmonary veins that accompany the bronchial tree. The veins leave the lungs at the hilum as right and left inferior and superior pulmonary veins. Each of these veins drains directly into the left atrium.

Oxygenation of blood in the alveoli

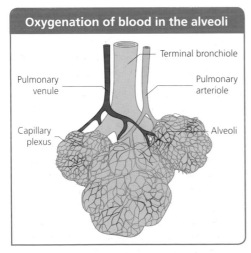

Figure 1.10 Alveoli receive deoxygenated blood from the pulmonary arterioles. Oxygenated blood leaves the alveoli through the pulmonary venules.

Pulmonary circulation

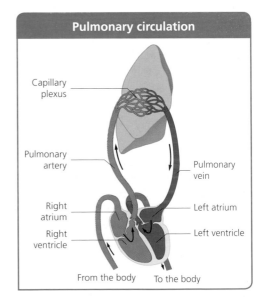

Figure 1.11 The pulmonary circulation. Blood supply to the alveoli is separate from that to the rest of the body. The pulmonary artery carries deoxygenated blood from the right ventricle to the lungs. Oxygenated blood returns to the left atrium through the pulmonary vein.

> **Major haemoptysis is the coughing up of large amounts of blood.** The condition is often caused by bleeding from a bronchial artery that has enlarged in response to lung disease, rather than bleeding from the low-pressure pulmonary circulation.

> **The pulmonary artery and pulmonary vein are unique.** The pulmonary artery is the only artery in the body to carry deoxygenated blood. The pulmonary vein is the only vein to carry oxygenated blood.

Anatomically, there is some overlap between the bronchial and pulmonary circulation; there are regions of the lung that both circulations supply. However, they differ physiologically. The arterial side of the bronchial circulation carries oxygenated blood at the same pressure as the rest of the systemic circulation. In contrast, the pulmonary artery carries deoxygenated blood at about a quarter of the pressure of the systemic circulation.

Deoxygenated blood in the bronchial circulation of the smaller bronchi drains to the pulmonary venous system. Thus the system is a minor arteriovenous shunt (a small hole between the arterial and venous systems). Bronchial veins supplying the larger airways drain into the azygous (right side) or hemiazygous (left side) veins.

Nerve supply

At each hilum is a pulmonary plexus with efferent and afferent autonomic nerves (**Table 1.4**). The plexus comprises branches of the vagus nerve and sympathetic trunk. The nerve supply runs down the bronchial tree, with little input to the alveoli. The walls of the alveoli contain stretch receptors, which are mechanoreceptors that respond when the lungs expand.

Lymphatics

Fluid in the air spaces of the alveoli is absorbed through the alveolar walls into the interstitium. From here, fluid travels along the bronchioles to lymph vessels (**Table 1.5**). These vessels merge as they follow the line of the bronchial tree to the hilum. They go through successive collections of lymph nodes before draining into the thoracic duct.

Histology

The walls of alveoli consist of a single-cell layer of squamous epithelium over a thin elastic basement (**Figure 1.12**). They are supported by extracellular matrix and capillaries. Alveolar walls contain holes that connect alveoli and terminal air ducts; these are the pores of Kohn.

The luminal surfaces of alveoli and the bronchial tree contain alveolar macrophages. When two or more alveoli have a common entrance, they are called an alveolar sac.

From the alveolar air space to the blood plasma are four layers. These layers are the respiratory membrane, across which oxygen must diffuse.

- Type 1 and type 2 pneumocytes (alveolar wall)
- Epithelial cell basement membrane
- Capillary basement membrane
- Capillary endothelium.

The respiratory membrane is $0.5\,\mu m$ thick.

The interstitium surrounding alveoli is sparse to allow efficient gas exchange. However, it does contain collagen and elastin fibres. Expansion of the interstitial space is the major pathological change in interstitial lung diseases.

Alveolar epithelium consists of two types of cell: type 1 and type 2 pneumocytes.

- Type 1 pneumocytes (squamous alveolar cells) are the main structural cells of the alveoli. They form a simple squamous epipthelial layer that covers 90% of the alveolar surface. Their large surface area and thin cytoplasmic layer allow rapid diffusion of oxygen into the blood
- Type 2 pneumocytes are ciliated, more cuboid cells. They tend to occupy the corners of alveoli and secrete surfactant. Their surface contains microvilli, which increase the surface area of the cell.

Respiratory system lymphatic drainage

Structure	Location	Afferents	Efferents to	Region(s) drained
Bronchomediastinal trunk	Along course of brachiocephalic vein	Paratracheal, parasternal and anterior mediastinal nodes	Left: thoracic duct Right: right lymphatic duct	Thoracic wall and viscera Medial parts of mammary glands
Bronchopulmonary and hilar nodes	Hilum of lung	Pulmonary lymphatics	Tracheobronchial nodes	Lungs
Anterior mediastinal nodes	Along brachiocephalic vessels and aorta	Anterior and middle mediastinum	Bronchomediastinal trunk	Thymus Anterior diaphragm Anterior pericardium and heart
Posterior mediastinal nodes	Along azygos veins and oesophagus	Posterior mediastinum and chest wall	Thoracic duct Inferior and superior tracheobronchial nodes	Posterior mediastinum, heart and pericardium Posterior diaphragm
Paratracheal nodes	Along trachea and oesophagus	Superior tracheobronchial nodes	Bronchomediastinal trunk	Trachea Upper oesophagus Lower larynx Upper lungs
Pulmonary nodes	In lungs	Lung parenchyma lymphatics	Bronchopulmonary and hilar nodes	Lung parenchyma and bronchi
Tracheobronchial nodes (inferior and superior)	Around tracheal bifurcation and right and left main bronchi	Bronchopulmonary nodes and lung lymphatics*	Bronchomediastinal lymph trunk Tracheobronchial and paratracheal nodes	Lungs, visceral pleura and bronchi Lower trachea Heart Oesophagus Middle and posterior mediastinum

*Left inferior tracheobronchial nodes drain into right inferior tracheobronchial nodes.

Table 1.5 Lymphatic drainage of the respiratory system

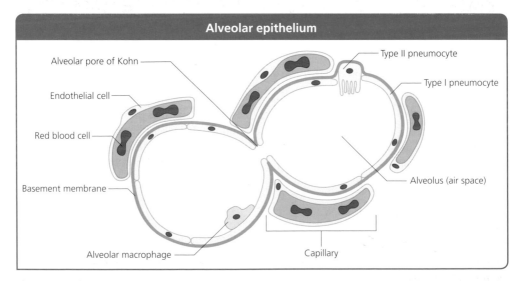

Alveolar epithelium

- Alveolar pore of Kohn
- Endothelial cell
- Red blood cell
- Basement membrane
- Alveolar macrophage
- Type II pneumocyte
- Type I pneumocyte
- Alveolus (air space)
- Capillary

Figure 1.12 The alveolar epithelium.

Some diseases reduce movement of gases across the respiratory membrane.

- Idiopathic pulmonary fibrosis and sarcoidosis scar the lung parenchyma and thicken the interstitium
- Pulmonary oedema in heart failure, and inflammation in hypersensitivity pneumonitis, cause swelling of the interstitium.

Thoracic wall

The thoracic wall is the outer margin of the thorax. The skin and muscle of the thoracic wall attach it to the shoulder girdle and trunk. The bony parts of the thoracic wall form the thoracic cage (**Figure 1.13**). The thoracic wall consists of:

- the thoracic part of the vertebral column posteriorly
- the sternum and costal cartilages anteriorly
- the ribs and intercostal spaces laterally
- the suprapleural extension superiorly
- the diaphragm inferiorly

The thoracic cavity is lined by the parietal pleura.

Thoracic vertebrae

The thoracic spine has an anterior concave curve. It comprises 12 thoracic vertebrae and intervertebral discs (**Figure 1.14a**). Each vertebra has a heart-shaped body from which a long spinous process descends.

Either side of the vertebral body are the costal facets. The superior and inferior costal facets are the sites at which each vertebra forms joints with the head of a rib. At the transverse costal facet, the transverse process articulates with the tubercle of a rib (**Figure 1.14b** and **c**).

Ribs

Ribs are long, curved, flat bones with a smooth upper border and a sharp thin inferior border (**Figure 1.14c**). The costal groove sits in the inferior border of the rib and contains the intercostal vessels and nerve (**Figure 1.15**). Each rib has a head, neck, tubercle, shaft and angle.

The 12 pairs of ribs are attached posteriorly to the thoracic vertebrae. Hyaline cartilages called costal cartilages connect the upper seven ribs to the lateral aspects of the sternum, and the 8th to 10th ribs to the cartilage immediately above. The costal cartilages of the 11th and 12th ribs are freestanding, with no anterior attachment. Costal cartilages provide the thoracic cage with its elasticity and mobility.

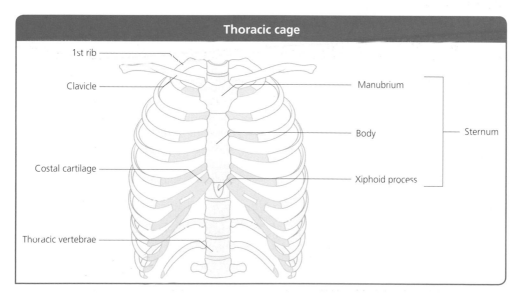

Thoracic cage

1st rib

Clavicle

Costal cartilage

Thoracic vertebrae

Manubrium

Body

Xiphoid process

Sternum

Figure 1.13 The thoracic cage.

Thoracic vertebrae

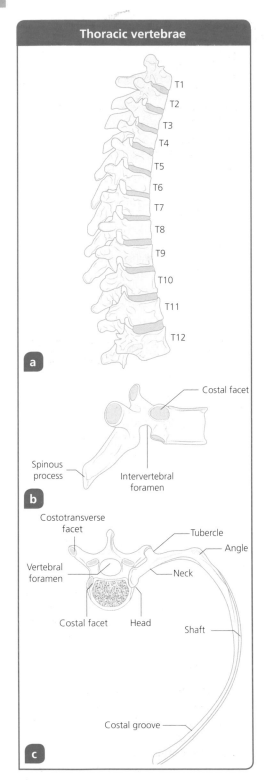

Figure 1.14 The thoracic vertebrae. (a) The 12 thoracic vertebrae. (b) Lateral view. (c) Axial view.

Intercostal space

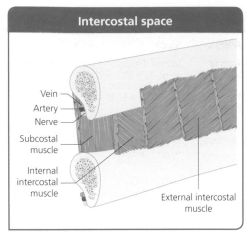

Figure 1.15 The intercostal space. The vein, artery and nerves make up the neurovascular bundle.

> The vertebrae and ribs are common sites of disease that cause chest pain. These diseases include vertebral collapse resulting from osteoporosis, spinal tuberculosis and metastases from lung or other cancers.

Sternum

The sternum is a flat bone in the midline of the anterior chest wall (**Figure 1.13**). From superior to inferior, the sternum comprises the manubrium sterni, the sternal body and the xiphoid process.

■ The manubrium connects to the clavicles and part of the second costal cartilages on each side. It sits opposite the 3rd and 4th thoracic vertebrae.
■ The sternal body connects to the manubrium superiorly with a fibrocartilaginous joint called the sternal angle.
■ The xiphoid process is a thin hyaline cartilage at the inferior end of the sternal body. It ossifies in adulthood.

Blood supply

The sternum receives blood from the sternal branches of the internal thoracic artery (**Tables 1.6** and **1.7**).

Nerve supply

The sternum and ribs are innervated by intercostal nerves. These arise from the thoracic

Arteries supplying the thoracic wall			
Artery	Source	Branches	Supply
Anterior intercostal	Internal thoracic musculophrenic	Unnamed muscular branches	Intercostal muscles anteriorly Skin over intercostal muscles
Highest intercostal	Costocervical trunk	Posterior intercostal artery	Intercostal muscles of intercostal spaces 1 and 2 Vertebral column and deep back muscles
Posterior intercostal	Highest intercostal and descending thoracic aorta	Posterior Spinal Anterior Collateral Lateral cutaneous	Intercostal muscles Spinal cord and vertebral column Deep back muscles Skin and fascia over intercostal spaces
Musculo-phrenic	Internal thoracic	Anterior intercostal arteries	Anterior diaphragm and anterior intercostal spaces 7–10 or 11
Internal thoracic	Subclavian	Pericardiacophrenic Anterior intercostal arteries Musculophrenic Superior epigastric	Mediastinum Anterior thoracic and abdominal wall Diaphragm

Table 1.6 Arteries supplying the thoracic wall

Veins draining the chest wall			
Veins	Tributaries	Drains into	Regions drained
Posterior intercostal	Lateral cutaneous	Brachiocephalic Superior intercostal veins Azygos vein Hemiazygos vein	Intercostal space, including skin Muscles and adjacent ribs Spinal cord at that segmental level and corresponding vertebra
Superior intercostal	2nd to 4th posterior intercostal veins	Arch of azygos and brachiocephalic veins	Intercostal spaces 2–4

Table 1.7 Veins draining the chest wall

nerve roots and run in the neurovascular bundle under each rib. The intercostal nerves also supply the overlying skin, the intercostal muscles and the underlying parietal pleura.

Histology

The sternum contains osteocytes and bone marrow. Osteocytes are cells that form hard bone. Bone marrow produces blood cells.

> **The neurovascular bundle is the artery, vein and nerve that run along the lower border of each rib.** To avoid this structure during procedures such as pleural aspiration or chest drain insertion, insert the needle into the thoracic cavity just above a rib.

Muscles of the thoracic cage

The main muscles of the thoracic cage are shown in **Table 1.8** and **Figure 1.16**. Each inter-costal space contains external and internal intercostal muscles and transverse thoracic muscle, and is lined by the endothoracic fascia and parietal pleura.

- The fibres of the external intercostal muscles run down and forwards from the inferior border of the rib above to the superior border of the rib below.
- The internal intercostal muscles form the middle layer of muscle. The fibres of the internal intercostal muscles run down and backwards from the subcostal groove of

Muscles of the thoracic wall

Muscle	Origin	Insertion	Action	Innervation	Artery or arteries
External intercostal	Lower border of rib	Upper border of rib below	Respiration: increases anteroposterior diameter of the chest	Intercostal nerves (T1–T11)	Intercostal artery
Internal intercostal	Upper border of rib	Lower border of rib above	Respiration: pulls ribcage down	Intercostal nerves (T1–T11)	Intercostal artery
Serratus posterior inferior	Thoracolumbar fascia, spines of vertebrae T11–T12 and L1–L2	Ribs 9–12	Respiration: pulls down lower ribs	Branches of ventral primary rami of spinal nerves T9–T12	Intercostal, subcostal and lumbar arteries
Serratus posterior superior	Ligamentum nuchae, spines of vertebrae C7 and T1–T3	Ribs 1–4	Respiration: elevates upper ribs	Branches of ventral primary rami of spinal nerves T1–T4	Posterior intercostal artery
Subcostalis	Angle of ribs	Angle of a rib two or three ribs above origin	Forced expiration	Intercostal nerves	Intercostal artery
Transversus thoracis	Posterior surface of sternum	Inner surfaces of costal cartilages 2–6	Forced expiration	Intercostal nerves 2–6	Internal thoracic artery

Table 1.8 Muscles of the thoracic wall

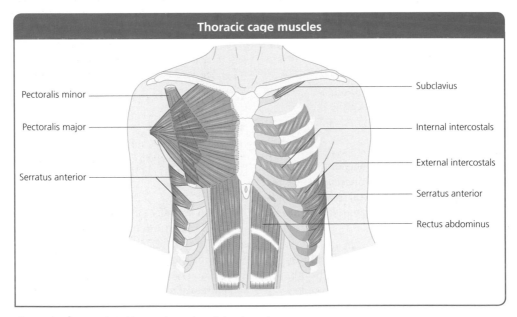

Figure 1.16 External and internal muscles of the thoracic cage.

the rib above to the upper border of the rib below.

The transverse thoracis forms the innermost muscle layer. This incomplete muscle layer crosses more than one intercostal space. Underneath it are the endothoracic fascia and parietal pleura.

The intercostal nerves and blood vessels run along the costal groove between the internal intercostal and transverse thoracis muscle layers. Superiorly to inferiorly, they are arranged vein, artery and nerve.

> **On rare occasions, weakness of the respiratory muscles causes respiratory failure.** This failure is caused by either nerve damage (e.g. in Guillain–Barré syndrome) or muscle damage (e.g. in muscular dystrophies). Respiratory muscle weakness is difficult to detect clinically but is confirmed by specialised pulmonary function tests.

Blood supply

Each intercostal space has a posterior intercostal artery arising from the subclavian artery or thoracic aorta. Each space also has two small anterior intercostal arteries, which are branches of the internal thoracic artery. The intercostal arteries supply the intercostal muscles, the overlying skin and the parietal pleura.

The posterior intercostal veins drain into the azygos or hemiazygous veins. The anterior intercostal veins drain into the internal thoracic and musculophrenic veins.

Nerve supply

The intercostal muscles are supplied by the corresponding intercostal nerves, which are formed by the anterior rami of the first 11 thoracic spinal nerves.

These nerves enter the intercostal space between the parietal pleura and the posterior intercostal membrane. They run forwards inferiorly to the intercostal vessels in the subcostal groove of the corresponding rib.

Lymphatics

Lymph drainage of the chest wall is into sternal and intercostal glands at the anterior and posterior ends of the intercostal spaces, respectively. These glands drain into the thoracic duct or directly into the internal jugular or subclavian veins of intercostal spaces.

Diaphragm

The diaphragm is a dome-shaped muscular and tendinous structure that separates the thorax from the abdomen (**Figure 1.17a and b**). It is the primary muscle of respiration.

The diaphragm has a peripheral muscular component arising from the margins of the thoracic outlet. This muscle is roughly divided into three parts:

- The sternal part arises from the posterior surface of the xiphoid process and consists of a small right and left muscular slips.
- The costal part arises from the deep surfaces of the lower six ribs and corresponding costal cartilages.
- The vertebral part arises from the arcuate ligaments.

The muscular components of the diaphragm are inserted into a central tendon. The diaphragm curves up into right and left domes, level with the upper border of the 5th rib on the right and lower border of the 5th rib on the left.

The level of the diaphragm varies with the phase of respiration. On inspiration, the diaphragm contracts and pulls downwards, thus increasing the diameter of the thorax. As well as acting as a muscle of inspiration, the diaphragm is a muscle of abdominal straining, assists with weight lifting and, as a thoracoabdominal pump, facilitates blood flow.

The diaphragm has three main openings:

- the aortic opening for the aorta, thoracic duct and azygous vein
- the oesophageal opening for the oesophagus, vagus nerve and gastric vessels
- the caval opening for the inferior vena cava and right phrenic nerve

> **Herniation of abdominal organs through the diaphragm into the thoracic cavity causes abnormal X-ray appearances.** The commonest example is a hiatus hernia, in which the stomach herniates through the oesophageal opening. Rare congenital defects of the diaphragm and trauma can result in small and large bowel herniation into the thoracic cavity.

Blood supply

The diaphragm is supplied by the pericardiacophrenic and musculophrenic branches of

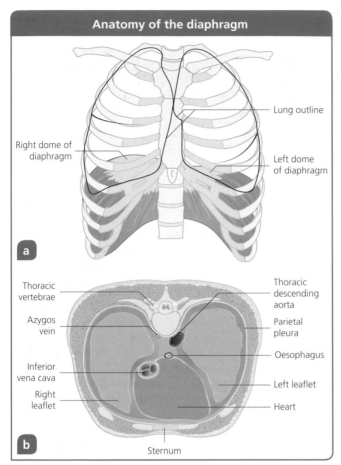

Figure 1.17 The diaphragm. (a) The diaphragm sits inferior to the lungs and attaches to the ribs and vertebrae. (b) Cross-section of the diaphragm. The central tendon consists of the right and left leaflets.

the internal mammary artery, as well as the inferior phrenic arteries, which arise from the aorta. Drainage is by the superior and inferior phrenic veins.

Nerve supply

The right and left phrenic nerves supply the diaphragm on each side. The phrenic nerves arise from the 3rd, 4th and 5th cervical nerve roots in the neck. They then pass anterior to the subclavian arteries into the mediastinum. Next, they pass anterior to the lung root, over the pericardium.

The right phrenic nerve crosses the diaphragm through the inferior vena cava orifice. In contrast, the left phrenic nerve penetrates the diaphragm directly.

Lymphatics

Diaphragmatic lymph vessels drain into the thoracic duct.

Pleurae

There are two pleurae: the parietal pleura and the visceral pleura, which are both serous membranes that line the thorax (**Figure 1.18**).

- The parietal pleura lines the thoracic wall and covers the thoracic surface of the diaphragm and the lateral aspect of the mediastinum. It then extends upwards into the neck to line the undersurface of the suprapleural membrane at the thoracic inlet.
- The visceral pleura covers the outer surfaces of the lungs and extends into the interlobar fissures.

The lungs are almost totally surrounded by the pleurae. Therefore lung surgery or biopsy entails penetration of the pleura. If air then enters the pleural space, the condition is known as a pneumothorax.

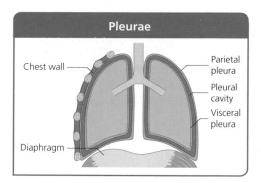

Figure 1.18 The pleurae. The pleural cavity separates the parietal pleura and the visceral pleura. It also contains a small amount of fluid that allows the two pleurae to move.

The visceral and parietal pleurae are separated by the pleural cavity. The pleural cavity contains only a few millilitres of fluid, which forms a thin film covering the surfaces of the pleurae. This film of fluid allows the two pleurae to move over each other.

The visceral and parietal pleurae join around the lung roots.

Blood supply

The parietal pleura is provided with blood from the intercostal arteries supplying the thoracic wall. The visceral pleura receives blood from the bronchial arteries.

Nerve supply

The parietal pleura is supplied by intercostal nerves and the phrenic nerves, and is very sensitive to pain. The visceral pleura is supplied from the pulmonary plexus.

> **Inflammation of the pleura causes a characteristic type of chest pain called pleuritic pain.** The commonest causes are lung infection ('pleurisy') or pulmonary infarction resulting from a pulmonary embolus.

Lymphatics

Pleural fluid is produced by the intercostal arteries and is absorbed by the lymphatic system, in a constant state of production and absorption. Pleural lymphatics cycle pleural fluid at an hourly rate of 0.4 mL/kg.

- In the parietal pleura, the lymphatics run along the intercostal spaces. They drain towards nodes along the internal thoracic artery and internal intercostal lymph nodes
- The visceral pleura is richer in lymphatic vessels. It has a network of vessels covering the lung surface and parenchyma, which drain into the hilar nodes.

Histology

Each pleura has five layers. The inner layer lines the pleural cavity; it is formed by a monolayer of flattened, squamous-like epithelial cells termed the *mesothelium*. The mesothelial layer is supported by a connective tissue layer, an elastic layer, another looser connective tissue layer and a fibroelastic layer.

Ventilation and respiration

Starter questions

Answers to the following questions are on page 58.

8. What is the difference between ventilation and respiration?
9. What role do the pleura play in ventilation?

Respiration is the process of gas exchange. The process has three steps (**Figure 1.19**).

1. The mechanics of ventilation: inhalation and expiration ('breathing')

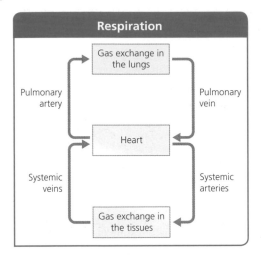

Figure 1.19 Respiration

2. Gas exchange between alveoli and blood (see page 29)
3. Gas exchange between systemic capillaries and the tissues and cells (see page 31)

The mechanics of ventilation: breathing

Air enters the lung through the trachea and bronchial tree. The elasticity of the tracheal wall allows it to stretch during swallowing, so that food can pass through the oesophagus.

Curved rings of hyaline cartilage prevent the trachea from collapsing during inspiration. The hyaline rings are incomplete, which allows the trachealis muscle to control the diameter of the trachea.

Like the rest of the bronchial tree, the tracheal and bronchial epithelium is coated in a film of mucus that traps dust and inspired particles. The trapped dust and particles are then beaten upwards by cilia on the surface of the epithelium towards the larynx (see section 1.8). Once they reach the larynx, larger particles are expelled by coughing and smaller ones are tipped into the oesophagus.

Air flows from the atmosphere into the alveoli because of pressure differences created by the contraction and relaxation of the respiratory muscles.

■ When air pressure inside the lungs is less than that of the atmosphere, air moves into the lungs.

■ When air pressure outside the lungs is less than that inside, air moves out.

Breathing in is called inspiration and breathing out, expiration.

Air movements during respiration follow Boyle's law: the volume of a gas is inversely proportional to the pressure of the gas. Just before inhalation, air pressure in the lungs is equal to atmospheric pressure. For air to flow into the lungs, their size must increase. Expansion of the lungs increases the volume of the alveoli. This increase in alveolar volume reduces alveolar pressure to below that of the atmosphere, and it is this pressure difference that forces air into the lungs.

The reverse happens during expiration, which forces air out of the lungs.

For the lungs to expand on inspiration, the diaphragm and external intercostal muscles contract (**Figure 1.20**). Contraction of the diaphragm flattens it, and the vertical diameter of the thoracic cage is increased. When the external intercostal muscles contract, the ribs are elevated and the lateral and anterior-posterior diameter of the chest increases.

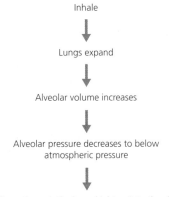

The pressure difference that occurs is about 2 mmHg, which is transmitted to the lungs by creating a negative pressure in the pleural space. As a result, about 500 mL of air is inhaled during resting inspiration. In active or forced breathing, the pressure difference is greater, around 100 mmHg, and 2-3 L of air is inhaled. In more active breathing, the accessory muscles, including the sternocleidomastoids, trapezii, scalenes and pectoralis minor

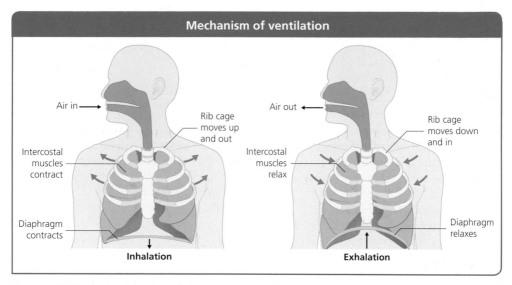

Figure 1.20 The mechanism of ventilation. The intercostal muscles and diaphragm contract, increasing the size of the thoracic cavity and drawing air into the lungs. Relaxation of the muscles and the elastic recoil of the chest wall reduce the size of the thoracic cavity and forcing air out of the lungs.

(**Figure 1.16**), help to elevate the sternum and ribs.

> **The diaphragm is the main muscle of respiration.** Unilateral paralysis of the diaphragm as a result of a phrenic nervy palsy causes dyspnoea. However, bilateral paralysis (e.g. caused by a high transection of the cervical cord) is quickly fatal because of the resultant respiratory failure.

Expiration increases the pressure in the lungs over atmospheric pressure by a passive process, and no muscle contraction is necessary. The inspiratory muscles relax, and elastic recoil of the wall of the chest and the lungs, supported by the inward pull of the surface tension of the alveolar air-fluid interface, reduces the volume of the thoracic cavity. The air pressure in the alveoli is higher than that of the atmosphere, so air moves up the trachea and out of the lungs. During this process, the diaphragm moves up, and the ribs move down, returning to their pre-inspiration positions.

Air can be forced from the lungs by a more active process called exhalation: contraction of the internal intercostal muscles and abdominal muscles. This causes the inferior ribs

to move down, the diaphragm to move up, and the spaces between the ribs to contract, thus increasing abdominal and thoracic pressure.

The maximum inspiratory pressure that can be generated is 100 cm H_2O. Maximum expiratory pressures are 150–200 cm H_2O.

The following factors affect the mechanics of ventilation.

- Pressure differences generated by movement of the diaphragm and chest wall
- The surface tension of the air-fluid interface in the alveoli: alveolar surface tension
- The resistance to gas flow through the bronchial tree: the airway resistance, measured as the pressure drop along the bronchial tree required to produce a given flow rate
- The elasticity of the lung, known as lung compliance, measured as the change in volume of the lung per unit change in distending pressure

Alveolar surface tension and surfactant

The fluid surrounding the air in the alveolus produces an inward force termed surface tension. Surface tension increases the work of breathing required to distend the alveoli. However, the surfactant phospholipid secreted by type 2 pneumocytes has major effects on the surface tension properties of alveolar lining fluid.

- Surfactant reduces surface tension more than saline alone, especially when compressed in the expiratory phase. This decreases the work required to distend alveoli and expand the lungs during inspiration.
- The effects of surfactant on surface tension stabilise alveoli; they also prevent inspiration drawing interstitial fluid into them (**Figure 1.21**).

Airway resistance

Airway walls resist the flow of air in and out. Airway resistance is directly proportional to the length of the tube, and inversely proportional to the 4th power of the radius. Therefore small changes in airway diameter have a marked effect on airway resistance. The major sites of airway resistance are the larger airways up to the 7th generation of bronchial divisions.

> **In emphysema, elastic tissue is lost, which increases lung compliance.** Therefore patients with emphysema have no problem inhaling, but extra effort is needed to exhale. In contrast, patients with lung fibrosis have decreased lung compliance; their 'stiff lungs' must work harder to inhale a given volume of air.

Compliance

Compliance is the effort needed to stretch the lungs and chest wall. An increase in compliance means an increase in lung distension at a given pressure. Conversely, a decrease in compliance is a decrease in lung distension at a given pressure.

Compliance depends on both surface tension and elasticity. Elastic fibres in the lungs stretch easily, helping to increase compliance.

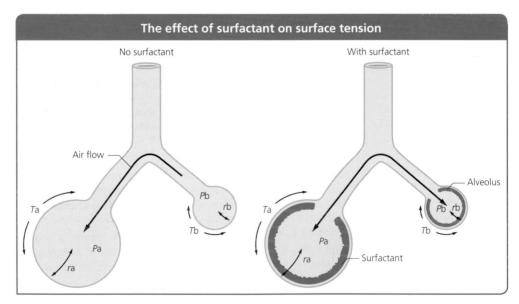

Figure 1.21 The effect of surfactant on the surface tension of two alveoli (a and b). The Law of Laplace describes the relationship between surface tension, (T); the radius of the alveolus, (r); pressure within the alveolus (P), and is $P = 2Tr$. Without surfactant $Ta = Tb$, therefore $Pa < Pb$ and the pressure difference leads to air flow from b to a and collapse of the smaller alveolus. With the addition of surfactant $Ta > Tb$, so $Pa = Pb$ and there is no air flow, so small alveoli remain stable and do not collapse.

In laminar flow, air molecules move in parallel down the bronchi. This movement results in less resistance than turbulent flow, in which air molecules move in a disordered fashion.

- Gas density and viscosity. Increased gas density or viscosity increases airway resistance. This is why breathing heliox (helium mixed with oxygen, which is less dense than air) can benefit patients with upper airways obstruction.
- Dynamic airways collapse (**Figure 1.22**). During expiration, the generation of a positive pressure drives air out of the alveoli but also acts on the bronchial tree. This compresses the tubes when the intraluminal pressure falls below pleural pressure. Dynamic collapse is an important cause of airways obstruction in emphysema.

> **The respiratory system contains a large number of airways <2 mm in diameter, but they contribute only about 20% of airway resistance.** This is why mild small airways obstruction (e.g. caused by early chronic obstructive pulmonary disease, COPD) is not readily detected by normal pulmonary function tests.

The following affect airway resistance.

- Lung volume. Bronchi are supported by the surrounding lung tissue, so their diameter decreases at low lung volumes during expiration. Conversely, the airways enlarge and resistance decreases during inspiration.
- Bronchial smooth muscle tone. Contraction of bronchial smooth muscle constricts the airways. The sympathetic nerves help relax smooth muscle, thus increasing bronchial diameter and decreasing resistance.
- Type of air flow. Resistance is affected by the type of airflow down the bronchi.

Lung volumes

Air movements during inspiration and expiration are divided into several different lung volumes (**Figure 1.23**).

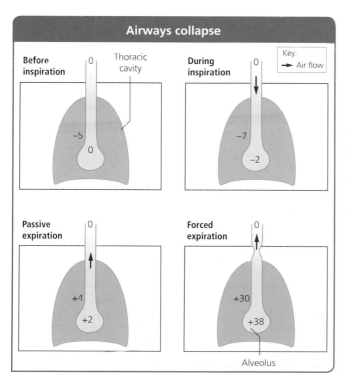

Airways collapse

Before inspiration — Thoracic cavity — 0 — −5 — 0

Key: → Air flow

During inspiration — 0 — −7 — −2

Passive expiration — 0 — +4 — +2

Forced expiration — 0 — +30 — +38 — Alveolus

Figure 1.22 Pressure changes in the airways. Intrathoracic and intraluminal pressures are shown (in mmH_2O). In each case, the lung volume is the same. During inspiration, the intrathoracic airways tend to be distended, lowering airway resistance. In passive expiration, a positive alveolar pressure is generated by elastic recoil of the lung. In forced expiration (exhalation), high intrapleural pressure and elastic lung recoil create a large positive alveolar pressure to drive flow; they also compress central airways, thus limiting flow.

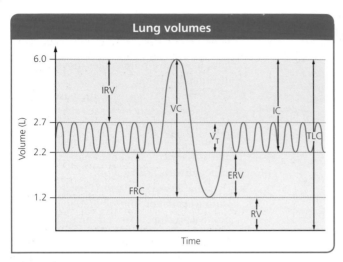

Figure 1.23 Lung volumes. ERV, expiratory reserve volume; FRC, functional residual capacity; IC, inspiratory capacity (the sum of tidal and inspiratory reserve volumes); IRV, inspiratory reserve volume; RV, residual volume; TLC, total lung capacity; V_T, tidal volume; VC, vital capacity.

- Total lung capacity (TLC): the largest amount of air contained by the lungs on full inspiration (on average, 6.0 L in men, 4.2 L in women).
- Residual volume (RV): the remaining air in the lung after a complete forced exhalation (on average, 1.2 L in both men and women).
- Vital capacity (VC): the greatest volume of air that can be inhaled and exhaled; in other words, the difference between TLC and RV (about 4.8 L in men and 3.0 L in women).
- Tidal volume (V_T): the volume of air inhaled and exhaled during a normal breath; about 10–15% of VC when at rest, increasing to up to 60% during exercise (normally about 0.5 L).
- Functional residual capacity (FRC): the volume of air left in the lung after expiration of a normal tidal volume breath, usually about 50–60% of VC. At FRC, the opposing forces of lung expansion from chest wall recoil and of the lungs to recoil inwards are balanced. FRC is altered by disease; for example, obesity reduces chest wall recoil and therefore decreases FRC, and emphysema increases lung compliance and reduces lung inward recoil, and therefore increases FRC. Pleural pressure at FRC is –5 cm H_2O; as a consequence of this negative pressure, a hole in the visceral pleura sucks air into the pleural space to cause a pneumothorax. Normal FRC is around 2.2 L in men and 1.8 L in women.

- Inspiratory and expiratory reserve volumes (IRV and ERV, respectively): the volumes of air that can be recruited to increase resting V_T. IRV is about 3.2 L in men and 2 L in women. ERV is around 1.0 L in men and 0.8 L in women.

When freedivers dive below 50 m, their lungs reduce to just a sixth of their normal volume. Lung collapse is prevented by blood moving into the thoracic cavity, which increases lung compliance. Other physiological adaptations, such as bradycardia and peripheral vasoconstriction, help people to survive longer without oxygen underwater than on dry land.

The work of breathing

Ventilating the lungs requires muscular effort to overcome airway resistance and to stretch the tissues of the chest wall, pleurae and lungs. Stretching of the tissues provides stored energy for expiration through elastic recoil. The work of breathing is at its least at FRC, and is only about 1-2% of a normal person's oxygen requirement at rest. However, the work of breathing increases substantially in lung diseases, because of the following factors (**Figure 1.24**).

- Lung volumes. With low lung volumes (e.g. in interstitial lung disease), the airways narrow, thus increasing airflow resistance. At high

Work of breathing

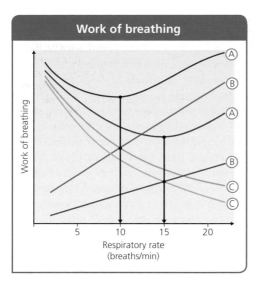

Figure 1.24 Work of breathing. Red, a patient with COPD. Blue, a normal patient. The total work done by the patient with COPD is higher than normal and the rate at which they are comfortable breathing is lower than normal [the minimal total work (arrows)]. A, total work of breathing; B, work to overcome airflow resistance; C, work to overcome elastic recoil.

lung volumes, the effort needed to stretch the chest wall a certain distance increases. Therefore patients with hyperexpanded lung as a result of COPD or severe asthma have an increased work of breathing.

■ Airways obstruction. This increases airway resistance and therefore the work of breathing.
■ Restrictive chest wall or lung diseases (e.g. obesity or extensive pleural thickening). These conditions increase the effort required to stretch the chest wall and thus also increase the work of breathing.

Take a large breath in so that you fully inflate your lungs. Then try to breathe in and out while maintaining a large lung volume. It requires much more effort than breathing at resting lung volumes. This partially replicates how patients with emphysema feel, having to breathe at a high FRC.

Distribution of ventilation

Although pleural pressure at FRC is on average -5 cm H_2O, this value varies from -8 cm at the top of the lung to -2 cm H_2O at the bottom. The lower negative pressure of the pleurae at the bases means that basal alveoli can distend more during inspiration. This effect, combined with their close proximity to the motion of the diaphragm, means that the alveoli in the bases of the lungs contribute a higher proportion of tidal volume than that of the alveoli in the apices. However, the lower pleural pressure in the bases causes the small airways to collapse, especially in obese patients. The higher negative pressure in the pleural space at the apices causes the alveoli at the top of the lungs to be more distended than those at the bottom. Therefore the upper parts of the lungs are common sites for spontaneous pneumothoraces.

Gas transfer in the lung (external respiration)

Ventilation is the main mechanism by which air containing oxygen enters the alveoli. Once oxygen reaches the alveoli, passive diffusion is the main mechanism by which it enters the capillary blood.

Oxygen is a gas, so it exerts a partial pressure determined by the atmospheric pressure. At sea level, atmospheric pressure is 760 mmHg and oxygen is 21% of air, therefore the partial pressure of oxygen in inspired air (FIO_2) is:

$$760\,\text{mmHg} \times 0.21 = 160\,\text{mmHg}$$

However, in this calculation the inspired air is assumed to be dry when it is, in fact, saturated with water vapour. At a body temperature of 37°C, the partial pressure of water vapour is 47 mmHg. Therefore the partial pressure of oxygen is recalculated as

$$(760\,\text{mmHg} - 47\,\text{mmHg}) \times 0.21 = 150\,\text{mmHg}$$

> **The main purpose of the cardiorespiratory system is to inhale and deliver oxygen to cells and to transport carbon dioxide to the lungs.** The respiratory system is efficient at delivering oxygen to the blood. However, the amount of oxygen that makes it into tissues is much less, as shown by looking at approximate oxygen partial pressures.
>
> - Inspired oxygen: 160 mmHg
> - Alveolar oxygen: 100 mmHg
> - Oxygen in the blood: 100 mmHg
> - Oxygen at tissue level: 10 mmHg

A further complication is that inspired air contains primarily oxygen and nitrogen, but moving down the bronchial tree to the alveoli, carbon dioxide is also present. This carbon dioxide affects the alveolar partial pressure of oxygen ($P\text{AO}_2$). The alveolar partial pressure of carbon dioxide ($P\text{ACO}_2$) is usually equal to the arterial partial pressure of carbon dioxide ($P\text{aCO}_2$) that can be measured by arterial blood gas tests. $P\text{AO}_2$ can then be calculated as follows.

$$P\text{AO}_2 = P\text{IO}_2 - P\text{ACO}_2/R$$

R is the respiratory quotient, which is the amount of carbon dioxide excreted for the amount of oxygen used and is usually quoted as 0.8. $P\text{IO}_2$ is the partial pressure of inspired oxygen.

Oxygen passively diffuses from the alveolus to the capillary blood. An oxygen molecule must pass through the alveolar and capillary walls, and through the plasma membrane and cytoplasm of a red blood cell, to combine with a haemoglobin molecule (**Figure 1.25**).

Normally, diffusion of both oxygen and carbon dioxide happens within 0.25 s. This is a third of the total transit time of a red blood cell through the pulmonary capillaries in normal lungs. However, in exercise the red blood cell transit time decreases to about 0.25 s. Therefore conditions such as interstitial lung diseases, which impair diffusion by increasing alveolar-capillary membrane thickness, may lead to a characteristic drop in arterial partial pressure of oxygen ($P\text{aO}_2$) on exercise.

Carbon dioxide in the blood is excreted by diffusion across the alveolar membrane; this process is more efficient than oxygen diffusion. Therefore respiratory diseases that inhibit oxygen diffusion, unless very severe, have no effect on the excretion of carbon dioxide.

> **Fick's law describes the factors that affect gas transfer across a membrane.** It states that V_gas is proportional to $A \times P/L$
>
> Gas transfer through a membrane (V_gas) is proportional to membrane surface area (A) and partial pressure across the membrane (P), but inversely proportional to thickness (L). Emphysema decreases A, and interstitial lung diseases increase L. This explains why pulmonary function tests for patients with emphysema and interstitial lung disease show reduced gas transfer.

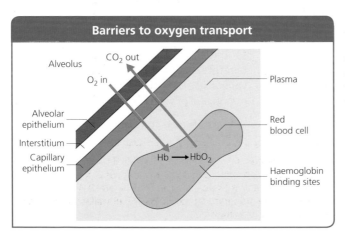

Barriers to oxygen transport

Alveolus — CO_2 out — O_2 in — Plasma — Alveolar epithelium — Interstitium — Capillary epithelium — Red blood cell — $Hb \longrightarrow HbO_2$ — Haemoglobin binding sites

Figure 1.25 Barriers to oxygen transport from the alveolus to the haemoglobin molecule. Diseases which increase the distance that O_2 and CO_2 have to travel across the barriers (e.g. interstitial lung disease or pulmonary oedema) will impair external respiration.

Gas transport in the blood

At the simplest level, the cells of the body take in fuel and make energy. This requires oxygen and produces carbon dioxide. These gases must therefore be transported between the pulmonary capillaries of the lungs, and cells located deep in distant tissues such as the liver, bowel, muscles and skin. Understanding why we breathe in oxygen and breathe out carbon dioxide requires knowledge of what happens within the cell, and particularly within the mitochondria where energy is created and stored.

Cellular metabolism

Cells need energy to function and survive. The mitochondria in the cells turn food into energy. They take glucose which is ingested in the diet, and use it to produce an energy form that can be used in processes that take place in all cells in the body. This chemical energy currency, without which cells would die, is ATP (adenosine triphosphate). An active cell will use approximately 2 million molecules of ATP a second. In order to produce ATP from glucose, the glucose molecule is sent through a series of reactions which strip it of electrons. These electrons are then sent through the electron transport chain within the mitochondria (**Figure 1.26**). The flow of electrons causes the proteins to act as pumps, pumping hydrogen ions from one compartment of the mitochondria to another. The stored up hydrogen ions are a source of potential energy. To create ATP, the hydrogen ions flow through ATP synthase which re-phosphorylates the ADP (adenosine diphosphate) molecule.

Oxygen is required for this process as it is electronegative and can pick up electrons. This is essential to maintain the flow of electrons through the electron transport chain and therefore continue the production of ATP. Each molecule of oxygen picks up 4 electrons and 4 hydrogen ions to form 2 molecules of water. The waste from this process is therefore a harmless biological substance.

In order for oxygen to get from the pulmonary capillaries to the mitochondria of the cell it must be transported through the blood. (**Figure 1.19** and **Figure 1.27**).

Oxygen transport

Oxygen is transported in the blood in two ways:

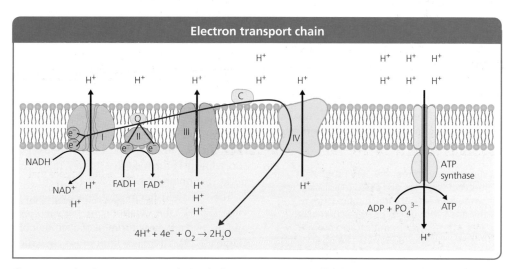

Electron transport chain

$$4H^+ + 4e^- + O_2 \rightarrow 2H_2O$$

Figure 1.26 The electron transport chain which generates energy in the form of ATP. NADH and FADH donate electrons. Oxygen acts as the 'terminal electron acceptor' producing water as the end product of the process. C, cytochrome C protein, which passes electrons from complex III to IV. FADH, flavin adenine dinucleotide. I–IV, protein complexes of the electron transport chain. NADH, nicotinamide adenine dinucleotide. Q, coenzyme facilitates the process of electron transfer.

Haemoglobin subunits

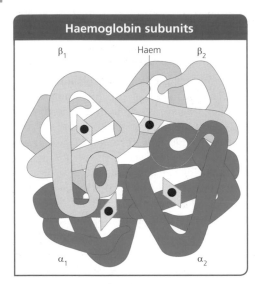

Figure 1.27 The haemoglobin molecule has four subunits. Each subunit contains a haem group that can bind to an oxygen molecule.

- as free dissolved oxygen (Pao_2) in the blood plasma
- as oxyhaemoglobin in red blood cells.

Oxygen in plasma

Oxygen is not very soluble in plasma, so only a small amount of the gas is transported this way under normal conditions. For each mmHg of Pao_2, 0.0031 mL of oxygen is dissolved in each 100 mL of blood. This value is calculated using Henry's law. With a normal cardiac output of 5 L/min, oxygen delivery by this method is only 15 mL/min – totally inadequate considering that tissue oxygen requirement at rest is about 250 mL/min. Pao_2 is measured by arterial blood gas sample.

Henry's law states that 'the number of molecules of gas dissolved in solution is proportional to the partial pressure of the gas.' This allows us to calculate the amount of oxygen and carbon dioxide dissolved in blood plasma at a given Pao_2.

In normal circumstances, most oxygen is transported bound to haemoglobin in red blood cells. However, in extreme circumstances the amount of oxygen dissolved in plasma becomes significant.

Oxyhaemoglobin in red blood cells

Each red blood cell contains around 250 million haemoglobin molecules. Since each haemoglobin molecule can carry 4 oxygen molecules this allows much greater transport of oxygen than is possible in plasma.

Haemoglobin is a molecule consisting of four protein subunits. Each subunit is a protein chain, folded to create a pocket containing a non-protein haem group. A haem group consists of a charged iron atom held in a ring structure – together known as porphyrin. When oxygen is not bound, the iron is in the Fe^{2+} state. When it binds, it oxidises iron to Fe^{3+}. Binding of oxygen causes a slight conformational shift in the protein which alters its relationship with the other protein subunits, and therefore the affinity of the haemoglobin molecule for oxygen. This is known as co-operativity (**Figure 1.28**).

In adults the haemoglobin molecule is usually made up of 2 alpha and 2 beta proteins (α2β2), together known as Haemoglobin A. Changing the protein ratio changes the affinity of the molecule as a whole for oxygen. In the foetus, haemoglobin F is α2γ2. In patients with sickle cell disease their haemoglobin molecules are usually α2βS2.

In the pulmonary capillaries, oxygen binds to the haem portion of the haemoglobin molecules within red blood cells. It remains bound until arrival at the tissues, where the conditions are optimal to cause release of oxygen from the haemoglobin. Such conditions include low partial pressure of oxygen (Po_2), low pH and, in active tissues, high temperature and high levels of 2–3-DPG.

The oxygen-haemoglobin dissociation curve shows the relationship between Po_2 and the percentage saturation of haemoglobin (**Figure 1.29**). There is a limit to Po_2, at which point the haemoglobin is fully saturated, with all haem binding sites occupied by oxygen. The curve shows that at a Po_2 of 60 mmHg haemoglobin is approximately 90% saturated. Increasing the Po_2 above this level will only increase the amount of transported oxygen by a

Haemoglobin co-operativity

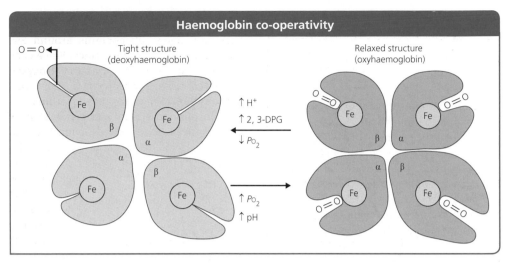

Figure 1.28 Haemoglobin co-operativity. As each sequential oxygen molecule binds to the tight state, it is easier to bind the next oxygen molecule, so that the molecule becomes progressively relaxed.

Oxygen dissociation curve

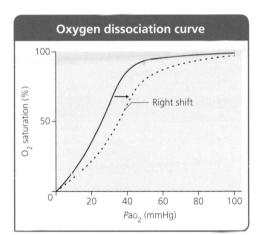

Figure 1.29 Oxygen dissociation curve. During right shift, haemoglobin's affinity for oxygen is reduced, allowing bound oxygen to be released from the blood into the surrounding tissues. Po_2, partial pressure of oxygen.

small amount. The percentage of haemoglobin saturated with oxygen can be measured using pulse oximeters. It is a non-linear relationship, as the conformation of the haemoglobin molecule depends on the number of molecules bound. This means that as one molecule of oxygen becomes unbound, the affinity for the others falls, and vice-versa. This is known as co-operativity. Below an arterial oxygen saturation (Sao_2) of 90%, small changes in Pao_2 cause

large differences in haemoglobin saturation. Various factors can shift the oxygen-haemoglobin dissociation curve to the right:

- lower pH
- higher $Paco_2$ (the Bohr effect)
- higher temperature
- higher concentrations of 2,3-diphosphoglycerate (DPG) in red blood cells

Moving the curve affects the relationship between Pao_2 and haemoglobin saturation. Highly metabolically active tissues undergoing anaerobic respiration are warm and acidotic, with higher $Paco_2$ and 2,3-DPG. These factors move the oxygen-haemoglobin dissociation curve to the right, facilitating the offloading of oxygen from haemoglobin and making the gas available to the tissues.

The total oxygen content of blood can be calculated using the following equations.

O_2 bound to haemoglobin = 1.34 × haemoglobin concentration in g/dL (Hb) × saturation

O_2 dissolved in plasma = 0.0031 × Pao_2 (mmHg)

The factor of 1.34 is used because each gram of haemoglobin can carry 1.34 mL of oxygen when fully saturated.

As an example, if a patient has a haemoglobin concentration of 14 g/dL and their oxygen saturation is 98% at a Pao_2 of 95 mmHg,

O_2 bound to haemoglobin $= 1.34 \times 14 \times 0.98 =$ 18.4 mL O_2/100 mL blood

O_2 dissolved in plasma $= 0.0031 \times 95 = 0.3$ mL O_2/100 mL blood

Therefore, the total is 18.7 mL O_2/100 mL blood. As can be seen from these formulae, the Pao_2 is not the sole determinant of oxygen content: the haemoglobin concentration is also critical. In anaemia, there are fewer binding sites for oxygen. Therefore the oxygen content of the blood decreases even though Pao_2 and oxygen saturations are unchanged. The actual delivery of oxygen to tissues (Do_2) is also determined by cardiac output (Q, measured in mL/min). The following formula builds on the above equations to show this.

$$Do_2 = [1.39 \times Hb \times Sao_2 + (0.003 \times Pao_2)] \times Q$$

Cardiac output is itself determined by stroke volume and heart rate. Both are increased on exercise as oxygen consumption increases. However, stroke volume reaches a maximum at relatively low levels of exercise, so further increases in cardiac output depend on heart rate alone.

Carbon dioxide transport

Carbon dioxide is transported in the blood (60% in plasma, 40% in red cells) in three ways (**Figure 1.30**):

- as bicarbonate, both in plasma and within red blood cells (81%)
- as free dissolved carbon dioxide (8%)
- as carbaminohaemoglobin (11%)

Bicarbonate in blood

Within the red blood cell carbon dioxide combines with water to form carbonic acid (H_2CO_3) in a reaction catalysed by the enzyme carbonic anhydrase.

This is a fast process and is essential to efficient transport of carbon dioxide. H_2CO_3 then dissociates to H^+ and HCO_3^-, which is bicarbonate. HCO_3^- then floods out of the cell and is

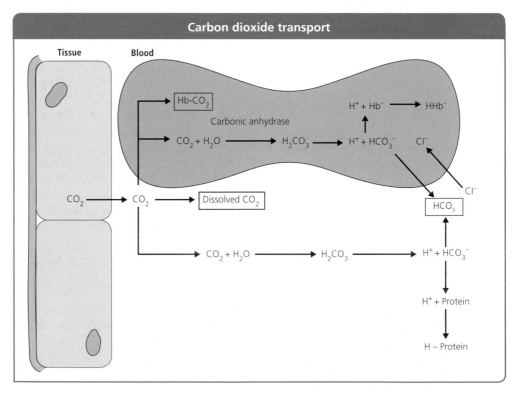

Figure 1.30 Carbon dioxide is transported in the blood in three ways: as bicarbonate, as freely dissolved carbon dioxide and bound to haemoglobin as carbaminohaemoglobin.

exchanged for chloride (Cl⁻). The H⁺ can combine with proteins, including haemoglobin itself, which leads to a change in the affinity for oxygen, the Bohr effect.

Alternatively, within the plasma the carbon dioxide can combine with water to produce carbonic acid (H_2CO_3) but this is a very slow process and would not allow adequate transport of carbon dioxide away from cells to be exhaled at the lungs. The free H⁺ combines with proteins within the plasma, to leave bicarbonate HCO_3^-:

$$H_2CO_3 \rightarrow H^+ + HCO_3^-$$

Bohr effect: increases in the concentration of carbon dioxide, or decreases in pH, result in a lower affinity of haemoglobin for oxygen, shifting the oxygen-haemoglobin dissociation curve to the right. This effect is due to H⁺ binding with haemoglobin leading to a conformational change in the protein which means the binding site binds oxygen less well. Higher concentrations of carbon dioxide lead to increased H⁺ due to carbonic anhydrase catalysing the reaction $CO_2 + H_2O \rightarrow H_2CO_3 \rightarrow HCO_3^- + H^+$.

Free dissolved carbon dioxide

Carbon dioxide is about 20 times more soluble in plasma than oxygen. Therefore about 8% of carbon dioxide is transported as the free dissolved gas, a much more significant proportion than for oxygen.

Haldane effect: binding of oxygen to haemoglobin promotes the release of carbon dioxide. This effect is through two mechanisms. Firstly, the binding of oxygen to haemoglobin induces a conformational change which reduces the affinity of haemoglobin for carbon dioxide in the form of carbaminohaemoglobin. In addition, oxygen binding to haemoglobin leads to release of bound H⁺ ions. They can then associate with HCO_3^- to produce carbon dioxide and water in a reversal of the reaction catalysed by carbonic anhydrase. This leads to carbon dioxide release in the pulmonary circulation and exhalation of carbon dioxide.

Carbaminohaemoglobin

Carbon dioxide combines with the terminal amine groups of haemoglobin to form carbaminohaemoglobin. The oxygenation status of haemoglobin has a significant effect on the amount of carbon dioxide that can be bound; deoxygenated haemoglobin has a greater affinity for carbon dioxide than that of oxygenated haemoglobin (the Haldane effect).

The result is that oxygen binding to haemoglobin in the pulmonary capillaries releases the carbon dioxide bound to the haemoglobin and therefore facilitates elimination of carbon dioxide by the lungs.

Gas transfer: blood and tissues (internal respiration)

Oxygen is delivered to the tissues by the circulation. It must then be extracted from the blood and find its way to the mitochondria, where it can be used in metabolism to generate ATP.

The amount of oxygen extracted at the level of the tissues, oxygen consumption (Vo_2), can be directly measured or calculated.

- Direct measurement requires knowing inspired and expired oxygen concentrations, as well as the expired minute volume (the volume of gas exhaled in one minute).
- To calculate Vo_2 indirectly, the Fick equation is used to quantify the oxygen lost between the arterial and venous sides of the circulation.

$$Vo_2 \, (O_2 \text{ consumption, mL } O_2/\text{min}) = Q \times (Cao_2 - Cvo_2)$$

Cao_2 is the oxygen-carrying capacity of arterial blood. Cvo_2 is the oxygen-carrying capacity of venous blood. This equation can be expanded to:

$$Vo_2 = Q \times [(1.34 \times Hb \times Sao_2/100) + 0.003 \times Pao_2] - [(1.34 \times Hb \times Svo_2/100) + 0.003 \times Pvo_2]$$

where Svo_2 is the venous oxygen saturation and Pvo_2 is the venous partial pressure of oxygen.

On average in a resting individual, Po_2 decreases to about 40 mmHg in venous blood after oxygen extraction in the tissues. This results in a haemoglobin saturation of about 75% in venous blood and the pulmonary artery.

> **Clinically, the mixed venous oxygen concentration, Svo_2, can be a useful indicator of oxygen consumption.** If Svo_2 is decreasing, then overall oxygen consumption is increasing. Of course, this does not indicate which tissues or organs have an increased oxygen requirement.

Oxygen arriving at the tissues must move from capillary blood to individual cells. This delivery is influenced by factors that affect diffusion, including:

- intercellular Po_2 diffusion gradient
- diffusion distance
- rate of oxygen delivery to the capillary (Do_2)

- position on the oxygen-haemoglobin dissociation curve
- rate of cellular oxygen use and uptake (Vo_2)

To illustrate the effects of such factors in a clinical context, consider what may occur in sepsis. Tissue oedema may develop because of increased vascular permeability or excessive fluid administration. This may lead to an increased diffusion distance and therefore impaired oxygen diffusion. In addition, the rate of cellular oxygen use may be decreased because of the effects of endotoxins and cytokines, further contributing to cellular hypoxia (lack of oxygen).

It is important to understand that supranormal levels of oxygen delivery cannot compensate for diffusion problems between capillary and cell, nor for metabolic failure within the cell. Therefore administration of high-flow oxygen (Fio_2) is not the sole answer to tissue hypoxia.

Control of ventilation

Starter questions

Answers to the following questions are on page 58.

10. Why do people with head injuries have abnormal breathing patterns?
11. How much conscious control do we have over breathing?
12. What makes it harder for the lungs to expand and contract, and in which conditions is this relevant?

Ventilation is controlled by respiratory centres in the brain stem. The rate and depth change in response to input from sensory receptors and other areas of the brain. By adapting to such input, the respiratory centres maintain oxygen delivery, carbon dioxide levels and acid–base balance within the strict levels that are compatible with life. This is an example of a homeostatic mechanism, and it depends on receptors, control centres and effectors.

The main factors that control respiration are $Paco_2$, Pao_2 and pH (**Figure 1.31**). These chemical factors are monitored by chemoreceptors (sensory receptors, **Table 1.9**) that provide input to respiratory centres. The respiratory centres send nerve impulses to effectors in the respiratory muscles that control their frequency and force of contraction, thus changing the rate and depth of breathing. Changes in $Paco_2$, Pao_2 or pH away from normal levels cause appropriate alterations in breathing patterns to normalise the biochemical changes.

Respiratory centres

The respiratory centres in the brain are in the medulla, pons and brain stem. The inspiratory centre, a paired set of neurones,

Control of ventilation

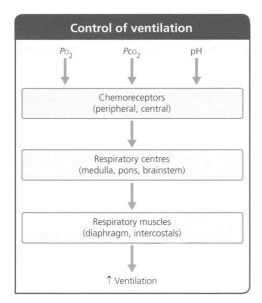

P_{O_2} P_{CO_2} pH

Chemoreceptors
(peripheral, central)

Respiratory centres
(medulla, pons, brainstem)

Respiratory muscles
(diaphragm, intercostals)

↑ Ventilation

Figure 1.31 Control of ventilation. Changes to the levels of arterial blood gases are detected by chemoreceptors. These activate the respiratory centres, which increase the respiration rate by stimulating the respiratory muscles. P_{aCO_2}, arterial partial pressure of carbon dioxide; P_{CO_2}, partial pressure of carbon dioxide; P_{aO_2}, arterial partial pressure of oxygen.

is in the medulla and sets the basic rhythm of automatically initiated inspiration. The inspiratory centre sends nerve impulses via the phrenic nerve to the diaphragm, and via intercostal nerves to the external intercostal muscles. This stimulates muscle contraction and thereby the process of inspiration.

The neurones then stop firing for a few seconds. In response, the respiratory muscles relax, elastic recoil of the lungs occurs and the chest wall contracts; these processes cause expiration. Automatic firing of the inspiratory centre produces a normal respiration rate of around 12 breaths/min.

The expiratory centre is in the medulla and works mainly in forced expiration (exhalation) to stimulate contraction of internal intercostal and abdominal muscles.

The respiratory centres in the pons modify inspiration, but their exact role is unclear.

Central chemoreceptors

Central and peripheral chemoreceptors modify the breathing rhythm initiated by the respiratory centres through changes in P_{aCO_2}, P_{aO_2} and pH.

■ Central chemoreceptors in the medulla monitor pH, which is directly related to P_{aCO_2} (see section 1.6).
■ Peripheral chemoreceptors in the aortic bodies in the aortic arch and in carotid bodies at the bifurcation of the common carotid arteries also monitor pH, P_{aCO_2} and P_{aO_2}. These feed information to the respiratory centres through the vagus and glossopharyngeal nerves.

The rate and depth of breathing are affected by the central chemoreceptor responding to changes in pH caused by alterations in P_{aCO_2}. Carbon dioxide diffuses from the blood into cerebrospinal fluid in the 4th ventricle, where it combines with water to form carbonic acid. This dissociates into hydrogen ions and bicarbonate ions:

$$CO_2 + H_2O \rightarrow H_2CO_3 \rightarrow H^+ + HCO_3^-$$

Receptors affecting ventilation			
Type	Location	Detects	Action on respiration rate
Peripheral	Aortic arch Bifurcation of common carotid arteries	↓ O_2 levels ↑ CO_2 levels ↓ pH	Increases
Central	Medulla	↑ CO_2 levels ↓ pH	Increases
Stretch	Lungs	Muscle use	Decreases
	Muscles	Muscle use	Increases
Irritant	Lungs	Dust and foreign particles	Increases

Table 1.9 Receptors affecting the rate of ventilation

The hydrogen ions stimulate the central chemoreceptors, which in turn send nerve impulses to respiratory centres in the medulla. Increasing carbon dioxide leads to a decrease in pH, so the central chemoreceptors fire more frequently and stimulate more impulses to respiratory muscles. This process increases the rate and depth of breathing, more carbon dioxide is expired and $Paco_2$ levels return to normal.

Peripheral chemoreceptors

Peripheral chemoreceptors detect increased $Paco_2$ through the associated decrease in the pH of arterial blood. The chemoreceptors respond by sending more impulses to respiratory centres to increase the rate and depth of breathing and improve excretion of carbon dioxide.

In exercise, the muscles produce lactic acid. The acid enters the blood, thereby increasing its concentration of hydrogen ions and decreasing its pH. Compensatory mechanisms increase ventilation in response. Breathing returns to normal as more carbon dioxide is expired and the blood concentration of hydrogen ions is lowered.

The Pao_2 is also monitored by peripheral chemoreceptors. However, Pao_2 needs to be very low before there is any change in ventilation. Also, the resulting increase in respiration has only relatively small effects on Pao_2.

The rate and depth of breathing can also be increased voluntarily, in response to pain or emotion, and by irritants such as dust or fumes.

Many drugs have sedative effects that can reduce respiratory drive. Such effects can cause a person with existing respiratory disease to develop type 2 respiratory failure. In contrast, only a limited number of drugs stimulate respiratory drive (e.g. doxapram); on rare occasions, these drugs can be used to treat type 2 respiratory failure.

Acid–base balance

Starter questions

Answers to the following questions are on page 58.

13. Why does the body need to regulate the acid-base balance so tightly?

14. What is a buffer and how is it involved in acid-base balance?

Normal body pH is tightly controlled between 7.35 and 7.45. The body can tolerate a range of pH of 6.8–7.7, which is equivalent to a hydrogen ion concentration of 20–160 nmol/L (an 8-fold absolute change). Therefore even slight changes in pH can have severe physiological effects.

Normal body metabolism leads to acid production (i.e. the production of hydrogen ions). Examples of acids produced by the body are lactic acid, phosphoric acid and sulphuric acid. When the production of such acids increases the concentration of hydrogen ions, the body must avoid a decrease in pH by:

- increasing the buffering of the acids
- excreting the acids

Control of the body's pH is termed acid base balance. pH control is effected by the kidneys, the lungs and different buffers. Arterial blood gas tests are used to assess acid-base balance in patients.

Buffer systems

A buffer is a substance that reduces changes in a solution's free hydrogen ions when acid or base is added. Thus, buffers maintain pH within the normal range.

The buffering system provides the body's first response to correcting body pH; the system acts within seconds or minutes. The key buffer is the bicarbonate carbonic acid system.

$$H^+ + HCO_3 \rightleftharpoons H_2CO_3 \rightleftharpoons CO_2 + H_2O$$

The conversion of carbonic acid to carbon dioxide and water is catalysed by carbonic anhydrase, a key enzyme for acid-base balance. This system prevents increases in metabolic acid. For example:

$$HCl + NaHCO_3 \rightarrow H_2CO_3 + NaCl$$

Non-carbonic buffers reduce acid production caused by increases in carbonic acid after rises in $Paco_2$ as a result of under-ventilation (respiratory acidosis). The most common non-carbonic buffer is haemoglobin.

Carbon dioxide enters red blood cells and combines with water to form carbonic acid. Deoxyhaemoglobin carries a negative charge, which attracts hydrogen ions from the carbonic acid to form a weak acid. This explains why red blood cells give up oxygen more easily when carbon dioxide levels are higher, shifting the oxygen haemoglobin curve to the right.

Respiratory system buffering

The respiratory system is the major factor controlling acid–base balance. The lungs excrete 99% of the carbonic acid produced daily. For comparison, the kidneys excrete only 1% (**Figure 1.32**).

The respiratory system can effect changes in pH within a couple of minutes, mainly by excreting carbon dioxide. Excess production of acid by metabolic processes (metabolic acidosis) increases carbonic acid. The carbonic acid then dissociates into carbon dioxide and water in a reaction catalysed by carbonic anhydrase. The carbon dioxide is eliminated by the lungs during expiration. Thus, increased respiration eliminates more acid. This process is controlled by the direct stimulation of chemoreceptors by reduced pH.

> **Measurement of arterial blood gases (ABGs) provides much useful information during an acute illness,** for example helping to identify respiratory failure (low Po_2), metabolic acidosis and cellular hypoxia (e.g. in sepsis, which requires intensive care). Ability to interpret ABGs rapidly is essential.

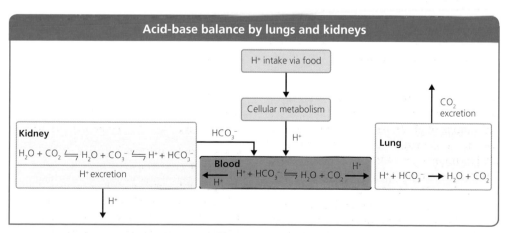

Figure 1.32 Acid–base balance by the lungs and kidneys. H^+ ions are produced as a result of cellular metabolism. They are buffered by HCO_3^- and by proteins such as haemoglobin so that they can be carried in the blood. They are also buffered by ammonia and other substances and excreted in the kidney. The kidney also replaces the supply of bicarbonate. In the lungs H^+ combines with HCO_3^- to produce CO_2 which is exhaled. The two excretion methods can be up or down regulated in response to changes in the overall acid–base balance.

Renal system buffering

The kidneys, as well as the respiratory system, have an important role in acid–base balance. However, unlike the respiratory system, the kidneys respond slowly to changes in pH.

The kidneys can compensate for decreases in pH by increasing the excretion of hydrogen ions and by conserving bicarbonate. These mechanisms can take several days to develop, so they do not usually completely compensate for the increase in acid. The extent of renal compensation can be judged by measuring base excess on blood gases; larger positive values suggest significant renal compensation for an acidosis.

If the levels of two of pH, bicarbonate and carbon dioxide have been measured, the Henderson–Hasselbalch equation allows the 3rd value to be calculated.

$$pH = 6.1 + \log_{10}(HCO_3^-)/(0.03 \times P\text{A}CO_2)$$

Disturbances of acid–base balance are discussed in Chapter 2.

Pulmonary circulation

Starter questions

Answers to the following questions are on page 58–59.

15. What is so special about the pulmonary circulation system?
16. Why do we need to breathe in oxygen, rather than another gas?
17. Why is blood in arteries red and blood in veins blue?

The role of the pulmonary circulation is to:

- supply deoxygenated blood to the lungs
- facilitate oxygenation of this blood by close interactions with alveoli
- transport oxygenated blood to the heart

Deoxygenated blood is delivered by the pulmonary arterial system, which arises from the right ventricle (**Figure 1.11**). The pulmonary artery walls are thin and contain only a small amount of smooth muscle. Therefore the system is a low-pressure one, with a mean systolic arterial pressure of about 25 mmHg. The low pressure of the pulmonary arterial system maintains the work of the right heart at a low level.

The pulmonary arteries divide to form an extensive interconnected capillary bed around the alveoli. When cardiac output increases, these capillaries almost completely cover the surface of the alveoli.

A red cell passes across several alveoli before returning to the pulmonary veins; its average transit time is 0.75 s under normal resting conditions. Because of gravity, lung perfusion by the pulmonary circulation is increased at the lung bases and reduced at the lung apices.

Both $P\text{A}O_2$ and $P\text{A}CO_2$ are key regulators of blood flow in the pulmonary circulation. Alveolar hypoxia or an increase in $P\text{A}CO_2$ causes vasoconstriction of the supplying pulmonary arterioles and arteries. This normal physiological response prevents ventilation–perfusion mismatches, in which deoxygenated blood passes through regions where oxygenation will not happen (**Figure 1.33** and **Figure 1.34**).

> The vasoconstrictive response of pulmonary arterioles to hypoxia is a physiological mechanism for matching ventilation with perfusion. However, persisting hypoxia in chronic lung diseases causes generalised pulmonary arteriole vasoconstriction that is pathological and results in pulmonary hypertension and right-sided cardiac failure (cor pulmonale).

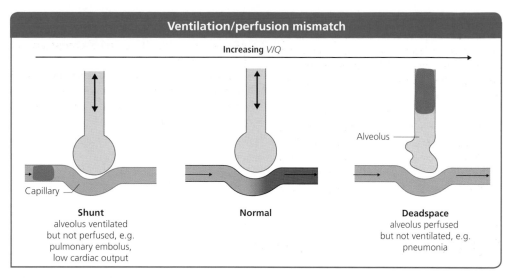

Ventilation/perfusion mismatch

Increasing *V/Q*

Alveolus

Capillary

Shunt
alveolus ventilated
but not perfused, e.g.
pulmonary embolus,
low cardiac output

Normal

Deadspace
alveolus perfused
but not ventilated, e.g.
pneumonia

Figure 1.33 Ventilation/perfusion mismatch. There are compensatory mechanisms to prevent V/Q mismatch significantly affecting overall lung function. For example hypoxic vasoconstriction means that blood flow is reduced to alveoli with a low *V/Q*.

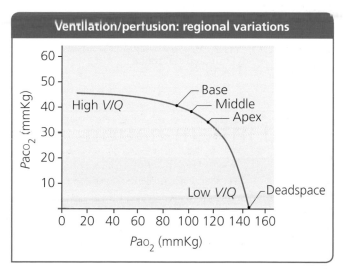

Ventilation/perfusion: regional variations

$Paco_2$ (mmKg)

High *V/Q*

Base
Middle
Apex

Low *V/Q*   Deadspace

Pao_2 (mmKg)

Figure 1.34 Regional variations in perfusion and ventilation lead to variations in *V/Q* ratio. Basal alveoli with lower *V/Q* ratios tend towards shunts, whereas apical alveoli with high *V/Q* ratios tend towards deadspace.

The bronchial circulation helps regulate temperature and humidity in the airways because of its anatomical configuration. It also supplies fluid for secretion into the airways in response to inflammation.

Lymphatic drainage from the lungs is normally <0.5 mL/min and is into the brachiocephalic veins. This flow can increase up to 10-fold when pulmonary oedema is present.

Additional functions of the pulmonary circulation

The main function of the pulmonary circulation is to move blood around to allow gas exchange within the lungs. Other functions include acting as a blood volume reservoir (**Table 1.10**). The lung can reduce pulmonary vascular resistance, because pulmonary

Respiratory system functions	
Respiration	Transfer of O_2 into the blood Excretion of CO_2 Control of acid–base balance
Immunological	Adaptive immunity to respiratory microorganisms Acting as a filter to remove invading pathogens from the blood
Pulmonary circulation	Blood volume reservoir Acting as a filter to prevent pulmonary emboli reaching the systemic circulation
Metabolic	Conversion of angiotensin-1 to angiotensin-2 Synthesis (e.g. coagulation factors) Inactivation of metabolic factors (e.g. histamine, bradykinin and serotonin)

Table 1.10 Functions of the respiratory system

artery pressures increase through recruitment and distension. This mechanism also allows the lungs to increase blood volume with small changes in pressures.

The lungs also filter blood passing from the venous to the arterial circulation, removing different types of emboli. For example, blood clots originating in the venous system are filtered out by the pulmonary capillary bed, preventing arterial thrombosis. Similarly, large numbers of white cells are sequestered within the pulmonary circulation, and transient bacteraemias are controlled before reaching the arterial circulation.

The lung also has metabolic functions. Angiotensin-1 is metabolised to the vasoconstrictor angiotensin-2 by angiotensin-converting enzyme in the pulmonary circulation. The pulmonary endothelium synthesises coagulation factors and metabolises histamine, bradykinin and serotonin.

Lung immunity and inflammation

Starter questions

Answers to the following questions are on page 59.

18. Why do patients with sepsis have a high respiratory rate even if they do not have a lung infection?
19. How does the immune system affect non-infectious lung diseases?
20. What types of vaccine are used to protect against respiratory infections?

The lungs are constantly exposed to inhaled air and aspirated contents of the nasopharynx, putting them at risk of infection by many different microorganisms. To prevent infection, the lungs have a complex immune defence including physical defences and innate and adaptive immune responses. However, lung tissue is delicate, and an excessive immune response could easily impair gas exchange.

Maintaining healthy lungs requires a balance between producing effective immune responses to pathogens, and minimising inflammatory responses to these pathogens as well as other inhaled proinflammatory substances (e.g. allergens, pollutants and noxious agents). Excessive immune and inflammatory responses are responsible for many of the clinical features of lung infections. These abnormal responses also cause many non-infective diseases of the lung (as well as other organs); for example they underlie the pathogenesis of asthma, COPD, acute respiratory distress syndrome and interstitial lung diseases.

Innate and adaptive immunity

Immunity to microbial pathogens is divided into innate and adaptive immune responses.

- Innate immunity consists of physical, mucosal and cellular defences that act rapidly to prevent all invading pathogens through non-specific responses to conserved microbial-derived molecules
- Adaptive immunity develops after exposure to an invading pathogen and takes days to develop. Pathogen molecules that cause an adaptive immune response are termed antigens; they are usually proteins but can be polysaccharides or lipids. Once present, an adaptive immune response can clear the invading pathogen and prevent subsequent infections by the same pathogen. The adaptive response is highly effective but very specific.

The immunological response to infection

The immunological response to a pathogen is divided into the following overlapping steps (**Figure 1.35** and **Table 1.11**).

1. Physical and mucosal defences; these usually prevent infection and the subsequent steps
2. Interactions with immune cellular responses: either innate alone (if this is the first exposure to the pathogen) or innate and adaptive (if there has been prior exposure to the pathogen)
3. Inflammation
4. Development of adaptive immune responses (which takes ≥ 5 days)
5. Clearance of the invading pathogen. Mechanisms required for the killing and clearance of examples of important type of respiratory pathogens are shown in **Table 1.12**
6. Resolution of inflammation

A similar stepwise response can also occur to non-infective stimuli such as inhaled allergens (e.g. pollen) or pro-inflammatory chemical substances (e.g. asbestos fibres).

Physical and mucosal defences

The respiratory system contains structural and mucosal barriers that:

- prevent microbes reaching the lung
- improve clearance of those that do

Physical barriers of the upper airways

Nasal hairs filter large particles (> 30 µm). The removal of smaller particles (10–30 µm) is

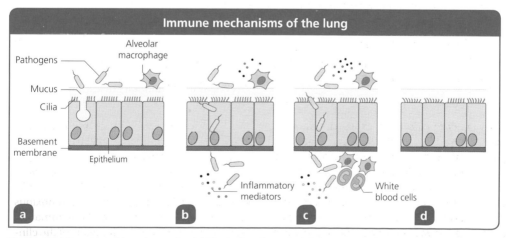

Figure 1.35 Overview of lung immunity. (a) Physical and mucosal defences provide a barrier to pathogens. (b) Invading pathogens trigger the immune response. (c) White blood cells are recruited by inflammation. (d) The pathogens are cleared and inflammation resolved.

Comparison of innate and adaptive systems		
	Innate	Adaptive
Evolution	All animals	Only found in jawed vertebrates
Specificity of response	Broad and not specific	Highly specific
	Depends on PAMPs	Depends on host recognition of antigen
	No immunological memory	Powerful immunological memory
Speed of response	Immediate, with recruitment of additional effectors within hours	Develops after 5 to 7 days
		Rapid during reinfection
Site	At epithelial surfaces and in blood	Antibodies: blood and lung epithelial lining fluid
	Some recruitment in response to inflammation e.g. neutrophils, extravasation of extracellular fluid containing complement	T cells: spleen, lymph nodes, BALT
		Recruited during infection into the lungs
Efficacy	Generally effective at preventing infection being established	Highly protective against some pathogens eg viral pathogens, systemic infection with bacteria
		Important for controlling pathogens that overcome innate immunity
Main lung effectors	Physical defences	Antibody and B cells
	Mucosal antimicrobial peptides, lysozyme, lactoferrin	Th1, Th2, Th17 CD4 cells
	Alveolar macrophages	CD8 cytotoxic cells (viruses)
	Complement	Amplified phagocyte and complement mediated immunity (bacteria)
	Neutrophils, eosinophils, basophils, mast cells	
	NK cells (intracellular pathogens)	
	Interferons (viruses)	

Table 1.11 Comparison of the innate and adaptive immune systems

improved by the increased air-mucosal contact produced by turbulent airflow through the nose.

The entire respiratory epithelium down to the alveoli and including the nasal passages is covered in a layer of mucus. The mucus traps particulate matter and microbes and thus facilitates their removal.

During infection or inflammation, vasodilation causes nasal congestion to narrow the nasal passages, thus limiting the number of particles or microbes entering the nose. Increased mucus production helps clear the nose of particles and microbes.

Coughing and sneezing

Stimulation of receptors in the nose, larynx and trachea triggers cough and sneeze to forcibly expel particles and improve mucociliary clearance. A cough has three phases:
1. an inhalation
2. a forced exhalation against a closed glottis
3. a sudden opening of the glottis, which releases air from the lungs through the mouth

A cough can be voluntary or involuntary. Involuntary coughs usually result from irritation of the respiratory mucosa. The average cough expels 3000 droplets of saliva at speeds of up to 80 km/h.

A sneeze is an explosive expulsion of air from the lungs though the nose and mouth. Sneezes are usually initiated by irritation of the nasal mucosa. A sneeze can expel 40,000 droplets at speeds of up to 320 km/h. Both coughs and sneezes can spread infectious re-

		Immune control of respiratory pathogens
Pathogen	Type of pathogen	Killing mechanisms
Streptococcus pneumoniae	Extracellular bacteria	Mucosal antimicrobial peptides, lactoferrin, lysozyme
		Opsonisation by complement and antibody
		Macrophage and neutrophil phagocytosis
Mycobacterium tuberculosis	Intracellular bacteria, infects macrophages	Mucosal antimicrobial peptides, lactoferrin, lysozyme
		Macrophage; requires T cell-mediated adaptive immunity to boost intracellular killing mechanisms
		Neutrophils
Influenza A	RNA virus, infects epithelial cells	Interferons by boosting cell resistance to viral infection and improving NK cell function
		Cytotoxic CD8 T cell (adaptive immunity) and NK cell (innate immunity) mediated lysis of infected cells
		Antibody (prevent viral adhesion to cells, and identifies virally infected cells for NK killing)
Aspergillus fumigatus	Extracellular filamentous fungi	Inhaled spores: phagocytosis by macrophages
		Hyphae: neutrophil degranulation over hyphal surface (too large to be phagocytosed)

Table 1.12 Immune mechanisms involved in control of important respiratory pathogens

spiratory diseases, particularly those caused by viruses.

The glottis

Closure of the glottis during eating and drinking prevents ingested material from entering the lungs. The glottis also bars vomitus from the lungs.

Airway branching

The change in airflow at airway branch points increases contact between particulate matter and the respiratory epithelial mucous layer. As airflow is reduced, particles of >2 μm settle because of the effect of gravity. Particles 0.2–0.5 μm in size are usually exhaled. However, particles between 0.2 and 2 μm, which include most bacteria and some fungal spores, can reach the alveoli.

Mucociliary escalator

The mucous layer covering the bronchial epithelium contains mucopolysaccharides produced by submucous glands in the large airways, and goblet and club (Clara) cells in the smaller airways. The apical surfaces of epithelial cells of the bronchial tree are covered in hair-like projections into the mucous layer; these are called cilia. There are about 200 cilia

per cell. The ciliated cells extend from the trachea to the terminal bronchioles.

Cilia are 6–8 μm long. They consist of proteins organised into outer and central bundles (**Figure 1.36**), the contraction of which causes the cilia to beat in a coordinated fashion. This movement propels mucus up and out of the airways and into the oesophagus, thereby clearing the lungs of microbes and particulate matter trapped in the mucus (**Figure 1.37**).

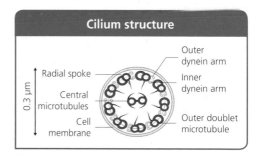

Figure 1.36 Cross section of a cilium. There are 9 outer pairs of microtubules, 1 central pair connected by nexin bridges (between the outer microtubules) and radial spoke proteins (outer to inner microtubules). The short inner and outer dynein arms power the movements of the cilium. The majority of mutations causing primary ciliary dyskinesia affect the dynein arms. Cilia are 6–8 μm in length and 0.3 μm in diameter.

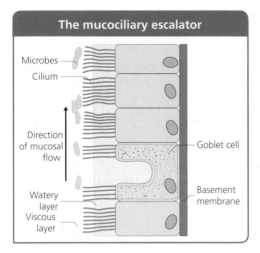

The mucociliary escalator

Microbes
Cilium

Direction of mucosal flow

Goblet cell

Watery layer
Viscous layer

Basement membrane

Figure 1.37 The mucociliary escalator. The mucus that coats the airways has two layers: an upper viscous layer and a watery sublayer. The viscous layer is moved upwards by the force of the strokes of the cilia. Their movement carries microbes and foreign bodies trapped in the mucus out of the airways.

> **Patients with genetic defects of the cilia (primary ciliary dyskinesia) develop recurrent lower respiratory tract infections and bronchiectasis,** which demonstrates the importance of the mucociliary escalator for preventing lung infection.

Epithelial barrier function

Intercellular tight junctions between epithelial cells and the basement membrane prevent the passage of molecules and microbes past the epithelium. Endothelial cells also have an external basement membrane that helps prevents microbial invasion of the blood.

Soluble mediators of immunity

As well as mucus, the airway-lining fluid contains a wide range of soluble mediators of immunity that inhibit or kill microbial pathogens. These soluble mediators of immunity are produced by the epithelium and include lactoferrin, antimicrobial peptides (e.g. defensins and LL-37), secretory leucocyte protease inhibitor and lysozyme.

Soluble immune effectors present in the blood and, to a lesser extent, in airway-lining fluid can also coat invading pathogens.

These soluble immune effectors can then be recognised by receptors on the cell surface of phagocytes to improve the efficiency of phagocytosis in a process called opsonisation. This group of soluble immune effectors include the following.

- Surfactant
- Blood acute phase reactants such as C-reactive protein
- The complement system: a proteinase cascade that opsonises invading pathogens with the powerful opsonin C3b and iC3b, and produces proinflammatory mediators (C3a and C5a); complement can also kill some bacteria directly through punching holes in their cell membranes by forming the membrane attack complex
- Antibody (as part of the adaptive immune response): antibody improves opsonisation directly by binding to Fc-γ receptors on the surface of white cells, or indirectly by increasing opsonisation of the pathogen with complement

Cellular immune effectors

Microbes penetrating the body's physical and mucosal defences then interact directly and indirectly with immune effector cells, which include dedicated immune effector cells such as a range of different types of white cells, and cells with other functions that can contribute to the immune response such as epithelial cells (**Table 1.13**). The range of white cells involved in immune interactions varies with the type of invading organism and the site of infection.

Important white cell types are:

- alveolar macrophages
- neutrophils
- monocytes
- dendritic cells
- mast cells
- eosinophils
- lymphocytes (B cells, T cells, γδ cells)
- natural killer cells

Alveolar macrophages

Alveolar macrophages are long-lived cells resident within the lung (with a lifespan measured in at least months) in the lumen of the

Lung immune effector cells			
Cells	Site	Role(s) as or in	Relevance in disease
Epithelial cells	Bronchial tree Alveoli	Barrier to pathogens Mucociliary clearance of pathogens Production of soluble antimicrobial products Inflammatory responses to infection	Target cells for respiratory viral infections Inherited ciliary dyskinesia results in bronchiectasis Epithelial damage drives lung fibrosis
Alveolar macrophages	Bronchial lumen Alveoli	Phagocytosis and killing of pathogens Inflammatory responses to infection	Important for preventing pneumonia Target cell for intracellular pathogens (e.g. tuberculosis)
Dendritic cells	Respiratory mucosa	Antigen presentation	Development of adaptive immune responses
Neutrophils	Bone marrow Blood Alveoli (if inflamed) Bronchi (if inflamed) Lung interstitium (if inflamed)	Phagocytosis and killing of pathogens (extracellular bacteria and fungi)	Important for preventing pneumonia COPD and bronchiectasis characterised by neutrophilic infiltration of the airways Neutrophil proteases cause emphysema Sputum purulence is caused by neutrophil content
Mast cells	Respiratory mucosa	Release of histamine and IL-4	Important for immunity to parasites Important for pathogenesis of allergic asthma
Eosinophils	Blood, lymph nodes and BALT Respiratory epithelium during inflammation	Activation by IgE Release of histamine, major basic protein, reactive oxygen species and IL-4	Important for immunity to parasites Important for pathogenesis of allergic asthma
B cells	Lymph nodes, spleen and BALT	Production of antibody (humoral adaptive immunity)	Antibody deficiency syndromes result in respiratory tract infections and bronchiectasis
T cells (cell-mediated immunity)	Lymph nodes, spleen and BALT Respiratory epithelium, interstitium and brochoalveolar lavage fluid during inflammation	CD8 cells: kill virally infected and tumour cells CD4 Th1: boost inflammatory responses and macrophage killing of intracellular pathogens CD4 Th2: improve antibody responses CD4 Th17: improve mucosal immunity Tregs: anti-inflammatory NK cells: kill host cells	CD8 cells increase epithelial damage during influenza Th1-mediated inflammation important in control of tuberculosis and for pathogenesis of COPD and sarcoidosis Th2 important for pathogenesis of asthma Th17 possibly important for pathogenesis of neutrophilic asthma Tregs important for preventing autoimmune disease NK cells kill virally-infected and tumour cells

BALT, bronchus-associated lymphoid tissue; COPD, chronic obstructive pulmonary disease; Ig, immunoglobulin; IL, interleukin; Tregs, T regulatory cells.

Table 1.13 Key effector cells of lung immune response

alveoli and bronchi, where they provide a key line of defence against microbial invasion. They are the predominant cell found in fluid recovered from deep within the respiratory tract during bronchoscopy (bronchoalveolar lavage fluid, BAL), and express a large range of surface proteins that bind to microbial products and immune mediators (**Figure 1.38**).

Alveolar macrophages are phagocytic. Phagocytosis is the process by which white cells actively ingest and kill invading microbes. During phagocytosis, microbes are internalised by the macrophage in a membrane-lined vacuole called a phagosome. The phagosome then merges with another cellular vesicle, the lysosome, to form a phagolysosome, in which the microbes are killed by:

- proteases
- antimicrobial proteins and peptides
- superoxide and nitric oxide

As well as phagocytic and microbicidal functions, alveolar macrophages secrete inflammatory mediators and can present microbial antigens to lymphocytes (see page 54).

Similar macrophage populations are present in other organs. For example, in the spleen and liver macrophages phagocytose microbes that have entered the blood.

Neutrophils

Neutrophils are short-lived (with a lifespan measured in days) circulating white cells with a characteristic multilobed nucleus. They are phagocytic, and their main role is to kill invading microbes, especially extracellular bacteria.

During infection, the bone marrow produces large numbers of neutrophils. Consequently, the blood's white cell count is increased (leucocytosis). Neutrophils migrate from the blood to sites of infection and inflammation in the lung. For example, during pneumonia neutrophils migrate into the alveoli. Therefore, during infection they are often the dominant cell type in sputum or fluid obtained by bronchoalveolar lavage.

Monocytes

Monocytes are the largest circulating white cells and have a notched or bean shaped nucleus that replenish and support tissue macrophage populations. They migrate to the lungs in response to infection and inflammation. The process of migrating into the lungs stimulates monocytes to mature into phagocytic macrophages or into dendritic cells.

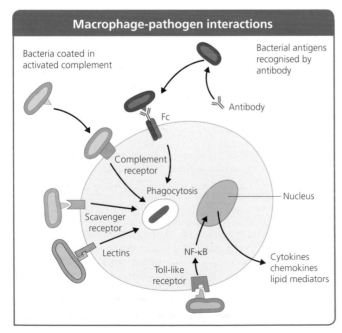

Figure 1.38 Macrophage interactions with pathogens. Five main types of receptor on macrophages interact with pathogens: complement receptors, Fc receptors, lectins, scavenger receptors and Toll-like receptors. Binding of a pathogen to one of these macrophage receptors stimulates phagocytosis and the release of various inflammatory mediators.

Macrophage-pathogen interactions

Bacteria coated in activated complement

Bacterial antigens recognised by antibody

Antibody

Fc

Complement receptor

Phagocytosis

Nucleus

Scavenger receptor

Lectins

NF-κB

Toll-like receptor

Cytokines chemokines lipid mediators

Dendritic cells

Dendritic cells are resident cells in the mucosa of the lung. Their main role is not to kill microbes but to stimulate an adaptive immune response to infection. To this end, dendritic cells have long cellular extensions that sample airway contents. They then migrate to lung lymph nodes to present to lymphocytes microbial antigens from degraded microbes.

Mast cells

Mast cells are present in the lung mucosa, and bind IgE, a type of antibody central to allergic reactions, to their surface. Mast cells respond to molecules that induce allergic responses as they are recognised by cell-surface bound IgE, releasing inflammatory mediators, especially histamine and interleukin (IL)-4 which cause vasodilatation (dilatation of the blood vessels) and lymphocyte recruitment to the affected area.

Mast cells have a central role in allergic responses.

Eosinophils

Eosinophils are uncommon white cells (<6% of all white cells) found in the blood, lymph nodes and lymph tissue that is closely associated anatomically with the respiratory mucosa. Eosinophils are similar to mast cells in that they release histamine and IL-4 when activated by antibodies, a process called degranulation. They are also activated by the chemokines eotaxin and RANTES. Another cytokine, IL-5, is important for maintaining eosinophils at sites of inflammation.

Eosinophils have a central role in killing parasites. They are also key cells in the pathogenesis of asthma.

Lymphocytes

Lymphocytes are small white cells with large nuclei and a thin layer of cytoplasm found in the blood, spleen, lymph nodes and tissue associated lymphoid tissue such as bronchus associated lymphoid tissue (BALT), and at sites of inflammation. This type of cell has several subsets largely defined by their function rather than anatomical appearance, each with distinct functions in the immune response.

B cells

When activated, B cells differentiate into plasma cells and produce antibodies. B cells are essential for antibody-mediated adaptive immunity (humoral immunity).

T cells

T cells are essential for cell-mediated adaptive immunity (adaptive immune effector responses mediated directly by cells) and also for many antibody responses.

T cells are divided into two main types.

- CD8 cytotoxic cells kill virus-infected cells and tumour cells
- CD4 cells are further subdivided into T helper (Th) cells; Th1, Th2 and Th17 subsets each stimulate different aspects of the adaptive immune response

Another T-cell subset is the γδ T cells, which release cytokines as part of the innate immune response.

T regulatory cells (Tregs)

T regulatory cells, also known as Tregs, modulate inflammatory responses by producing anti-inflammatory cytokines (defined below) and prevent immune-mediated damage to the host. Tregs are important for preventing autoimmune diseases, such as rheumatoid arthritis.

Natural killer cells

Natural killer cells are lymphocytes that kill cells infected with viruses or other intracellular pathogens and tumour cells as part of the innate immune response or after target cells are recognised by a specific antibody.

Inflammation

A key feature of the innate immune response is the generation of inflammation in response to invading pathogens (**Figure 1.39**).

Induction

In the lungs, inflammation due to infection depends on the recognition of microbes by alveolar macrophages and epithelial cells, which is achieved with the following molecules:

- Host cell membrane receptors called pathogen associated molecular patterns

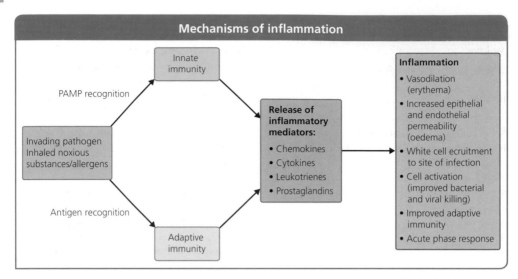

Figure 1.39 Mechanism of inflammation generation. Inflammation can be generated by both the adaptive and the innate immune system. PAMP, pathogen-associated molecular pattern; Th, T helper.

(PAMPs), which bind to a range of molecules that are conserved between microbial pathogens. These can respond to molecules expressed on the surface of the pathogen or released into host fluids. The most important PAMPs are the toll-like receptors (TLRs), e.g. TLR-4 recognition of lipopolysaccharide, a conserved component of many bacterial cell walls

■ Cell surface receptors for proinflammatory cytokines (e.g. IL-1 and tumour necrosis factor-alpha) and products of the activated complement and clotting pathways

■ Intracellular receptors that recognise microbial PAMPs found inside the cell (e.g. Nod-like receptors) recognise peptidoglycan released from bacterial cell-walls after bacteria have been killed and degraded in phagosomes

Mediators

The identification of microbes by these receptors causes the cells to produce proinflammatory mediators either through changes to gene transcription or altering activity of key enzymes responsible for mediator synthesis. Inflammatory mediators include:

■ Cytokines: proteins that bind to cell surface receptors on other cells and thereby influence their behaviour, for example by activating neutrophils so that they are more able to phagocytose invading bacteria

■ Chemokines: proteins that cause other cells to migrate to the site of infection, usually by exiting the blood; in the lung, the migrating cells must penetrate endothelial cells to reach the lung interstitium, and epithelial barriers to enter the lumen of the alveoli and bronchi

■ Lipid mediators of inflammation: the leukotrienes and prostaglandins

Increased expression of chemokines and cytokines is controlled by cellular transcription factors, the most important of which is NF-κB. Some key inflammatory mediators for lung disease are listed in **Table 1.14**.

Effects

The consequences of inflammation are as follows.

■ Vasodilation, which increases blood flow to the site of infection and therefore assisting white cell recruitment and providing a source for the increase in extracellular fluid

■ Increased vascular and epithelial permeability, which increase the amount of extracellular fluid in the interstitium

Inflammatory mediators for lung disease		
Mediator	Role or effects	Example(s) of clinical relevance
NF-κB	Transcription factor	Controls increased expression of cytokines and chemokines during inflammation
Histamine	Vasodilation Stimulation of lymphocyte migration	Important for allergic reactions and hay fever; inhibited by antihistamines
IL-1	Proinflammatory cytokine	Causes pyrexia, important for immunity to infection
IL-6	Proinflammatory cytokine Causes acute phase response	Causes pyrexia, important for immunity to infection Anti-IL-6 treatment for rheumatoid arthritis predisposes to infection
IL-8	Neutrophil chemokine	Major role for neutrophil infiltration of the lung during infection
Tumour necrosis factor α	Proinflammatory cytokine Inhibits development of CD4 Th2 cells	Causes pyrexia, important for immunity to infection Anti-tumour necrosis factor treatment used for sarcoidosis and rheumatoid arthritis, but predisposes to infection (e.g. tuberculosis)
IL-10	Anti-inflammatory Inhibits development of CD4 Th1 cells	Important for control and resolution of inflammation during infection
Transforming growth factor-β	Anti-inflammatory Induces fibrosis	Important for development of pulmonary fibrosis
IL-4	Increases development of CD4 Th2 cells B-cell activation (to produce IgE)	Important for allergic asthma
IL-5	Promotes eosinophil survival	Important for allergic asthma
IL-13	B-cell activation (to produce IgE)	Important for allergic asthma
Eotaxins and RANTES	Induce eosinophil migration and activation	Important for allergic asthma
Interferon-γ	Increased macrophage killing capability	Has been used during treatment of some chronic infections
Interferon-α and interferon-β	Inhibit viral replication in the cell Activate natural killer cells	Important for immunity to viral infections
Leukotrienes	Increase smooth muscle contraction, vascular permeability and mucus production	Antileukotrienes (e.g. montelukast) used to treat asthma
Prostaglandins	Pro- and anti-inflammatory	Target for non-steroidal anti-inflammatory drugs (e.g. ibuprofen)

IL, interleukin.

Table 1.14 Key inflammatory mediators for lung diseases

and alveoli. This increases the amount of antibody and complement present at the site of infection, so improving microbial killing
■ Migration and extravasation of white cells (neutrophils, monocytes and lymphocytes) to the site of infection
■ Activation of the clotting pathway with fibrin deposition, forming an extracellular protein barrier layer to prevent bleeding and migration of microbes into the blood

■ A systemic acute phase response characterised by rapid increases in circulating blood concentrations of a range of plasma proteins called acute phase reactants (e.g. C-reactive protein and ferritin) which can help inhibit microbial survival in the blood. The acute phase response is largely driven by the cytokine IL-6, which acts on the liver and is recognised clinically by the presence of fever (temperature > 37.5 °C), high C-reactive protein and increased erythrocyte sedimentation rate

- Enhanced phagocytic function of macrophages and neutrophils, improved cellular antiviral defences (mainly mediated by interferons), and activation of natural killer and mast cells
- Improved cellular antiviral defences. These are mainly mediated by interferons (IFNs), which have complex effects on host cells that reduce their susceptibility to viral infection including decreasing protein synthesis, degrading RNA, and inducing cell death by apoptosis
- An improved adaptive immune response, resulting in more effective antibody and/ or cellular immunity to the causative pathogen

> **Blood tests that help in recognising and monitoring inflammation** include C reactive protein (CRP) (e.g. >100 mg/L in bacterial pneumonia versus the normal <5 mg/L), and erythrocyte sedimentation rate (ESR) (less sensitive than CRP). White cell count also rises (due to increased circulating neutrophils) and serum albumin falls, but these are not reliable markers of inflammation. In chronic inflammation haemoglobin concentration falls and platelet count rises (thrombocythaemia).

Clinical effects

Inflammation is essential for the control of invading pathogens but is also directly responsible for some of the clinical features of infection (**Table 1.15**). For example, the leak of fluid and migration of white cells into the alveoli causes consolidation, the cardinal feature of pneumonia. Hence the effects of inflammation on alveoli impair gas exchange and can result in hypoxia. Excessive inflammatory responses to infections can also inhibit myocardial and renal function, cause systemic hypotension and result in widespread endothelial leak throughout both lungs. These effects can cause septic shock and acute respiratory distress syndrome (see Chapter 11). As a consequence there are powerful mechanisms involved in controlling inflammation in the lungs in response to invading microbes or physical insults. These include the release of anti-inflammatory cytokines such as interleukin-10 (IL-10) by macrophages and Tregs, and by apoptosis and macrophage ingestion of recruited white cells which counterbalance pro-inflammatory stimuli.

Once an infection is controlled, similar mechanisms promote inhibition of inflammation and allow the affected tissue to return too normal. Failure of these poorly understood regulatory mechanisms will promote prolonged inflammation and damage to the host tissues.

> **Inflammation associated with infections, even severe pneumonias, usually resolves completely with little or no persisting lung damage.** However, some infections result in destruction of lung tissue, caused either directly by the pathogen or indirectly by the inflammatory response; lung cavitation is the consequence. Lung repair after infection by other pathogens (e.g. tuberculosis) causes a fibrotic reaction; an excess of extracellular matrix proteins are formed, which distort the lung tissue.

Inflammation due to non-infective stimuli

Lung inflammation is also caused by inhaled non-infective stimuli. These include cigarette smoke, pollution and mineral dusts which cause inflammation by similar processes as microbes. These non-infective stimuli cause inflammation by physical damage to host cells releasing 'danger associated molecular patterns' (DAMPs) rather than PAMPs. In addition, lung inflammation can be caused by antigens that cause an allergic inflammatory reaction, i.e. an inflammatory response to a usually harmless molecule which damages the host.

The four main types of allergic response (allergy, antibody-dependent cytotoxicity,

Immune- and inflammation-mediated respiratory diseases

Disease	Immune mechanisms
Immune responses to infection	
Respiratory viruses	Epithelial cell death Mucosal damage Increased risk of secondary bacterial infections
Pneumonia	White cell recruitment Extracellular fluid leak into alveoli to form consolidation and cause hypoxia
Tuberculosis	CD4 Th1-mediated response with associated lung damage (cavitation, bronchiectasis and focal lung fibrosis), lymphadenopathy and pleural effusions Mantoux (or Heaf) test: type 4 hypersensitivity reaction to tuberculosis antigens
Acute respiratory distress syndrome	Excessive inflammation causing generalised extracellular fluid leak into alveoli and severe hypoxia
Septic shock	Excessive inflammation causing hypotension and multiorgan failure
Bronchiectasis	Previous pneumonia or viral infections causing bronchial wall damage that impairs immunity and allows chronic bacterial infection
Empyema	White cell recruitment and extracellular fluid leak into the pleural space Formation of fibrinous adhesions that create pleural loculations
Abnormal immune responses	
Anaphylaxis	Type 1 hypersensitivity reaction with IgE-mediated mast cell degranulation
Hay fever	Type 1 hypersensitivity reactions to pollen etc.
Asthma	CD4 Th2, eosinophils, IgE, IL-4, IL-5 and IL-13-mediated allergic airways inflammation CD4 Th17 responses possibly important for neutrophilic forms of asthma
Chronic obstructive pulmonary disease	CD4 Th1-mediated neutrophilic airways inflammation
Pulmonary fibrosis	Abnormal tissue repair with increased formation of extracellular matrix
Sarcoidosis	CD4 Th1-mediated granulomatous inflammation
Hypersensitivity pneumonitis	Type 3 and type 4 hypersensitivity reactions to inhaled antigens
Vasculitis	Type 3 hypersensitivity reaction caused by autoantibodies to neutrophils or basement membrane proteins

Ig, immunoglobulin; IL, interleukin.

Table 1.15 Examples of immune- and inflammation-mediated respiratory diseases

Hypersensitivity reactions

Type	Name	Mechanism
1	Allergic responses	Immunoglobulin E-mediated activation of mast cells, basophils and eosinophils CD4 Th2 responses
2	Antibody-dependent cytotoxicity	Antibody binding to host cells causes cell death through activation of complement, natural killer cells and macrophages
3	Immune complex disease	Antibody binds to soluble antigens to form antibody–antigen complexes that deposit in tissue to cause inflammation
4	Delayed type hypersensitivity	Antigen recognition by CD4 Th1 or Th2 cells and cytotoxic CD8 cells Independent of antibody Takes 2–14 days to develop

Table 1.16 Types of hypersensitivity reaction

immune-complex disease, and delayed type hypersensitivity) are described in **Table 1.16**. Allergic inflammatory responses to inhaled non-infective stimuli and allergens underlie episodes of acute lung inflammation (e.g. acute hypersensitivity pneumonitis and exacerbations of asthma and COPD) and persisting chronic inflammation leading to irreversible lung damage (e.g. in COPD and pneumoconiosis). Abnormal lung healing after poorly defined insults causes interstitial lung diseases, both those with an excessive fibrotic response driven by fibroblasts (pulmonary fibrosis) and those associated with poor resolution of lung inflammation (e.g. organising pneumonia).

Mechanisms of adaptive immune responses

The adaptive immune response requires precise recognition by the immune system of specific molecules expressed by the target pathogen. On first exposure to a particular pathogen, a subset of the body's T cells, B cells or both develops an adaptive response to antigens expressed by this pathogen. This process allows the adaptive immune mechanisms to specifically target this particular pathogen.

Importantly, the ability to recognise an antigen persists. This 'immunological memory' prevents subsequent infections with pathogens expressing the same antigen. An adaptive response is powerful but very specific, and it does not usually prevent infections with a different pathogen or sometimes even different strains of the same pathogen. For example, an adaptive response against one strain of influenza A stimulated by previous infection or vaccination does not prevent infection with other strains. An adaptive immune response also affects the inflammatory response to a pathogen, altering the nature and strength of the resulting inflammation.

> **Vaccination exploits the adaptive immune response (usually antibody) to artificially create immunity to pathogens**. Exposure to purified antigen or a live non-virulent or dead form of the pathogen prevents infection with that pathogen thereafter. Vaccines are available for common respiratory pathogens, including influenza A and *S. pneumoniae* (**Table 1.17**).

Development of adaptive immunity

Adaptive immune responses develop

Vaccines for respiratory pathogens			
Target pathogen or infection	Antigen	Efficacy	Target group(s)
Influenza A	Viral surface proteins	Very effective but highly strain specific, so needs a new formulation each year	People >65 years old People with chronic disease Everyone during pandemics
S. pneumoniae	Capsule polysaccharide	Unconjugated*: good against septicaemia, weak against pneumonia, ineffective in infants Conjugated*: very effective against vaccine serotypes	Unconjugated*: people >65 years old or with chronic disease Conjugated*: all infants
Tuberculosis (*M. tuberculosis*)	Bacille Calmette–Guérin: attenuated *M. bovis*	Relatively weak	Infants in high-risk areas
Whooping cough (*Bordetella pertussis*)	Killed or live attenuated *B. pertussis*	Effective	Infants
Diptheria (*Corynebacterium diphtheriae*)	Diptheria toxin	Very effective	Infants

*Unconjugated: capsule polysaccharide alone. Conjugated: capsule polysaccharide attached to a carrier protein.

Table 1.17 Vaccines for important respiratory pathogens

through the presentation of antigens to T and B cells by antigen-presenting cells.

- CD4 T cells are stimulated by professional antigen-presenting cells, mainly dendritic cells and macrophages
- CD8 cells are stimulated by antigens from intracellular pathogens that are displayed on the surface of the infected cell
- B cells are stimulated by soluble antigens encountered in the blood and by antigens presented on dendritic cells within the lymph nodes. B cells also present antigen to CD4 cells to stimulate cytokine responses that improve B cell maturation into antibody secreting plasma cells

The loss or impaired function of professional antigen-presenting cells, T cells or B cells results in defects in adaptive immune responses.

The different mechanisms of adaptive immunity are shown in **Figure 1.40** and methods of antigen recognition in **Table 1.18**.

> **Like inflammation, adaptive immune responses can also be harmful to the host.** CD4 Th1 responses can increase inflammation-mediated tissue damage. Also, antibody responses to otherwise harmless antigens can cause allergic responses.

Role of antibody

B cells recognising a specific antigen differentiate into plasma cells that produce antibodies (also called immunoglobulins, Igs) that bind to that antigen. Antibodies consist of two heavy and two light chains, and are one of the main effectors of the adaptive immune response.

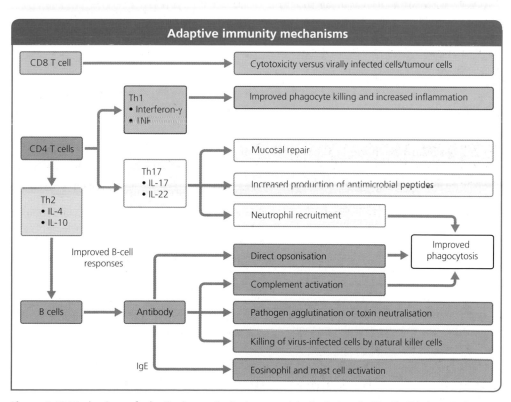

Figure 1.40 Mechanisms of adaptive immunity. Ig, immunoglobulin; IL, interleukin; Th, T helper; TNF, tumour necrosis factor.

Antigen recognition mechanisms	
Method of antigen recognition	Role(s)
Secreted antibody (site of main activity)	
IgA (secreted into mucosal fluids)	Complement fixation, antigen neutralisation, Fcγ receptor mediated phagocytosis, pathogen agglutination, NK recognition of infected cells
IgG (blood and lung epithelial lining fluid)	Complement fixation, antigen neutralisation, Fcγ receptor mediated phagocytosis, pathogen agglutination, NK recognition of infected cells
IgM (blood, secreted into mucosal fluids)	Complement fixation, antigen neutralisation, Fcγ receptor mediated phagocytosis, pathogen agglutination, NK recognition of infected cells
IgE (blood and lung epithelial lining fluid, surface of mast cells)	Mast cell and eosinophil activation for parasite killing, allergy and anaphylaxis
IgD (unknown)	Unknown
B-cell receptor (B cell surface, identical structure to antibody)	Stimulate antibody production and B cell maturation
T cell receptor (surface of T cells)	CD4 cells: stimulate production of immunomodulatory cytokines (examples given in brackets): Th1: promote macrophage functions (IFγ) Th2: promote antibody production and immunity to parasites (IL4) Th17: neutrophil recruitment, promote mucosal immunity (IL17) T regs: control of inflammation (IL10, TGFβ) CD8 cells: recognition and killing of cells infected by intracellular pathogens

Table 1.18 Antigen recognition mechanisms of the adaptive immune response

Antibodies have a very variable antigen binding site head that recognises and binds to microbial antigens, and a non-variable portion that binds to Fcγ cell surface receptors. Antibodies circulate in the blood and are secreted on to mucosal surfaces including those in the lungs. Antibodies bound to their target antigen mediate an immunological response by:

- direct opsonisation of pathogens for phagocytosis via Fc-γ receptors
- indirect opsonisation by increasing complement deposition on pathogens
- neutralisation of antigen function (e.g. antibodies to diphtheria toxin prevent its toxic effects)
- agglutination, which causes pathogens to clump together, thus inhibiting their growth and making them more readily phagocytosed
- activating mast cell and eosinophil degranulation (important for killing parasites)
- improving the recognition and killing of virus-infected cells by natural killer cells

Different functional classes of antibody are recognised (**Table 1.18**). IgA is secreted on to mucosal surfaces. IgG, IgM and IgE are found in the circulation. IgG is also found in airway and alveoli lining fluid, especially during infections, when the integrity of the alveolar epithelium breaks down as a result of inflammation.

Mechanisms of cell mediated immunity

CD4 Th1, Th2 and Th17, and CD8 cytotoxic T cells, all provide specific mechanisms of cell-mediated immunity that are effective against different types of pathogens (**Figure 1.40**).

- CD4 Th1 cells produce the cytokines interferon-γ and tumour necrosis factor-α. These cytokines improve neutrophil, macrophage and natural killer cell antibacterial functions, resulting in more efficient killing of pathogens that specialise in living inside macrophages. For example, Th1-mediated responses allow macrophages to kill *M. tuberculosis* (the cause of tuberculosis) residing in phagolysosomes. Th1 responses tend to cause an increase in inflammation

■ CD4 Th2 cells produce the cytokines IL-4, IL-5 and IL-10. These cytokines help induce strong antibody responses that protect against extracellular bacteria, viruses and parasites. IL10 is also anti-inflammatory and Th2 responses tend to reduce inflammation.

■ CD4 Th17 cells produce the cytokines IL-17 and IL-22. These cytokines improve mucosal immunity by stimulating epithelial cells to produce the chemokine IL-8, which recruits neutrophils to the site of infection. Th17 cytokines also improve respiratory epithelium repair and secretion of antibacterial peptides. CD4 Th17 responses help protect mucosal surfaces such as the upper respiratory tract and lung from infection by extracellular bacteria

■ CD8 cytotoxic T cells are important for adaptive immune responses to viruses.

When cytotoxic T cells recognise foreign antigens on the surface of virally infected host cells they release intracellular granules containing perforin and granzymes. These punch holes in the target cell membrane and kill the cell. They can recognise and kill tumour cells by the same mechanism.

A low level of bacterial colonisation is normally present in the bronchial tree: this is the lung microbiome. The microbiome changes during disease, with increased levels of pathogenic bacteria such as *Haemophilus influenzae*. The gut microbiome has a role in regulating inflammation and epithelial repair, but the role of the lung microbiome remains unclear.

Answers to starter questions

1. The respiratory system plays a vital role in the transfer of oxygen to blood and the excretion of carbon dioxide. It also helps control acid–base balance and protect the body from infection.

2. Our respiratory system is not very efficient. Because the same 'pipes' are used to breathe air in and out, this creates an anatomical dead space that reduces efficiency. It also means we inhale air that is always a mixture of exhaled gases in the air we are breathing in, reducing diffusion gradients. The most efficient vertebrate respiratory system is found in birds, which have a system of air sacs that fill and empty differentially during inspiration and expiration, with air travelling in one direction.

3. The respiratory system does not contribute to gas exchange until after birth. In the womb, the foetus receives oxygen from the mother through the umbilical cord. Carbon dioxide is excreted through the cord too. From 9 weeks onwards the foetus does make breathing-like movements, as a practice for birth.

4. Severe respiratory system abnormalities are fatal for the developing fetus. However, a number of abnormalities of lung development are compatible with life. Bronchogenic cysts arise from abnormal budding of the ventral foregut, pulmonary hypoplasia results from incomplete development of the distal lung and in pulmonary sequestration a bronchopulmonary mass forms without a normal bronchial communication. Children who survive often suffer breathlessness, recurrent infections and disability.

5. The nose has several key functions for respiration.

   ■ The nose warms and moistens inhaled air before it reaches the lungs
   ■ Hair and mucus in the nasal cavity act as a filter for larger particles
   ■ The mucous layer also captures microbes
   ■ The nasal mucosa is the first site of immune defence

   Sneezing is an effective way of ridding the respiratory tract of potentially dangerous particles in the air before they reach the lungs

Answers *continued*

6. The trachea branches into the right and left main bronchi. These primary bronchi divide into secondary bronchi. Further branching produces tertiary bronchi, then bronchioles and eventually terminal bronchioles. The terminal bronchioles at the end of the bronchial tree open into small cavities in the lung parenchyma: the alveoli. Each terminal bronchiole supplies several alveoli. Alveoli are much smaller than bronchioles and have a different function.

7. The average TLC for a middle-aged healthy man is 5–6 L. Regular training improves the exercise capacity of athletes partly by increasing their lung capacity. A higher lung capacity allows more oxygen to be delivered to the blood per breath, thus helping support the vastly increased oxygen consumption that occurs during exercise. The largest lung capacity officially recorded is that of British rower Peter Reed, with an amazing 11.68 L recorded in 2006 while he was training for the Olympic Games.

8. Ventilation is the whole process of inspiration and expiration; respiration refers specifically to gas exchange within the lungs.

9. The pleurae are membranes that line the thorax. They can move over each other facilitated by the small amount of fluid in the pleural space, making it easier for the lungs to expand and contract when breathing.

10. Breathing is controlled by respiratory centres in the brainstem. Severe head injuries can lead to direct damage to these centres or secondary damage due to increased intracerebral pressures. This can lead to Cheyne-Stokes breathing, irregular breathing or tachypnoea. All are poor prognostic signs in traumatic brain injury.

11. Breathing is controlled consciously and unconsciously. People can learn to increase the conscious element using meditation, yoga, vocal training or in sports such as swimming. This requires impulses from the cerebral cortex to affect the brainstem. It is usually associated with changes in heart rate too. There is a limit to conscious control and unconscious systems usually kick in when carbon dioxide or oxygen levels fall outside of the normal range (to prevent unconsciousness).

12. The ability of the lungs to move is partly determined by compliance. Compliance is the effort needed to stretch the lungs and chest wall, and depends on both tissue elasticity and surface tension in the alveoli. Some lung diseases alter lung compliance; for example, emphysema increases compliance and interstitial lung disease decreases it. Both conditions make ventilation of the lungs difficult.

13. It is essential that the lungs and kidneys regulate the pH of the blood within a narrow range of pH 7.35–7.45. Outside of this, many physiological processes do not work. Severe alkalosis can cause muscle weakness and low calcium levels resulting in tetany. Severe acidosis can lead to coma and death.

14. A buffer reduces changes in a solution's free hydrogen ions when acid or base is added, therefore preventing a sudden and dramatic change in pH. The key buffer in the human body is the bicarbonate carbonic acid system.

15. The major role of the pulmonary circulation is to supply deoxygenated blood to the lungs, facilitate oxygenation of this blood through close interactions with alveoli, and then transport the oxygenated blood to the heart. Deoxygenated blood is delivered by the pulmonary arterial system, which arises from the right ventricle. This is a low-pressure system and the only place in the body where deoxygenated blood is carried by arteries.

Answers *continued*

16. Oxygen is needed to accept the free electrons at the end of the electron transport chain in the mitochondria to allow production of the cell's energy, ATP. It is the only gas that can accept multiple electrons, and also mop up the additional free H^+ ions, and produce a safe compound as a result of this reaction. The entire system is critically dependant on the use of oxygen to produce ATP. After breathing just a few breaths of nitrogen or helium, a human would become unconscious and rapidly die from critical hypoxia.

17. The simple answer is that blood is never blue. All human blood is red, whether it is oxygenated in arteries or deoxygenated in veins. The colour comes from the complex formed between haemoglobin, iron and oxygen. The complex absorbs higher energy (shorter wavelength) light, therefore leaving longer wavelength red for our eyes to detect. Deoxygenated blood is darker red and oxygenated blood is bright red. Veins within the body, for example seen during surgery, are not blue. The only veins that appear blue are those in the skin of people with light skin. This is due to the relative amounts of blue and red wavelength light that is reflected by both skin and blood. There are animals with truly blue blood. One example is the Horseshoe crab whose blood is blue, because at the centre of the oxygen-carrying protein is copper, rather than iron.

18. A high respiratory rate is one of the earliest signs of sepsis. It occurs for local and central reasons; pyrexia, lactic acidosis and cytokines affect the respiratory control centre. Tissue oedema sometimes develops as a result of increased vascular permeability or excessive fluid administration increasing the diffusion distance for oxygen. This can lead to hypoxia and a high respiratory rate.

19. Most non-infectious lung diseases are associated with or caused by abnormalities of the immune system. Allergy to inhaled antigens causes some types of asthma, allergic bronchopulmonary aspergillosis and hypersensitivity pneumonitis. Inhalation of cigarette smoke or mineral dusts causes the excessive localised inflammation in the lungs that results in COPD and different types of pneumoconiosis. Pulmonary vasculitis and interstitial lung diseases associated with connective tissue diseases and rheumatoid arthritis are caused by autoimmunity; in these conditions, the immune system directly attacks the lungs. Even lung cancer has some immunological basis; it is a failure of the host immune system to recognise and kill abnormal host cells at an early stage, before they grow into tumours.

20. The original vaccine was an attenuated live virus: cowpox. The cowpox vaccine induced an immune response that prevented infection with a related aggressive viral pathogen: smallpox. Similarly, the vaccine for tuberculosis, bacillus Calmette–Guérin, is an attenuated live derivative of the pathogenic organism *M. tuberculosis*. A killed whole-cell organism can also be used as a vaccine. For example, killed *B. pertussis* bacteria are used as one type of vaccine against whooping cough. Vaccines are also made of single or multiple types of specific molecules from a microorganism. Examples of these subunit vaccines include the diphtheria toxin, surface proteins of influenza A and the capsular polysaccharide of *S. pneumoniae*.

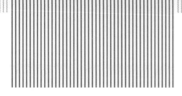

Chapter 2
Clinical essentials

Introduction

Many respiratory diseases are readily diagnosed by using information obtained in a thorough history, supported by the clinical examination. A good clinical assessment reduces the number of investigations necessary to achieve a diagnosis. Furthermore, knowledge of the clinical context is essential for the accurate interpretation of abnormalities found on diagnostic testing.

The ability to take a detailed history and perform an effective clinical examination remains an essential skill for the clinician, despite the increasing power of diagnostic investigations.

Epidemiology and patient demographics

Which respiratory diseases are likely in particular patients greatly depends on epidemiological factors. Both age and sex affect the probability of disease (**Tables 2.1** and **2.2**). For example:

■ cystic fibrosis is unlikely to present in an elderly person; conversely, chronic obstructive pulmonary disease (COPD) or lung cancer are rare in young adults
■ pneumothorax is more common in men, but primary pulmonary hypertension is more common in women

Ethnicity and country of birth also have powerful effects on the probability of contracting specific diseases (**Table 2.3**). Therefore to accurately define the potential differential diagnosis for each clinical presentation, clinicians need to know how the patient's age, sex, ethnicity, and country of birth or areas of former residence affect the epidemiology of respiratory diseases.

Effect of age on probabaility of respiratory diseases			
Probability	Young adult (18–45 years)	Middle age (46–75 years)	Elderly (> 75 years)
Common	Asthma	Obstructive sleep apnoea COPD Asthma Lung cancer	COPD CAP Lung cancer Pleural disease
Less common	Hyperventilation Pneumothorax CAP Pulmonary embolism Cystic fibrosis Sarcoidosis Bronchiectasis	Interstitial lung disease CAP Pulmonary embolism Bronchiectasis Sarcoidosis Pleural disease Pneumoconiosis	Interstitial lung disease Asthma Pulmonary embolism Bronchiectasis

CAP, community-acquired pneumonia; COPD, chronic obstructive pulmonary disease.

Table 2.1 Examples of the effect of age on the epidemiology of respiratory diseases

Gender differences in respiratory diseases	
More common in men	More common in women
COPD Lung cancer Interstitial lung diseases Obstructive sleep apnoea Pneumoconiosis Mesothelioma Pneumothorax	Asthma Bronchiectasis Obesity hypoventilation Pulmonary embolism Primary pulmonary hypertension Lung complications of rheumatological conditions Lymphangioleiomyomatosis*

*Women only.

Table 2.2 Examples of effects of gender on the epidemiology of respiratory diseases

Associations of ethnic origin/country of birth and respiratory diseases	
Caucasian	Cystic fibrosis
Afro-Caribbean	Sarcoidosis
Born in Eastern Europe, Asia or Africa	Tuberculosis
Born in a developing country	Tuberculosis, bronchiectasis
Born in sub-Saharan Africa	Tuberculosis, HIV infection

Table 2.3 Associations between ethnicity and geographical factors and common respiratory diseases

Common symptoms and how to take a history

Starter questions

Answers to the following questions are on page 137–138.

1. What types of chest pain are most likely to have a serious underlying cause?
2. Why does the presence of non-respiratory symptoms matter?
3. What are the most relevant aspects of the social history for respiratory disease?
4. What are the most relevant aspects of the past history for respiratory disease?
5. How do you assess the severity of a chronic respiratory disease?

Common symptoms differ depending on whether the disease is acute or chronic.

- In acute respiratory disease, the most common presenting symptom is shortness of breath (dyspnoea); less common acute presentations include haemoptysis and chest pain
- In chronic respiratory disease, patients usually present with a cough or dyspnoea, and less commonly with sputum production, haemoptysis (coughing up blood) or chest pain

Another frequent reason for referral for a respiratory opinion is an abnormal chest X-ray. Abnormalities on chest X-ray are often not associated with any symptoms.

History taking for respiratory patients starts with the standard format for a clinical assessment.

1. Patient's age and gender
2. Presenting complaint(s)
3. History of presenting complaint

   i. Define the presenting complaint in detail. The following should be asked about each symptom: What has been the duration of the symptom? How did it start, e.g. insidiously or suddenly, after a defined event? What has the pattern been over time, e.g. slowly progressive, acute then constant, episodic? What makes it worse? What things/which drugs can make it better? Are there any associated symptoms?
   ii. Define any additional respiratory symptoms: dyspnoea, cough, sputum, wheeze, chest pain and ankle oedema
   iii. Define any additional extrathoracic symptoms relevant to the current presentation

4. Past medical history. Ask about:
   i. Asthma
   ii. Hay fever or eczema (atopy)
   iii. Tuberculosis
   iv. Thoracic surgery
   v. Other specific medical problems that could be relevant to the current presentation

5. Family history
6. Social history. Ask about:

   i. Smoking
   ii. Use of recreational drugs and alcohol
   iii. Present and previous occupations
   iv. Pet ownership, hobbies and travel history
   v. Place of birth

7. Review of symptoms (general overview of non-respiratory symptoms)
8. Treatment history

   i. Present medications
   ii. Known allergies
   iii. Previous treatments, if relevant (e.g. previous radiotherapy or cytotoxic chemotherapy)

The past medical and social history questions should be targeted according to the presenting complaint. For example, ask a patient presenting with haemoptysis specifically about previous tuberculosis infection and whether anyone in their family has had tuberculosis, and ask a patient presenting with pleuritic chest pain about risk factors for pulmonary embolism.

For each specific symptom, examples of the most important questions to ask patients are given under the appropriate headings. Exactly how these questions are worded can vary as long as they are easily understood by the patient.

Dyspnoea

Dyspnoea means difficulty breathing and is one of the most common symptoms of respiratory disease. However, dyspnoea is also a common symptom of cardiac disease and anaemia, which must always be considered in the differential diagnosis of patients presenting with this symptom.

Tachypnoea is an increased respiratory rate, which is an examination finding. Orthopnoea is shortness of breath when lying down, and is common for most causes of dyspnoea, if severe enough; the patient may describe having to sleep propped up in bed or even sleeping in a chair to avoid lying down. Paroxysmal nocturnal dyspnoea is a subclass of orthopnoea that describes episodes of sudden waking with severe dyspnoea that resolves quickly when the patient sits up; the condition is usually caused by left ventricular failure rather than lung disease.

Dyspnoea is a technical term that is not used by patients. Instead, they describe the symptom in terms of having shortness of breath, difficulty in breathing and chest tightness. Therefore use these descriptions when asking patients about dyspnoea.

When a patient complains of difficulty in breathing, the answers to these questions will define the problem in more detail and suggest the differential diagnosis.

- 'How long have you been suffering from shortness of breath?'
- 'Is the breathlessness constant or does it come and go? If it is constant, is it getting worse with time?' (i.e. what is the pattern of the dyspnoea?)
- 'What does your breathlessness stop you doing?' (i.e. how severe is the dyspnoea?)

'How long have you been suffering from shortness of breath?'

The duration of dyspnoea identifies likely causes (**Table 2.4**). For example, a pulmonary embolus and a pneumothorax both cause sudden onset dyspnoea, but COPD usually has a history of worsening dyspnoea over several years. Many chronic respiratory diseases start insidiously, and the patient may not realise that mild dyspnoea on exertion some time before the current presentation is clinically significant. Therefore the patient should be asked specifically about their past exercise tolerance before the time they thought their symptoms started.

'Is the breathlessness constant, or does it come and go?'

With chronic presentations, the pattern could be one of three main types (**Table 2.4**).

- Progressive, as in COPD and interstitial lung disease
- Constant, as in pleural thickening and stable COPD
- Intermittent with periods of normality, as in asthma

Determine whether the dyspnoea dates from a specific event or particular circumstances (e.g. an empyema that has left pleural thickening or from a known pulmonary embolism).

Patients with progressive and constant patterns of breathlessness frequently also suffer from exacerbations. Exacerbations are additional intermittent periods of deterioration lasting for days or even weeks. Exacerbations of COPD and asthma frequently follow viral upper respiratory tract infections.

Patterns of dyspnoea			
Sudden onset	Episodic	Progressive (over weeks)	Progressive (over months or years)
No warning:	Normal between episodes:	Pleural effusion	COPD
Pulmonary embolism	Asthma	Lobar collapse[†]	Interstitial lung disease
Pneumothorax	Hyperventilation	Pulmonary embolism	Pulmonary embolism (months rather than years)
	Ischaemic heart disease	Cardiac failure	'Chronic' asthma
		Neuromuscular disease	Bronchiectasis
Preceding symptoms:	Persisting dyspnoea between episodes:	Extensive malignancy	Pneumoconiosis
Asthma	COPD	Lymphangitis carcinomatosis	Chest wall disease
Lobar collapse*	'Chronic' asthma	Anaemia	
Pulmonary embolism	Cardiac failure		
Pulmonary oedema	Valvular heart disease		

COPD, chronic obstructive pulmonary disease.

*Caused by inhalation of a foreign body or sputum plug.

†Caused by benign or malignant bronchial tumour.

Table 2.4 Patterns of common causes of dyspnoea

In many chronic respiratory diseases (e.g. COPD and asthma), dyspnoea varies significantly from day to day. For example, breathlessness may worsen temporarily with poor weather or increased pollution. In contrast, an exacerbation is a sustained period of deterioration that is generally more severe.

MRC dyspnoea scale	
Score	Degree of breathlessness
0	Normal
1	Able to walk and keep up with people of similar age but not when walking up hills or stairs
2	Able to walk 1.5 km on the level at own pace but unable to keep up with people of similar age
3	Able to walk about 100 m on the level without stopping
4	Breathless at rest or on minimal effort (e.g. when undressing or moving around a room)

Table 2.5 The Medical Research Council scale for dyspnoea

'What does your breathlessness stop you doing?'

This is a vital question for chronic presentations. It establishes the present severity of dyspnoea, which indicates how advanced a disease is. Knowing the present severity of dyspnoea also allows comparison with past and future severity, thereby enabling the rate of progression of the disease to be determined.

Severity of dyspnoea is judged by identifying the level of exercise at which the patient becomes short of breath.

- In mild dyspnoea, the patient notices that they are breathless only when climbing stairs or walking up steep inclines, but they walk as far as they like on the level
- More marked dyspnoea is noticed when the patient is walking fast or talking at the same time, going up slight inclines, doing housework or carrying shopping
- With more severe dyspnoea, the patient is able to walk only a limited distance on the level before stopping
- Patients with very severe respiratory disease are breathless on moving around their own house, and even at rest

If the patient has been breathless for some time, judge the speed of deterioration by asking about changes in exercise tolerance over time (e.g. 'How far could you walk 6/12/24 months ago before becoming breathless?'). The Medical Research Council dyspnoea scale is used to assess breathlessness (**Table 2.5**).

Cough

A persistent cough is one of the most frequent presenting symptoms in the respiratory outpatient department. Potential common causes are listed in **Table 2.6**.

In a patient with a significant smoking history (> 20 pack-years), the important diagnoses to exclude are lung cancer and COPD, but most cases are due to simple chronic bronchitis. In young or non-smoking patients, the most common causes of a persistent cough are asthma, gastro-oesophageal reflux and chronic upper respiratory tract disease (sinusitis and rhinitis), often associated with a post-nasal drip. Treatment with angiotensin-converting enzyme inhibitors is a frequent cause of chronic cough; such cases are easily rectified by stopping the drug.

Many causes of cough have associated symptoms that make the diagnosis more obvious. For example, cough with progressive dyspnoea makes COPD or interstitial lung disease more likely. However, some causes of cough are associated with only minimal other symptoms. For example, up to half of patients with asthma present with cough and no other symptoms.

Ask the following specific questions about the cough.

- 'How long have you had the cough?'
- 'Does the cough ever disappear completely for days or weeks at a time?'
- 'Are there any associated upper respiratory symptoms, such as runny nose, nasal stuffiness, face pain?'
- 'What time of day is the cough at its worse?'

Causes of persisting cough		
Frequency	With no or minimal sputum	With sputum
Common	Asthma Post-nasal drip Gastro-oesophageal reflux Cough habit Smoking	Asthma (yellow sputum) Smoking COPD
Less common	Lung cancer Interstitial lung disease Whooping cough Foreign body inhalation Mediastinal lymphadenopathy or lesions Occupational dust exposure	Lung cancer Bronchiectasis* Interstitial lung disease Lung abscess* Occupational dust exposure

*Can be purulent phlegm.

Table 2.6 Common causes of persisting (>4 weeks) cough with or without sputum production

- 'What makes the cough worse?'
- 'Does the cough produce phlegm?'
- 'Do you suffer from heartburn or acid taste in the mouth?' (to identify symptoms of gastro-oesophageal reflux)

'How long have you had the cough?'

Upper respiratory tract and lung infections are common causes of a new cough. However, they usually settle within 2–3 weeks and are initially associated with other symptoms of infection.

Patients with an infective cough usually present to hospital only if the cough is associated with a severe infection or an exacerbation of chronic lung disease. A smoker with a cough persisting for ≥4 weeks requires a chest X-ray to look for a potential lung cancer, especially if they are older than 50 years.

Cough caused by asthma, chronic bronchitis related to smoking, gastro-oesophageal reflux, upper respiratory tract disease and, less commonly, bronchiectasis can be present for years before presentation.

Cough is a common presentation of lung cancer; however, it is also common in patients with COPD without cancer. A history of a new type of cough or a cough that is more persistent than normal in a present or previous smoker could indicate lung cancer, which must be investigated by chest X-ray

'Does the cough disappear completely for days or weeks at a time?'

Cough associated with asthma and upper respiratory tract disease is usually highly variable, with prolonged periods of no cough followed by periods of severe cough. The latter are often precipitated by a viral upper respiratory tract infection. In contrast, cough caused by bronchiectasis, chronic bronchitis and COPD are less variable, although there are often periods when the cough is worse or better than usual.

'Are there any associated upper respiratory symptoms?'

Chronic rhinitis and sinusitis are common causes of chronic cough. Their symptoms are persistent nasal stuffiness, nasal discharge, facial pain and headaches. Ask the patient specifically whether they feel fluid dropping down the throat from the back of the nose; this is a post-nasal drip. Post-nasal drips result from upper respiratory tract disease and cause a persistent cough.

'What time of day is the cough at its worse?'

In asthma, the cough is characteristically at its worst when the patient gets up in the morning. Coughs caused by asthma also tend to wake patients in the middle of the night.

'What makes the cough worse?'

Knowing factors that exacerbate the cough help in diagnosis.

- Cough caused by oesophageal reflux is worse after eating or lying down.
- Cough caused by asthma is frequently exacerbated by viral upper respiratory tract infection, exposure to smoke or dust, and changes in air temperature. Exposure to specific allergens can also worsen coughs in people with asthma. These allergens include cat dander, occupational allergens, and particles released by pollen grains during thunderstorms.

'Does the cough produce phlegm?'

This is an essential question when evaluating a presenting complaint of cough. The patient may also describe coughing up blood (haemoptysis).

'Do you suffer from heartburn or acid taste in the mouth?'

Gastro-oesophageal reflux is a common cause of isolated cough. The patient may have:

- heartburn; burning retrosternal chest pain caused by acid reflux into the oesophagus (especially after meals or on lying down)
- an intermittent acid/sour taste in the mouth
- non-painful regurgitation of stomach contents

> **A patient complaining that every cold makes them cough for weeks may have asthma.** Viral upper respiratory tract infection causes the initial cough but also exacerbates the underlying asthma. This causes the cough to persist long after the infection has been cleared.

Sputum

Production of sputum indicates active inflammation of the airways or alveoli, and should not occur in patients with a normal respiratory tract. Common causes of sputum production are listed in **Table 2.6**. Sputum can be characterised as follows.

- Mucoid: white or clear phlegm. Causes include acute viral infections and chronic diseases such as COPD and interstitial lung disease. This type of phlegm is also produced between exacerbations in mild cases of bronchiectasis.
- Purulent: green or brown sputum that is very thick and tenacious. Purulent phlegm is often caused by bacterial infection of the lower respiratory tract. Such infections can be either acute (bronchitis, pneumonia or lung abscess) or chronic (bronchiectasis). The hallmark of bronchiectasis is chronic daily purulent phlegm production, often in large volumes.
- Mucopurulent: white phlegm mixed with purulent phlegm or only mildly discoloured phlegm. Mucopurulent phlegm is present in milder bacterial infections or during recovery from infection.
- Yellow phlegm: this may be due to sputum eosinophilia. This suggests asthma but can also be produced during acute and chronic infections.

Ascertain the duration of sputum production. A short history suggests an acute infection, whereas a history over months or years suggests chronic bronchitis or bronchiectasis. Chronic bronchitis is defined as sputum production on most days over three consecutive months for two successive years.

Exacerbations of chronic lung disease associated with phlegm production (e.g. COPD and bronchiectasis) temporarily increases sputum volume and perhaps purulence. The volume of sputum production is easily estimated by asking the patient how many teaspoonfuls of sputum they produce over a day.

- Patients with bronchiectasis produce much larger daily volumes, frequently two to three tablespoonfuls or even a cupful or more daily
- Patients with allergic bronchopulmonary aspergillosis (ABPA) can cough up firm cylindrical lumps called sputum plugs or bronchial casts

Haemoptysis

Haemoptysis is production of sputum containing blood. This symptom can indicate severe disease, such as lung cancer or tuberculosis.

It is sometimes difficult to determine the source of the blood; it can originate from the lungs, the upper respiratory tract or the mouth. If the lung is the source, then the blood is produced by coughing. However, if the upper airways are the source, the patient often first describes a feeling of something pooling at the back of the throat.

Specific questions that need to be asked of a patient presenting with haemoptysis are as follows.

- How much blood have you coughed up? Is it pure blood or blood mixed with phlegm?
- How long have you been coughing blood?
- What colour is the blood?

'How much blood have you coughed up? Is it pure blood or blood mixed with phlegm?'

Small specks of blood mixed with mucoid or purulent phlegm are common in patients with COPD and other lung diseases causing significant cough. They are relatively reassuring but still require investigation.

Pneumonia infrequently causes haemoptysis combined with purulent phlegm ('rusty' phlegm). Pulmonary oedema occasionally causes pink frothy sputum resulting from the mixing of small amounts of blood with mucoid phlegm. Larger quantities of frank fresh bright red blood require detailed investigation to exclude potentially serious causes (**Table 2.7**).

Major haemoptysis is defined as >200 mL (about a cup of blood) in 24 h and is a potentially life-threatening medical emergency (see Chapter 11).

'How long have you been coughing blood?'

Haemoptysis of short duration could be the first presentation of a chronic condition or a rapidly progressive severe disease such as cancer or tuberculosis (**Table 2.7**). Haemoptysis that has been present for months or years is unlikely to be cancer or tuberculosis; in such cases, bronchiectasis and mycetomas are the main causes that need to be considered.

Causes of haemoptysis	
Minor haemoptysis	**Major haemoptysis***
Common	Common
Acute bronchitis	Lung cancer
Chronic bronchitis	Bronchiectasis
Lung cancer	Aspergilloma
Bronchiectasis	Tuberculosis
Pneumonia ('rusty' sputum)	
Cryptogenic (no cause in 40%)	
Less common	Rare
Pulmonary embolism	Vascular-bronchial fistula
Pulmonary oedema (pink and frothy sputum) and valvular heart disease	Pulmonary arteriovenous malformations
Aspergilloma	Lung abscess
Tuberculosis	
Vasculitis	
Pulmonary haemorrhage	
Trauma to the chest	
Lung abscess	
Lung metastases	
Clotting disorders	
*Over 200 mL in 24 h.	

Table 2.7 Causes of haemoptysis

'What colour is the blood?'

Continued production of fresh red blood indicates active bleeding in the lungs. After the active bleeding point has stopped, the patient will often cough up darker altered blood for a day or two as the lungs are cleared of residual blood.

Chest pain

A presenting complaint of chest pain needs to be defined in detail in the same way as pain affecting any other part of the body.

The acronym SOCRATES is often used to structure a focused chest pain history:

- **Site:** 'Where do you feel pain?'
- **Onset:** 'When did the pain start?'
- **Character:** 'Is the pain sharp, dull, cramping or burning?'
- **Radiation:** 'Does the pain move to affect other areas?'
- **Alleviating factors:** 'What makes the pain better?'
- **Time course:** 'How long does the pain last? Is it intermittent, constant, progressive or variable?'
- **Exacerbating factors:** 'What makes the pain worse?'
- **Severity:** 'What would you rate the pain on a scale of 1 to 10 (10 being the worst pain you have ever felt)?'

The main types of chest pain related to the respiratory system are:

- musculoskeletal or chest wall pain
- pleuritic chest pain
- pain caused by cancer
- chest pain from other causes

Their common causes are listed in **Table 2.8**.

Musculoskeletal or chest wall pain

This type of chest pain is common. It is similar to pleuritic chest pain in that it usually affects only one side of the lung, is sharp in nature and is worsened by deep breaths. However, the relationship to deep breathing and coughing is less acute, and musculoskeletal chest pain is also often exacerbated by movement (e.g. twisting from side to side). In addition,

Causes of respiratory chest pain	
Nature of pain	**Common causes**
Musculoskeletal type	Post-exercise
	Post-coughing or attack of dyspnoea
	Bronchiectasis
	Chronic pleural disease
	Trauma
	Costochondritis
	Lobar collapse
	Pneumothorax
Pleuritic	Pneumonia
	Pleural infection
	Pulmonary embolism
	Dressler's syndrome
	Inflammatory effusions (rheumatoid arthritis and systemic lupus erythematosus)
Constant or progressive	Tumour invasion of chest wall or mediastinum
	Lung cancer
	Mesothelioma
	Post-thoracotomy
Other	Osteoporosis with vertebral collapse
	Shingles
	Thoracic root pain

*Central chest pain suggests a cardiac cause (angina) or an oesophageal cause and is rarely the result of lung disease.

Table 2.8 Causes of a respiratory pattern of chest pain*

musculoskeletal chest wall pain moves to different sites over the chest wall and is often associated with focal tenderness. Pain from a torn muscle or fractured rib usually has a clear precipitating event (e.g. a coughing fit or a fall). Similar chest wall pains are common in various lung diseases, such as pleural thickening and exacerbations of bronchiectasis. Pneumothorax and lobar collapse can also cause sudden onset chest pain of a similar nature to musculoskeletal chest pain.

Pleuritic chest pain

Pleuritic chest pain is caused by inflammation of pleura. This type of pain localises to the precise spot where the pleura is inflamed, usually unilaterally over the lateral aspect of the chest wall. It is sharp in nature and characteristically exacerbated by taking a deep breath or coughing, therefore the patient often takes only shallow breaths. Diaphragmatic pleuritic pain is occasionally referred to the abdomen or to the shoulder tip.

Pain from a fractured rib is similar to pleuritic chest pain. However, it is associated with a history of trauma or severe coughing, and usually has a sudden onset and marked local tenderness.

Pain caused by cancer

Infiltration of the chest wall and mediastinum by malignant tumours causes chest pain that is localised to the affected area, constant (unless the patient is given painkillers) and often described as gnawing in nature. Cancer pain slowly becomes more severe over time.

> **Any history of progressively worsening persistent pain over days or weeks, no matter where it is, suggests the possibility of cancer.** This type of pain must be investigated accordingly.

Other causes of chest pain

Central chest pain is only rarely caused by respiratory disease. Possible causes are angina, pericarditis, oesophageal reflux and oesophageal spasm. Acute tracheitis causes a raw feeling on inspiration over the central chest. Chest wall and lung surgery can cause persisting pain for years over or near the scar site, probably related to damage to intercostal nerves (post-thoracotomy syndrome).

Herpes zoster reactivation in a thoracic root (shingles) causes pain radiating down the dermatome supplied by the affected root; the pain and hypersensitivity of the skin precedes the characteristic vesicular rash. Collapse of thoracic vertebral bodies as a result of osteoporosis or infiltrations such as metastatic cancer or myeloma can also cause root pain radiating around the chest wall, as well as pain localised over the thoracic spine.

Wheeze

A history of wheeze suggests airways obstruction caused by:

- COPD
- Asthma
- Focal bronchial obstruction
    - Lung cancer
    - Foreign body
    - Tracheal/bronchial stenosis
- Bronchiolitis (in children)
- Bronchiectasis
- Left ventricular failure (cardiac asthma)

If the wheeze is louder on inspiration, it may be a symptom of upper airways obstruction. Wheeze is usually a highly variable symptom. It is often made worse by exercise and during exacerbations of the underlying lung disease.

Systemic symptoms

An important general question when deciding the differential diagnosis of patients presenting with respiratory disease is whether the patient has symptoms suggesting a systemic disturbance. These are:

- poor appetite (anorexia)
- unintended weight loss
- fevers
- night sweats
- fatigue
- malaise

Symptoms of systemic disturbance suggest infection, cancer or (less commonly) non-infective inflammatory disorders (e.g. acute sarcoid, acute hypersensitivity pneumonitis and vasculitis) (**Table 2.9**).

If the patient has lost weight, ask how much has been lost over how long. Slow weight loss with a preserved appetite is not uncommon in chronic respiratory disease, especially in COPD patients with emphysema. In contrast, rapid weight loss and anorexia strongly suggest a potentially serious new problem requiring investigation; important causes are cancer and tuberculosis.

A history of recurrent fever requires confirmation by the patient recording their own temperature at home. Night sweats can be

Respiratory diseases causing systemic disturbance		
Frequency	Acute (days)	Subacute or chronic (weeks or months)
Common causes	Viral upper respiratory tract infection Acute bronchitis or flu Pneumonia	Lung cancer Tuberculosis Sarcoidosis
Less common causes	Empyema Hypersensitivity pneumonitis Acute eosinophilic pneumonia	Other malignancy (e.g. lymphoma) Other chronic infections (chronic aspergillosis, *Nocardia*, non-tuberculous mycobacteria infection) Lung abscess or empyema Vasculitis

*Generally mild systemic symptoms.

Table 2.9 Respiratory diseases causing symptoms of systemic disturbance

pathological but are not uncommon in middle-aged patients without disease. Fatigue occurs in most chronic respiratory diseases but is also a common symptom in healthy people. Malaise is when the patient feels ill rather than just tired; it is a more specific indicator than fatigue of infective or neoplastic disease.

Other symptoms

Other symptoms may be relevant when taking a history.

Ankle swelling

Ankle swelling (oedema) is an important symptom in respiratory medicine.

- Bilateral swelling could be caused by cor pulmonale, the name for right-sided heart failure caused by pulmonary hypertension resulting from chronic hypoxic lung disease.
- Unilateral ankle and calf swelling, often with calf pain, is a symptom of a deep vein thrombosis and indicates that the patient is at risk of pulmonary embolism.

Upper airways symptoms

Upper airways symptoms are commonly associated with respiratory tract diseases such as asthma, vasculitis and bronchiectasis. Common symptoms include nasal stuffiness and discharge (rhinitis), as well as facial pain and a feeling of congestion (sinusitis).

Symptoms suggestive of atopy

Symptoms suggesting atopy, a tendency to allergic diseases such as allergic rhinitis (hay fever) and eczema, are common in patients with asthma. Hay fever presents with attacks of sneezing, red itchy eyes and rhinitis, usually in spring and early summer.

Symptoms of multisystem disease

Symptoms of multisystem disease, such as lung cancer, sarcoidosis and tuberculosis, frequently affect extrathoracic sites and present with non-respiratory symptoms. Lung diseases can also be manifestations of systemic autoimmune disease. For example, ask patients presenting with interstitial lung disease about pain and swelling affecting their joints; they may have rheumatoid arthritis.

Identification of extrathoracic involvement can provide the clue to a respiratory diagnosis or help target a diagnostic biopsy to a more accessible site than the lung. For example, a new neck lump could be caused by lung cancer metastases or tuberculosis, and is readily biopsied to confirm either diagnosis.

Past medical history

Aspects of the past medical history are relevant when certain lung diseases are being considered (**Table 2.10**). Ask the patient about asthma, tuberculosis, hay fever, eczema, and cardiac disease.

Asthma

Childhood asthma often resolves in young adulthood but returns later in life.

Tuberculosis

A history of tuberculosis identifies a patient who could have reactivation disease. In addition, previous tuberculosis infection frequently causes chronic lung damage and disease, such as bronchiectasis, chronic restrictive or obstructive lung function impairment, pleural thickening and cavities that are sometimes colonised by the fungus *Aspergillus* (mycetoma).

Key elements of the past medical history in respiratory disease	
History	**Relevance**
Preterm birth or low birthweight	Can result in bronchodysplasia and chronic lung function defects
	Low birthweight is associated with chronic lung diseases generally
Childhood infections (e.g. whooping cough, pneumonia, tuberculosis and measles)	Predispose to bronchiectasis and bronchiolitis obliterans
Childhood asthma	May return in adulthood
Eczema, hay fever, nasal polyps or rhinitis	Suggest atopy, so patient at risk of asthma
	Post-nasal drip can cause chronic cough
Chronic sinus disease	Associated with bronchiectasis
	Post-nasal drip can cause chronic cough
Gastro-oesophageal reflux	Can cause chronic cough
Previous tuberculosis (or family history of tuberculosis)	Can cause bronchiectasis, mycetomas, pleural thickening and restrictive or obstructive lung defects
	Suggests latent tuberculosis, so patient at risk of reactivation disease and increased risk of pneumonia
Rheumatoid arthritis	Associated with pulmonary fibrosis, bronchiectasis, nodules and bronchioloitis obliterans
	Treatments cause interstitial lung disease and increase risk of lung infection
Other autoimmune conditions	Associated with interstitial lung disease
	Treatments cause interstitial lung disease and increase risk of lung infection
Extrathoracic cancers	Potential causes of lung metastases, pleural effusions, lymphangitis and mediastinal lymphadenopathy
	Chemotherapy or radiotherapy may cause interstitial lung disease and increased risk of pneumonia
Throat and mouth cancer	Identifies patients at high risk of lung cancer
Ischaemic heart disease, hypertension, diabetes or rheumatic fever	Risk factors for cardiac failure and valvular heart disease (important differential diagnosis for respiratory causes of dyspnoea)
Previous chest X-ray	Old chest X-rays are helpful for assessing whether an abnormality is new (and therefore potentially serious) or old (likely to be a less serious problem)
Previous chest surgery	Current presentation may be a recurrence of previous disease or a complication of chest surgery

Table 2.10 Key elements of the past medical history for respiratory disease

Hay fever and eczema

A past history of hay fever or eczema suggests atopy, which would support a diagnosis of asthma.

Cardiac disease

Heart problems are important alternative causes for dyspnoea and chest pain. For patients presenting with dyspnoea, it is important to identify whether they have risk factors for cardiac causes of dyspnoea such as impaired left ventricular function (hypertension, ischaemic heart disease or diabetes) or valvular heart disease (rheumatic fever).

Family history

The relatives of patients with familial respiratory diseases are at increased risk of also being affected. These diseases include asthma, cystic fibrosis and emphysema resulting from alpha-1 antitrypsin deficiency.

A family history of tuberculosis identifies patients who are likely to have latent tuberculosis, and whose present symptoms could be caused by reactivation of the disease. Patients with a family history of tuberculosis may also have lung damage as a result of previous subclinical tuberculosis infection.

Social history

The lungs are particularly susceptible to environmental exposures. Therefore several aspects of the social history are crucial for a thorough clinical assessment.

- Smoking history
- Use of recreational inhaled or injected drugs
- Occupation
- Alcohol use
- Place of birth and travel history
- Hobbies and pets
- Social circumstances

Smoking history

Cigarette smoking is a risk factor for many lung diseases (**Table 2.11**). It causes 90% of lung cancers and almost all cases of COPD in

Substance misuse and respiratory disease	
Substance	Disease
Cigarette smoking	COPD
	Asthma
	Community-acquired pneumonia
	Tuberculosis
	Pneumothorax
	Interstitial lung disease (idiopathic pulmonary fibrosis, histiocytosis X and pulmonary eosinophilia)
Alcohol	Community-acquired pneumonia
	Aspiration
	Pleural effusion (caused by cirrhosis)
Intravenous recreational drugs (e.g. heroin)	HIV infection
	COPD and emphysema
	Interstitial lung disease (talcosis)
	Tuberculosis
	Metastatic lung abscesses from right-sided endocarditis
Inhaled recreational drugs (e.g. crack cocaine, marijuana)	Asthma
	Pneumothorax and pneumomediastinum
	COPD and emphysema
	Bullous lung disease
	Community-acquired pneumonia
	Tuberculosis

COPD, chronic obstructive pulmonary disease.

Table 2.11 Respiratory diseases associated with smoking and recreational drug use

high-income countries. Taking an accurate smoking history is essential for identifying a patient's risk for different lung diseases. Furthermore, continued smoking is a common explanation for why a patient has poorly controlled or deteriorating chronic lung disease. Smoking history is measured in pack-years.

1 pack-year = smoking 1 packet of 20 cigarettes per day for 1 year

For example, a 48-year-old man who has smoked 30 cigarettes per day (1.5 packs) since the age of 20 (28 years of smoking) has 42 pack-years (1.5 × 28).

If the patient is an ex-smoker, ascertain how old they were when they stopped. The risk of smoking-related lung disease is much reduced if they stopped before the age of 35 years.

Use of recreational inhaled or injected drugs

Recreational inhaled and injected drugs predispose to lung infections, HIV infection, accelerated development of COPD, bullous lung disease and pneumothorax (**Table 2.11**). The use of recreational drugs may have been many years before presentation with COPD or bullous lung disease. Also, patients may not volunteer information on drug misuse.

> **Remember smoking habits vary significantly over time.** A patient who gradually cut down from 40 cigarettes/ day and finally stopped a month ago may answer 'No' when asked 'Do you smoke?' When asked, 'How many were you smoking when you gave up last month?' they may answer 'Five a day', the number just before they stopped.

Occupation

A patient's occupation can expose them to environmental agents causing a wide range of lung diseases (**Table 2.12**). The most important of these are exposure to:

- asbestos (causes a pneumoconiosis and mesothelioma, a malignant pleural tumour)
- mineral dusts (can also cause pneumoconiosis)
- hypersensitivity pneumonitis (an allergic form of interstitial lung disease caused by exposure to a specific antigen)
- occupational asthma

The delay between occupational exposure and subsequent respiratory disease is often many years. Therefore the patient's previous occupations are as relevant as their present one.

Alcohol use

Excess alcohol consumption is an major risk factor for community-acquired pneumonia (because it impairs the immune response) and aspiration (due to its sedative effects associated with vomiting).

Place of birth and travel history

A patient's risk of tuberculosis is related to their place of birth (**Table 2.3**). Other lung pathogens have restricted geographical distribution, and a recent travel history to specific countries may provide a clue to infection with an unusual microorganism. Recent long-distance travel is a key risk factor for pulmonary embolus. Furthermore, travel by plane often causes infective exacerbations of underlying lung diseases.

> **Asking patients about recreational drug use, alcohol intake and sexual history (relevant for assessing HIV risk) is difficult and requires tact.** These questions need a private environment with the patient unaccompanied by their partner or relative.

Hobbies and pets

Allergy to cats or other pets are common reasons for poorly controlled asthma. Pigeon fancier's lung is a hypersensitivity pneumonitis caused by exposure to pigeons and other pet birds (e.g. parrots). Pet birds occasionally cause a rare form of community-acquired pneumonia called psittacosis.

Social circumstances

A description of the patient's home circumstances is needed for those with debilitating disease and who have restricted exercise tolerance because of dyspnoea. Knowing whether the patient lives alone, how many stairs they have to climb to reach their home or within the home, and whether they already have help with housework and shopping helps

Occupational respiratory diseases	
Disease	Relevant occupations and groups of workers
Pleural disease	Asbestos exposure: building trade (e.g. plumbers, carpenters, builders and tilers) boiler workers and pipe fitters dockworkers and ship workers engineers
Asthma	Work with animals (e.g. veterinary surgeons exposed to animal dander) Bakers Spray painters Cleaners Woodworkers Solderers
COPD	Coal miners (and other workers exposed to industrial dusts) Exposure to solid fuel smoke (in low- and middle-income countries)
Lung cancer	Asbestos exposure
Interstitial lung disease	Asbestos exposure
Pneumoconiosis	Coal miners and quarry workers Sandblasters Stone workers Metal workers
Hypersensitivity pneumonitis	Farm workers Pigeon fanciers Occupations exposing workers to any of a wide range of rare causes (e.q. malt worker's lung)
Pneumonia	Local epidemics (e.g. in a barracks) Welders Work with animals (e.g. shop workers handling pet birds for psittacosis, and farm workers with sheep for Q fever)
Obstructive sleep apnoea (affects patient's occupation)	Public transport workers* Taxi drivers* Drivers of heavy goods vehicles*

COPD, chronic obstructive pulmonary disease.

*Obstructive sleep apnoea can cause somnolence (the state of near-sleep) while driving; the patient must inform the appropriate driver-licensing authority (in the UK, the Driver and Vehicle Licensing Agency) of this diagnosis.

Table 2.12 Common respiratory diseases related to or affecting occupation

identify patients who need additional social or community support to cope with their illness.

> **Many aspects of social or occupational history affect respiratory disease, more than can easily be discussed in one consultation.** Identify the main differential diagnoses and tailor the questions accordingly.

Treatment history and allergies

Compile a full list of present prescription medications and any over-the-counter or alternative therapies that the patient is using regularly. Doing so helps identify drugs that are potentially relevant for the presenting complaint (**Table 2.13**). For example,

Drug therapies and respiratory diseases

Frequency	Disease or respiratory effects	Drug(s)
Common	Asthma	Beta-blockers (deterioration in symptoms)
		NSAIDs (causes exacerbations in 5%)
		Muscle relaxants
	COPD	Beta-blockers (deterioration in symptoms)
	Angiotensin-converting enzyme inhibitors	Dry cough
	Increased risk of pulmonary embolism	Oral contraceptive pill
		Tamoxifen
	Increased risk of infection	Corticosteroids (oral and inhaled)
		Biological therapies (infliximab and rituximab)
		Immunosuppressants (e.g. sirolimus, tacrolimus and cyclosporine)
		Chemotherapy (e.g. by causing neutropenia)
	Respiratory depression	Opiates
		Antianxiolytics (e.g. benzodiazepines)
		Antidepressants
		Antipsychotics
Uncommon	Interstitial lung disease	Amiodarone
		Cytotoxic chemotherapy (e.g. bleomycin. melphalan, cyclophosphamide, methotrexate and busulphan)
		Gold
		Nitrofurantoin
	Pulmonary eosinophilia	Nitrofurantoin
		Sulfonamides
		Sulfasalazine
		Chlorpropamide
	Non-cardiogenic pulmonary oedema	Opiates
		NSAIDs
	Pleural disease	Practolol
		Methysergide
		Bromocriptine
	Lupus-like syndrome (with pleuropulmonary involvement)	Hydralazine
		Isoniazid
		Procainamide

COPD, chronic obstructive pulmonary disease; NSAID, non-steroidal anti-inflammatory drug.

Table 2.13 Examples of medications relevant for respiratory diseases

angiotensin-converting enzyme inhibitors such as lisinopril frequently cause chronic cough. The process also helps identify health problems the patient may have not mentioned when asked about their medical history.

Ask patients with chronic respiratory disease about treatments tried before but no longer prescribed, as well as their relative efficacy. Assessing the patient's adherence to their prescribed treatments is important. For example, poorly controlled asthma often results from irregular or ineffective use of preventive inhalers. Ask the patient specifically about any allergies to medicines, especially antibiotics if they need treatment for an infection.

> **Recognition of drug-related lung disease requires a thorough drug history and awareness that drugs are always a potential cause of inflammatory lung conditions,** including airways diseases, interstitial lung disease, pleural effusions and lung infiltrations.

Common signs and how to examine the patient

Starter questions

Answers to the following questions are on page 138.

6. Is examining patients important when imaging tests are widely available?
7. Do all cases of haemoptysis require extensive investigation?
8. What are the causes of dullness to percussion over the chest wall?

A physical examination is used to identify signs that support specific diagnoses suggested by the history, and to exclude unexpected findings that suggest other medical problems. A systematic approach to the examination is necessary to ensure that all components are properly assessed.

1. General inspection
   i. Does the patient look systemically unwell? Do they have pyrexia (increased body temperature or fever)?
   ii. Is the patient's level of consciousness affected? Are they confused?
   iii. Is the patient dyspnoeic at rest? What is their breathing pattern?
   iv. Is the patient using their accessory muscles for respiration?
   v. Is there intercostal recession or tracheal tug?
   vi. What is the body habitus: cachexic (unnaturally underweight) or obese?
   vii. Is there chest wall deformity? Are there any visible thoracic scars?

2. Hands
   i. Are there any nail abnormalities? Does the patient have finger clubbing?
   ii. Is there peripheral cyanosis (bluish discoloration of the fingertips)?
   iii. Is there any evidence of arthritis or rash?
   iv. Is there an essential or a carbon dioxide retention tremor (asterixis)?
3. What is the pulse rate and rhythm?
4. What is the respiratory rate?
5. Head and neck
   i. Is there central cyanosis (bluish discolouration of the lips and tongue)?
   ii. Does the patient have a Horner's syndrome? (Very rare)
   iii. Is the jugular venous pressure increased?
   iv. Are there enlarged palpable cervical lymph nodes?
   v. Is the trachea central?
6. Is chest expansion on inspiration reduced (bilaterally or unilaterally)?
7. What is the position of the apex beat?

8. Is the percussion note normal?
9. Is tactile vocal fremitus normal?
10. Auscultation
    i. What is the relative ratio of inspiration to expiration?
    ii. What is the intensity of the breath sounds?
    iii. Are there any added sounds (wheeze, crepitations or pleural rub)?
11. Is vocal resonance normal?
    Repeat expansion, tactile vocal fremitus, percussion, auscultation and vocal resonance on the posterior chest. Finish by checking for any ankle or sacral oedema and inspecting any sputum

Full clerking of a patient presenting to the emergency department with a respiratory symptom requires examination of respiratory, cardiovascular, abdominal and neurological systems. In practice, a combined rapid cardiovascular and respiratory examination are done first; the rest of the examination is delayed until the patient is stable. In the outpatient department, reserve a neurological examination for selected patients with potentially multisystem disease (e.g. lung cancer) or with combined respiratory and neurological presenting complaints.

Surface markings of the lung

Knowledge of the surface markings of the lungs helps ensure accuracy when interpreting clinical examination findings and when doing invasive procedures. Several vertical lines are drawn across the chest wall to act as landmarks for underlying structures (**Figure 2.1**).

The sternal notch is at the level of the 2nd thoracic vertebral body, the sternal angle at the 4th and 5th, and the xiphoid process of the sternum at the 9th. The 1st to 7th ribs articulate with the sternum anteriorly. The costal margin consists of the anterior ends and cartilages of the 10th to 7th ribs. The 4th to 10th ribs can be palpated in the mid-axillary line. The 11th and 12th ribs have free lateral ends that can be palpated posteriorly in thin patients.

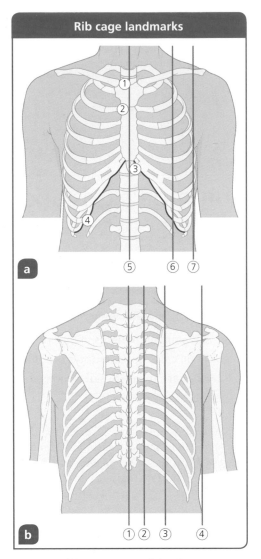

Rib cage landmarks

Figure 2.1 (a) Anterior view of the rib cage, showing the vertical lines used as landmarks. ①, Sternal notch; ②, sternal angle; ③, xiphoid process; ④, costal margin; ⑤, mid-sternal line; ⑥, mid-clavicular line; ⑦, anterior axillary line. (b) Posterior view. ①, Mid-vertebral line; ②, paravertebral line; ③ scapular line; ④, posterior axillary line.

Important dermatomes are C4 immediately below the clavicle, T2 at the sternal angle and T6 at the xiphisternum (**Figure 2.2**).

Surface markings of the borders of the lungs and pleurae are shown in **Figure 2.3**. The apex of the lung and its pleural covering project 2–3 cm above the medial 3rd of the clavicle. The lung borders then pass to the

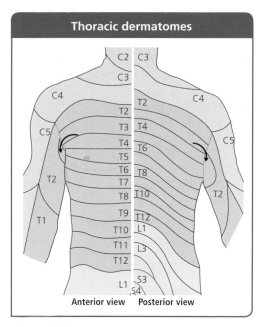

Thoracic dermatomes

Anterior view   Posterior view

Figure 2.2 Anterior and posterior view of the thoracic dermatomes.

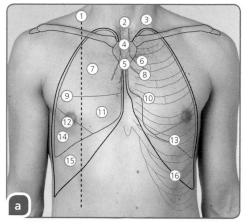

a

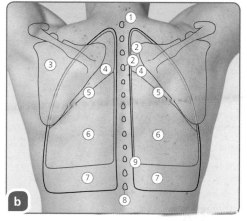

b

mid-sternal line at the sternal angle and continue inferiorly to the 6th costal cartilage; on the left side from the 4th to the 6th costal cartilages, the lung border is displaced leftwards by about 4 cm to accommodate the heart.

The lower border of the lungs and pleurae separate as they curve back to the posterior chest from the sternum. Their edges then run together up the paravertebral lines to the apices. The oblique fissures run from level with the 4th vertebral body posteriorly to a point between the 6th rib at the mid-clavicular line of sternum anteriorly. The horizontal fissure passes from the 4th costal cartilage at the sternum to the 4th rib in the mid-axillary line. As a consequence:

- examination of the anterior chest mainly assesses the upper lobes
- examination of the posterior chest mainly assesses the lower lobes

Signs originating in the middle lobe are best identified in the right lower anterior chest (**Figure 2.3**).

The trachea starts at the level of the 6th cervical vertebral body and bifurcates at the level of the sternal angle. During quiet respiration, the diaphragm reaches the level of the xiphisternal joint and the 5th rib in the mid-axillary line.

Figure 2.3 (a) Anterior surface markings of the lungs and pleurae. ① Mid-clavicular line ② trachea ③ lung apex ④ sternal notch ⑤ sternal angle–plane and tracheal bifurcation ⑥ 2nd costal cartilage ⑦ upper lobe of lung ⑧ left main bronchus ⑨ horizontal fissure ⑩ 4th costal cartilage ⑪ right middle lobe of lung ⑫ oblique fissure ⑬ 6th rib in mid-clavicular line ⑭ lower lobe of lung ⑮ costodiaphragmatic recess ⑯ inferior edge of pleura. (b) Posterior surface markings of the lungs and pleurae. ① C7 spinous process; ②, T3 spinous process; ③, scapula; ④, upper lobe of lung; ⑤, oblique fissure; ⑥, lower lobe of lung; ⑦, costodiaphragmatic recess; ⑧, T12 spinous process; ⑨ T10 spinous process.

The pleural spaces of the costodiaphragmatic recesses overlie both the kidneys and the liver. Therefore percutaneous biopsy of these organs can cause a pneumothorax by puncturing a pleura.

General examination and observation of the respiratory system

For the respiratory examination, the patient should be reclining at 45° in bed with their upper torso exposed. The patient must be warm and comfortable. If they are presenting with an acute illness, examination should be rapid and combined with a directed history while initiating immediate therapies. In an outpatient environment, or if the patient is less acutely ill, examination is usually delayed until after most of the history has been taken.

Assess the following aspects during the initial general inspection of the patient and their respiratory system.

- Does the patient look acutely unwell?
- Is the patient struggling to breathe?
- What is the patient's breathing pattern?
- Is the patient using their accessory muscles for respiration?
- Is there intercostal recession or tracheal tug?
- Is the patient's level of consciousness affected? Are they confused?
- Is the patient in pain?
- Does the patient have a temperature?
- Is there any evidence of weight loss? Does the patient look unusually thin?
- Are there any surgical scars over the thorax?
- Is there chest wall deformity?

Does the patient look acutely unwell?

Infective conditions and severe respiratory distress make the patient look acutely unwell. In contrast, patients presenting with chronic respiratory illness often look and feel perfectly well at rest.

Is the patient struggling to breathe?

Visible dyspnoea at rest is a sign of major cardiorespiratory impairment. Severe but less marked dyspnoea may be apparent only when the patient is walking into the consulting room.

What is the patient's breathing pattern?

Several different breathing patterns occur and suggest specific pathophysiological disorders.

Rapid shallow breathing

Patients with pleuritic chest pain avoid taking deep breaths. Patients with interstitial lung disease often have a characteristic rapid shallow breathing pattern. Rapid shallow breathing also occurs during hyperventilation episodes.

Prolonged expiratory phase

An expiratory phase that is prolonged suggests significant pulmonary airways obstruction, e.g. due to asthma or COPD.

Audible stridor

An audible inspiratory wheeze is called stridor. Stridor indicates potentially life-threatening upper airways obstruction.

Irregular breathing pattern

In severe respiratory failure, the patient's breathing slows and becomes irregular. This pattern suggests that respiratory arrest is imminent.

Kussmaul's respiration

This is a rapid deep sighing breathing pattern sometimes described as 'air hunger'. It is caused by acidosis, for example in cases of diabetic ketoacidosis.

Cheyne–Stokes respiration

This pattern of respiration is characterised by short periods of 5–30 s of no breathing (apnoea) followed by a period of increasing then decreasing respiratory rate. This type of breathing occurs in severe pulmonary oedema and brain stem lesions but is not usually a sign of lung pathology.

Excess abdominal movement on inspiration

The normal outward movement of the abdomen on inspiration is caused by the flattening of the diaphragm compressing the abdominal contents. This movement is often exaggerated in COPD.

Paradoxical breathing

This type of breathing occurs when diaphragmatic paralysis allows the negative pressure in the thoracic cavity during inspiration to suck abdominal contents upwards. This effect causes in-drawing of the abdomen on inspiration.

Is the patient using their accessory muscles for respiration?

Using the sternocleidomastoids, trapezius and latissimus dorsi during inspiration is a sign of respiratory distress.

Is there intercostal recession or tracheal tug?

Intercostal recession is in-drawing of the flesh between the ribs on inspiration and is a sign of respiratory distress. Tracheal tug is shortening of the distance between the suprasternal notch and cricothyroid cartilage during inspiration. Tracheal tug suggests that the lungs are hyperexpanded because of severe airways disease.

Is the patient's level of consciousness affected? Are they confused?

Marked hypoxia causes confusion. Increased $Paco_2$ also causes confusion as well as increasing drowsiness.

Is the patient in pain?

Pleuritic chest pain is frequently obvious because the patient winces on inspiration.

Does the patient have a temperature?

Pyrexia suggests active infection. However, it also occurs in inflammatory and neoplastic diseases.

Is there any evidence of weight loss? Does the patient look unusually thin?

Weight loss occurs in neoplastic disease and chronic infections, and sometimes in chronic respiratory disease.

Are there any surgical scars over the thorax?

Surgery and pleural procedures leave distinctive scars:

- Thoracotomies leave a lateral chest wall scar between the ribs that can be very long
- Video-assisted thoracoscopic surgery procedures usually leave two scars: a mini-thoracotomy scar about 8–10 cm long and nearby smaller scar (**Figure 2.4**)
- Pleural procedures leave small scars at the sight of chest drain insertion
- Mid-line sternotomy scars are largely the result of cardiac or (rarely) mediastinal surgery (e.g. thymectomy)
- Mediastinoscopy leaves a 3- to 4-cm horizontal scar over the suprasternal notch
- Mediastinotomy leaves a similar scar adjacent to the sternum

Is there chest wall deformity?

Reduced volume of the hemithorax

Previous extensive unilateral lung disease or lung surgery reduces the volume of the affected hemithorax. This is recognised by reduced movement of the affected side on breathing, visible tracheal deviation to the affected side, and flattening of the chest wall (especially anterior-superiorly).

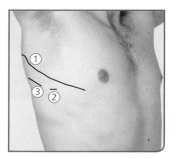
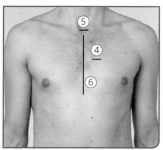

Figure 2.4 Thoracic surgery scars. ①, Thoracotomy scar; ②, pleural drain biopsy or video-assisted thoracoscopy (VATS) subsidiary port; ③, main VATs scar; ④, mediastinotomy; ⑤, mediastinoscopy; ⑥ sternotomy.

Hyperexpanded ('barrel') chest

Severe airways obstruction causes hyperinflated lungs with an increased anterior-posterior diameter and a more horizontal angle of the ribs.

Pectus excavatum

A recessed sternum is normally of no clinical consequence. However, the chest X-ray appearances of the mediastinum and cardiac borders maybe altered.

Pectus carinatum ('pigeon chest')

This is the name for a protruding sternum. Patients who had significant childhood asthma occasionally develop a pectus carinatum.

Visible chest wall masses

On rare occasions neoplastic lung disease erodes through the chest wall to cause a visible protruding mass that may ulcerate.

Kyphoscoliosis

Severe kyphosis (anteroposterior curvature of the spine) or scoliosis (lateral curvature of the spine) impairs the mechanical function of the lungs and can cause respiratory failure. Asymmetrical lung damage sometimes results in kyphoscoliosis, especially in children. Kyphosis occurs with thoracic spine involvement by tuberculosis and vertebral collapse due to osteoporosis.

Peripheral examination

Hands

Evidence of arthritis and rashes occur in systemic diseases that affect the lung. These diseases include rheumatoid arthritis, systemic sclerosis and sarcoidosis.

Nails

The nails should be inspected for clubbing, the causes of which are listed in **Table 2.14**. In clubbing, the nail develops a distinct curvature, with loss of the usual nail bed angle (**Figures 2.5** and **2.6**). On palpation, the nail bed feels spongy rather than firm. The distal phalanx may be expanded. Hypertrophic pulmonary osteopathy is severe clubbing associated

with symmetrical painful tender swelling of the wrists and ankles, caused by a periosteal reaction of the radii or tibia.

Yellow nails are a sign of yellow nail syndrome, a rare cause of bronchiectasis and pleural effusions. Blue discoloration of the fingers suggests peripheral cyanosis.

Tremor

Ask the patient to extend their arms in front of them. An essential tremor is a fine rapid regular tremor often caused by treatment with

Causes of finger clubbing	
Category	Causes
Respiratory	Lung cancer
	Bronchiectasis or cystic fibrosis
	Interstitial lung disease
	Lung abscess
	Empyema (prolonged)
	Chronic pulmonary tuberculosis
Cardiac	Bacterial endocarditis
	Cyanotic congenital heart disease
Other	Cirrhosis of the liver
	Inflammatory bowel disease
	Congenital (autosomal dominant)
	Idiopathic
*Cause unknown	

Table 2.14 Causes of clubbing

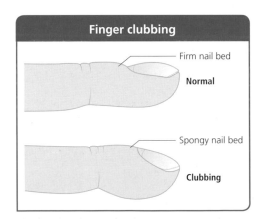

Finger clubbing

Firm nail bed

Normal

Spongy nail bed

Clubbing

Figure 2.5 Finger clubbing.

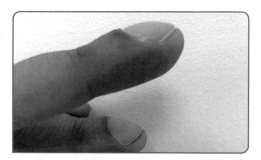

Figure 2.6 An example of finger clubbing.

β_2-agonists but also a sign of anxiety or thyrotoxicosis. Then ask the patient to bend their wrists up and spread their fingers; look for asterixis, a coarse irregular flapping tremor that is caused by increased $Paco_2$ or by hepatic failure.

Pulse rate (pulse)

A tachycardia suggests ill health, for example fever or respiratory distress, or anxiety. Increased $Paco_2$ causes a strong arterial impulse called a 'bounding' pulse. The pulse rate is irregular in atrial fibrillation. It is described as irregularly irregular because there is no regular component at all (unlike ectopic beats).

An irregular pulse also occurs in severe COPD due to multiple atrial ectopics (a wandering pacemaker).

Respiratory rate

Rate of respiration is an often forgotten but essential part of the respiratory examination. The usual adult respiratory rate is 12–16 breaths/min.

- A faster rate indicates that the patient is dyspnoeic
- A lower rate suggests that the patient is seriously ill and that intubation could be required

Some respiratory patterns suggest specific disorders (see page 80).

Blood pressure

Measurement of blood pressure is essential for patients presenting acutely to identify those with shock, for example caused by a tension pneumothorax or pneumonia. Hypertension causes cardiac impairment, a common differential diagnosis of chronic dyspnoea.

Eyes

Inspect the eyes for anaemia or jaundice. These signs are useful indicators of the patient's general health, although they are rarely related to respiratory disease.

Rarely, damage to the cervical sympathetic nerves, for example caused by lung cancer eroding through the apex of the lung and into the neck, causes Horner's syndrome. Horner's syndrome manifests with a combination of small pupil (meiosis), in-drawing of the eye (enophthalmos) and lowered eyelid (ptosis), with reduced sweating of the affected side of the face (**Figure 2.7**).

Lips and tongue

Inspect the lips and tongue for the blue discoloration of central cyanosis. If central cyanosis is present, the patient should also have peripheral cyanosis.

Cyanosis occurs when haemoglobin saturation decreases below 87%. Cyanosis is less obvious if the patient is anaemic. Conversely,

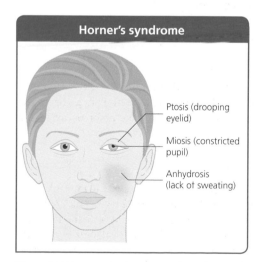

Figure 2.7 Horner's syndrome. The clinical features that are the result of an interruption to the cervical sympathetic chain: unilateral ptosis, meiosis and anhydrosis.

it is more apparent if they have polycythaemia (increased haemoglobin concentration).

Jugular venous pressure

Assess the jugular venous pressure (**Fig-ure 2.8**). Increased jugular venous pressure
is a sign of cor pulmonale, a relatively com-
mon complication of chronic lung disease, or
of acute right heart strain caused by pulmonary emboli. Severe cor pulmonale results in
tricuspid valve regurgitation, which causes
very prominent systolic s waves followed by a
rapid y descent in the jugular venous pressure
(**Figure 2.9**). Fixed dilated neck veins occur in
obstruction of the superior vena cava, which
also causes visible dilated veins over the
upper chest and severe oedema of the face or
arms.

Lymphadenopathy

Causes of generalised lymphadenopathy
include sarcoidosis, HIV infection, glandular fever, toxoplasmosis and systemic lupus
erythematosus. Localised lymphadenopathy
could be an indication of infection or malignancy affecting somewhere within the the

corresponding region of lymph drainage, or
lymphoma. For example:

- Cervical anterior and posterior lymph
  nodes may be enlarged in head and neck
  infections or malignancies, tuberculosis
  and lymphoma.
- Supraclavicular lymphadenopathy is
  associated with malignancy of the lungs,
  mediastinum and oesophagus or if on the
  left side, cancer of the stomach (Virchow's
  node).
- Axillary node enlargement indicates
  infection or malignancy of the arms,
  thoracic wall or breast.

Palpation

Trachea and apex beat

The position of the trachea and apex beat indicates whether mediastinal shift has occurred,
the causes of which are listed in **Table 2.15**.

- Collapse or loss of lung volume shifts the
  mediastinum, and therefore the trachea
  and apex beat, towards the affected side
- A large effusion or pneumothorax shifts
  them away from the affected side

The trachea should be checked for deviation.
There are several different methods for this; in
each, the examiner uses their fingers to com-
pare the position of the trachea to that of other
neck structures, such as the sternocleidomastoid muscles or their insertions (**Figure 2.10**).

The apex beat is defined as 'the most inferior and lateral site over the chest wall where
the cardiac impulse is palpable', which is
the mid-clavicular line in the 5th intercostal
space in normal subjects. The site of the apex
beat is identified by palpation of the chest
wall with the flat of the hand, moving from
a lateral inferior position more medially and
superiorly. The site of the apex beat is also
affected by cardiac disease, such as left ventricular dilation.

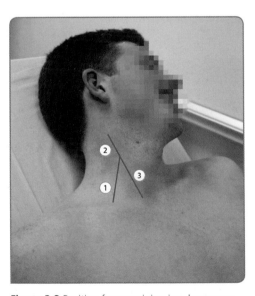

Figure 2.8 Position for examining jugular venous
pressure: head turned slightly to the left, patient
at 45°. ①, Clavicular head of sternocleidomastoid;
②, sternocleidomastoid; ③, sternal head of
sternocleidomastoid.

Chest expansion

Chest expansion is the increase in the size of
the thorax on inspiration and should be measured at the lung bases and the lung apices.

Jugular venous pressure waveforms

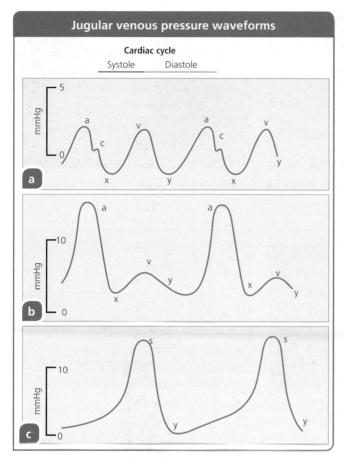

Figure 2.9 Jugular venous pressure waveforms in respiratory disease. (a) Normal jugular venous pressure. (b) Pulmonary arterial hypertension: increased a waves caused by increased end diastolic pressure in the right ventricle. (c) Pulmonary arterial hypertension with tricuspid regurgitation: ventricular systole causes massive s waves because of an open tricuspid valve. (a), Atrial systole; (x), x descent caused by ventricular filling; (c), closure of tricuspid valve at the start of systole; (v), filling of the right atrium during ventricular systole; (y), y descent caused by emptying of the right atrium into the right ventricle.

Causes of mediastinal shift	
Direction of shift	Causes
Towards affected side	Pneumonectomy or lobectomy
	Lobar collapse
	Previous severe destructive lung infection (e.g. tuberculosis)
	Chronic pleural disease
	Mesothelioma
Away from affected side	Pneumothorax
	Pleural effusion
	Massive lung or pleural tumour

Table 2.15 Causes of mediastinal shift

Expansion of the lung bases is measured by placing the fingertips on the ribs over the lateral chest wall in the axillae, bringing the thumbs together, asking the patient to take a deep breath, and measuring by eye the distance the thumbs move apart (**Figure 2.11**). The distance moved depends on the patient's size and age, but both sides should be equal and move at least 2–3 cm.

Expansion of the lung apices is measured by placing the flat of the hands on the superior chest wall anteriorly, with the thumbs parallel to each other. The key observation is whether the thumbs move up and away symmetrically.

When testing expansion, ensure that:

- the chest wall is not tender

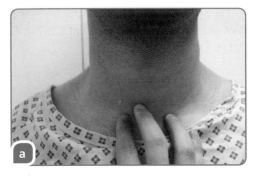

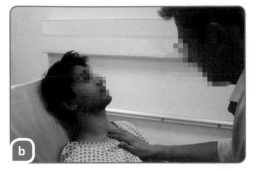

Figure 2.10 (a) Checking the position of the trachea. (b)The middle finger palpates the space either side of the trachea.

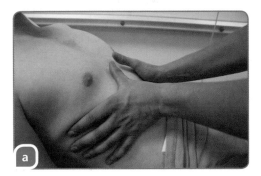

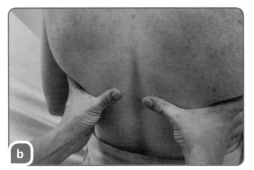

Figure 2.11 Testing lung expansion on inspiration (a) anteriorly and (b) posteriorly.

- the fingertips and hands are placed at the same level and symmetrically on either side of the chest
- the patient takes an adequately deep breath

Expansion of the chest is decreased by lung disease.

- Unilateral diseases (e.g. a pleural effusion) decreases expansion on the affected side only
- Bilateral diseases (e.g. COPD) decreases expansion evenly bilaterally

Tactile vocal fremitus

Tactile vocal fremitus is used to identify areas of the lung with reduced air entry. The edge of the hands or flat of the fingers is placed symmetrically over both sides of the chest wall. When the patient is asked to say '99', air entry is assessed by the degree of vibration felt in the examiner's fingers.

Tactile vocal fremitus is repeated in three or four places anteriorly then again posteriorly, moving from the top of the chest wall to the bottom and including both axillae (**Figure 2.12**). Causes of abnormal tactile vocal fremitus are listed in **Table 2.16**.

Percussion

Percussion is used to identify parts of the thoracic cavity that have become filled with fluid or solid. To percuss the chest, place the spread fingers of one hand firmly against the skin overlying the intercostal spaces. One finger (usually the middle finger) is then tapped sharply with a finger (again, usually the middle finger) from the other hand. The tapping hand uses a motion of the wrist, rather than the elbow, to generate the speed of the movement.

If percussion is done over an air-filled area, such as the normal lung, it generates a resonant noise suggesting a hollow area. In contrast, a fluid-filled or solid area produces a dull percussion note.

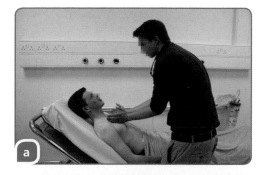

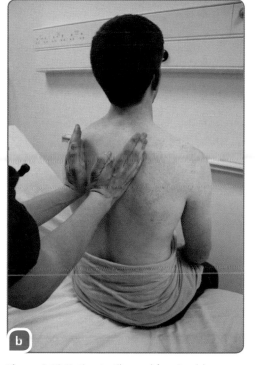

Figure 2.12 Testing tactile vocal fremitus (a) anteriorly and (b) posteriorly.

The percussed finger must be tightly pressed against the skin to generate a resonant note. Percussion should be done directly (with no underlying finger) on both clavicles, then using an underlying finger over the anterior chest at four or five sites (including the axillae) on alternate sides. The procedure is then repeated over the posterior chest four or five times (**Figure 2.13**), moving from the top of the chest wall to the bottom (**Figure 2.14**). Causes of abnormal percussion are listed in **Table 2.17**.

Causes of abnormal vocal resonance	
Vocal resonance	Causes
Increased (bronchial breathing)	Consolidation
	Over large cavities
	Top of a pleural effusion
	Over dense areas of local fibrosis
	Over lung apex if trachea is deviated to that side
Decreased	Pleural effusion
	Pneumothorax
	Lobar collapse or bronchial obstruction
	Pleural thickening
	Raised hemidiaphragm
	Pneumonectomy or lobectomy
	Bullae
	Severe airways disease (generalised)
	Obesity (generalised)

Table 2.16 Causes of abnormal vocal resonance, tactile vocal fremitus and breath sound intensity

Breath sounds

After percussion, the same sites over the chest wall, not forgetting the axillae, that were percussed should be examined using the stethoscope to listen to the breath sounds (auscultation) and then for vocal resonance (**Figure 2.14**).

The stethoscope is placed firmly on to the skin, and the patient asked to take deep breaths through their open mouth. The apices should be auscultated using the bell, and the rest of the chest using the diaphragm of the stethoscope.

Assess the following three aspects of the resulting breath sounds: ratio of inspiration to expiration, intensity of breath sounds, and the presence or absence of any added sounds.

Ratio of inspiration to expiration

In normal subjects, inspiration is slightly longer than expiration. However, in diseases causing lower airways obstruction, this is reversed as expiration becomes prolonged (**Figure 2.15**).

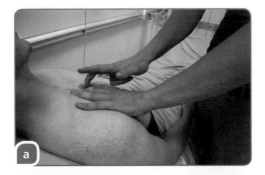

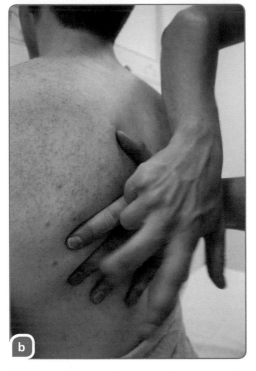

Figure 2.13 Percussion technique: (a) anterior and (b) posterior.

Intensity of breath sounds

Several conditions reduce the intensity of the audible breath sounds either unilaterally (e.g. in a pneumothorax) or bilaterally (e.g. in COPD). Dense consolidation increases the intensity of breath sounds and sometimes causes bronchial breathing. With bronchial breathing, breath sounds (and vocal resonance) have a specific, increased low-pitch quality which represents conduction of sounds generated by the large airways to the stethoscope.

Presence or absence of added sounds

Diagnosis of lung disease is often aided by identifying the presence or absence of added sounds (**Table 2.18**). Added sounds include the following.

■ Wheeze (also called rhonchi) is usually best heard during expiration, and is a sign of airways disease.
■ Crepitations (also called crackles or rhales) are a crackling noise usually best heard on inspiration. They generally indicate alveolar or interstitial disease, although exceptions are common.
■ Pleural rubs are usually best heard on inspiration and always indicate an abnormality or inflammation of the pleura. Pleural rubs are a creaky noise similar to the sound of walking in thick snow while wearing large boots. They are often transient and audible over very localised areas of the chest.

Other, but rare, added sounds include inspiratory and expiratory squeaks (which indicate small airways inflammation) and clicks (which are caused by pleural abnormalities).

Vocal resonance

Vocal resonance is used to assess breath sound intensity and confirm the results found during auscultation of breath sounds. The stethoscope is placed firmly on to the skin and the patient asked to say '99'. The intensity of the noise generated may be reduced or increased due to a similar range of causes that affect the intensity of breath sounds (**Table 2.16**). Bronchial breathing is occasionally accompanied by whispering pectoriloquy, which is when the patient whispers '99' and this is clearly audible during auscultation.

> **Bilateral lung abnormalities can be hard to detect with confidence, because there is no normal lung for comparison.** Examples are bilateral reductions in expansion and in breath sound intensity in patients with COPD.

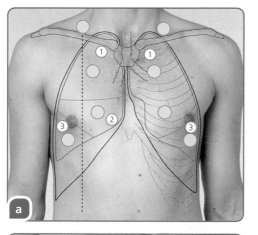

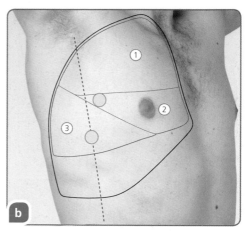

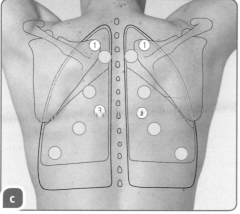

Figure 2.14 Placement of the stethoscope (blue circles) for auscultation, vocal resonance and percussion: (a) anterior, (b) axillae and (c) posterior ① upper lobes, ② middle lobe, ③ lower lobes.

Causes of abnormal percussion note	
Result	**Causes**
Increased dullness	Pleural effusion ('stony dull')
	Lobar collapse
	Dense consolidation
	Pneumonectomy
	Raised hemidiaphragm
	Pleural thickening
	Very large pleural or lung tumours
	Poor percussion technique
Increased resonance*	Pneumothorax
	Large bullae
	Large lung cavity

*Difficult to detect.

Table 2.17 Causes of abnormal percussion note

Additional features of the examination

The ankles and sacrum should be checked for pitting oedema, especially if the patient has central cyanosis or increased jugular venous pressure so may have cor pulmonale. Patients with suspected lung cancer or sarcoidosis should undergo abdominal examination to detect any hepatomegaly (enlarged liver) or splenomegaly (enlarged spleen). These patients should also have a neurological examination to find signs of any involvement of the nervous system. If the patient is producing sputum, this should be inspected to identify whether it is mucoid, purulent or mucopurulent, and whether it contains blood.

Common mistakes to avoid when examining the respiratory system include:

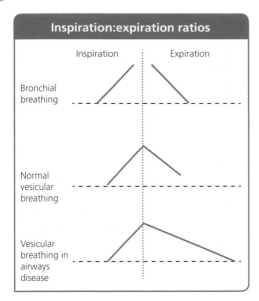

Inspiration:expiration ratios	
Inspiration	Expiration
Bronchial breathing	
Normal vesicular breathing	
Vesicular breathing in airways disease	

Figure 2.15 Breath sounds. The ratio of inspiration duration to expiration in normal breathing (vesicular), airways obstruction (e.g. due to COPD or asthma) and bronchial breathing (e.g. due to consolidation).

Causes of added lung sounds	
Lung sound	Causes
Wheeze	COPD
	Asthma (polyphonic)
	Viral lower airway infections
	Partial obstruction of a bronchus (monophonic)
	Upper airways obstruction (inspiratory: stridor)
Crepitations	Pulmonary oedema (fine)
	Pulmonary fibrosis and other interstitial lung diseases (fine)
	Pneumonia (coarse)
	Bronchiectasis (coarse)
Pleural rub	Pleural infection
	Over consolidation due to pneumonia
	Pulmonary embolism
	Dressler's syndrome
	Recently drained effusions
Squeaks (rare)	Bronchiolitis (inflammation of the bronchioles)
	Bronchiectasis

COPD, chronic obstructive pulmonary disease.

Table 2.18 Causes of added lung sounds on auscultation

- an inadequate general observation of the respiratory system
- forgetting to measure the respiratory rate, assess for tracheal deviation or check vocal resonance
- failing to place the fingers at the same level and symmetrically on the sides of the chest when testing expansion
- not percussing or auscultating as far down as the 10th thoracic vertebral body on the posterior chest
- forgetting to check for ankle and sacral oedema or to inspect the sputum

Examination features of common respiratory presentations

The clinical findings for specific clinical presentations are discussed below and summarised in **Table 2.19** (see pages 92 and 93).

Pneumothorax

A pneumothorax is air in the pleural space. It is usually a unilateral condition. Loss of negative pressure, combined with the increased volume of the hemithorax (caused by air in the pleural space), causes mediastinal shift away from the pneumothorax. Therefore the trachea and apex beat are deviated away from the affected side, unless the pneumothorax is small.

Chest expansion is reduced on the affected side, and percussion is resonant. There may be increased resonance (hyper-resonance) over the pneumothorax, although this is difficult to detect with certainty. The underlying lung collapses in response to the pneumothorax and is separated from the stethoscope by the pleural air. Consequently, breath sounds and vocal resonance are greatly reduced or absent. The air rises because of gravity, so the signs of a small pneumothorax are restricted to the apex of the lung.

Pleural effusion

Pleural effusions are fluid in the pleural space. Some findings are similar to those of a pneumothorax:

- the trachea deviated away from the affected side (with big effusions)
- reduced expansion of the affected side
- absent breath sounds and reduced vocal resonance over the effusion

However, in contrast to a pneumothorax, the presence of fluid in the pleural space makes the percussion note over the effusion very dull; it is often described as 'stony dull'. In addition, pleural fluid collects around the bottom of the lung, so effusions are detected at the lung bases. Sometimes there is a patch of bronchial breathing at the top of an effusion. With inflamed pleura, there is often a pleural rub at the points where the visceral and parietal pleurae become apposed again.

Consolidation

Diseases of the alveoli that replace air with an inflammatory exudate or more solid material cause patches of consolidation. The commonest cause is infection, termed pneumonia, which commonly affects entire lung segments or lobes. Patients with consolidation caused by pneumonia look ill, are pyrexial and have a tachycardia; these are signs of active systemic inflammation. With extensive consolidation patients have central cyanosis.

There is no mediastinal shift, so the trachea remains central. Expansion is reduced on the affected side. Over extensive dense consolidation, the percussion note is dull and there is bronchial breathing.

In practice, most pneumonia causes less dense consolidation, and the commonest sign is coarse inspiratory crepitations over the affected area, which in lobar pneumonia is asymmetrical in distribution. Bronchopenumonia causes widespread small patches of consolidation and causes widespread coarse inspiratory crepitations and harsh breath sounds.

Lobar collapse

Obstruction of a major airway (e.g. a lobar bronchus, the right intermediate bronchus, or the right or left main bronchus) causes resorption of the air in the alveoli and airways distal to the obstruction. This is called lobar collapse and has the following common causes.

- Lung carcinoma
- Less common lung tumours:
  - carcinoid
  - endobronchial metastases
- Sputum plugging:
  - asthma
  - bronchiectasis
  - ABPA
  - mechanically ventilated patients
  - postoperatively
- inhaled foreign body (e.g. or tooth or food)

The signs are similar to those of a pleural effusion, with reduced expansion, dullness to percussion, and reduced breath sounds and vocal resonance over the affected side. However, with lobar collapse lung volume is lost, so the apex beat and trachea shift towards the affected side. Pneumonectomy causes similar signs to total lung collapse but with a surgical scar.

Pulmonary fibrosis

With idiopathic pulmonary fibrosis, the commonest interstitial lung disease, the fibrosis starts in the lung bases and spreads up the lung as the disease progresses. There is no mediastinal shift, and expansion is reduced bilaterally. The lungs remain partially aerated, so percussion remains resonant. However, in severe disease lung volume is lost and the lungs end above the usual 10th thoracic vertebral body.

The most important sign is fine crepitations on inspiration over both lung bases, spreading to the whole lung in severe disease. The crepitations of pulmonary fibrosis are frequently distinctive: fine late inspiratory crepitations that occur in bursts and sound like Velcro being ripped apart.

About 10–15% of patients with pulmonary fibrosis have clubbed fingers or toes. Severely affected patients are cyanosed and may develop signs of cor pulmonale (see page 95). Patients with fibrosis associated with connective tissue disorders will have peripheral signs of the underlying disease (e.g. rheumatoid arthritis changes in the hands). Other causes of pulmonary fibrosis affect different parts of the lung, and the lung signs match this distribution. For example, radiotherapy

Examination findings for common respiratory presentations					
Respiratory presentation	Trachea	Expansion	Percussion	Auscultation	Vocal resonance
Pneumothorax	Central or deviated away, depending on size	Reduced on affected side	Hyper-resonant	Absent breath sounds No added sounds	Reduced or absent
Pleural effusion	Central or deviated away, depending on size	Reduced on affected side	Dull ('stony dull')	Absent breath sounds Pleural rub (sometimes) Bronchial breathing at the top (sometimes)	Reduced or absent
Lobar consolidation	Central	Reduced on affected side	Dull (if dense; resonant if less dense)	Bronchial breathing (if dense) Coarse crepitations	Increased or bronchial
Lobar collapse	Deviated towards	Reduced on affected side	Dull	Absent breath sounds No added sounds	Reduced

Table 2.19 Examination findings for common respiratory presentations. *Continued opposite.*

Examination findings for common respiratory presentations *continued*					
Respiratory presentation	Trachea	Expansion	Percussion	Auscultation	Vocal resonance
Pulmonary fibrosis	Central	Reduced bilaterally	Resonant	Fine inspiratory bibasal crepitations (Velcro crepitations)	Normal
Bronchiectasis	Central	Reduced bilaterally†	Resonant	Coarse inspiratory bibasal crepitations	Normal or increased
COPD or asthma	Central	Reduced bilaterally	Resonant	Prolonged expiration Quiet breath sounds throughout Expiratory wheeze	Normal or reduced throughout
Apical scarring (post-tuberculosis)	Deviated towards	Reduced unilaterally	Resonant or dull	Bronchial breathing (tracheal) Focal crepitations	Normal or increased

Table 2.19 Examination findings for common respiratory presentations (*continued*).

causes fibrosis in the radiotherapy field, and hypersensitivity pneumonitis and sarcoidosis cause mainly upper lobe disease.

Bronchiectasis

The main sign of bronchiectasis are coarse crepitations over the affected areas, with reduced expansion but usually a normal percussion note and vocal resonance. Like pulmonary fibrosis, bronchiectasis most commonly predominantly affects both lung bases symmetrically. However, bronchiectasis is often also localised to specific lobes either symmetrically or asymmetrically, with the signs distributed accordingly. Severe bronchiectasis causes progressive small airways obstruction resulting in additional signs similar to those seen in COPD.

> **A good presentation of the results of the respiratory examination needs to include the relevant negative and all the positive findings yet remain concise.** Try to avoid terms such as 'slight' or 'possible'. Finish with a sensible assessment of what the signs could mean. For example, a patient with basal dullness on percussion could have an effusion or lobar collapse but not a pneumothorax.

Chronic obstructive pulmonary disease

Overall, COPD causes more pronounced peripheral signs of lung disease than those detected using the stethoscope. Auscultation and vocal resonance may even seem normal. The lungs are hyperexpanded, but expansion on inspiration is markedly reduced bilaterally. With severe disease or during exacerbations patients are dyspnoeic at rest, using the accessory muscles of respiration with intercostal recession, a tracheal tug and pursed lip breathing. Pursing the lips together on exhalation generates intrinsic positive end-expiratory pressure that prevents dynamic airway collapse.

The percussion note is resonant and the usual areas of dullness are frequently lost over the liver and heart. The lower limit of the lungs posteriorly often descends below the 10th thoracic vertebral body as a result of lung hyperexpansion. On auscultation, the breath sounds and vocal resonance are quiet, the expiratory phase is prolonged and an expiratory wheeze may be heard. Severe COPD is often associated with non-specific indistinct bibasal crepitations.

Asthma

In asthma, the findings depend on the severity of the disease.

- Patients with controlled or mild asthma have no lung signs
- With more severe airways obstruction, there is hyperexpansion of the chest with bilaterally reduced expansion during inspiration. The trachea is central and the percussion note resonant. On auscultation, an expiratory polyphonic, often quite musical, wheeze is audible, as well as a prolonged expiratory phase
- In acute asthma, the patient is obviously short of breath, with increased respiratory and heart rate, intercostal recession, and an abnormally large decrease in systolic blood pressure on inspiration (> 15 mmHg, termed pulsus paradoxus)
- In life-threatening asthma, breath sounds are reduced on auscultation (a 'silent chest'), heart rate and respiratory rate decrease, and the patient's level of consciousness becomes impaired; these are clear signs of severe disease that needs immediate treatment to prevent respiratory arrest

Apical scarring

Previous tuberculosis results in asymmetrical lung scarring that usually affects the upper lobes. The most affected lung has marked volume loss, causing tracheal shift to the affected side. There can be dullness to percussion resulting from pleural thickening over the apex. On auscultation, bronchial breathing can be heard; this is caused by the presence of a large cavity or the tracheal shift.

Cor pulmonale

Chronic hypoxic lung disease eventually causes cor pulmonale. Therefore it is often associated with signs of right ventricular failure and pulmonary hypertension:

- a left parasternal heave caused by right ventricular hypertrophy
- increased jugular venous pressure with prominent a waves (**Figure 2.15**)
- a loud pulmonary component of the 2nd heart sound

- ankle oedema
- pleural effusions, ascites or both
- signs of tricuspid regurgitation (pansystolic murmur over the left parasternal 4th and 5th intercostal spaces, hepatomegaly that may be pulsatile and a jugular venous pressure with a prominent s wave and steep y descent) (**Figure 2.9**)

Investigations

Starter questions

Answers to the following questions are on page 138–139.

9. What is the alveolar/arterial gradient and why is it useful?
10. What investigations are useful for someone presenting with chronic dyspnoea?
11. How does the clinician decide on which biopsy method to use to obtain lung histology?
12. What are the advantages and disadvantages of using CT scans to assess lung disease?

Once a thorough clinical assessment has been made, selected investigations are needed to:

- confirm the suspected diagnosis
- exclude the important differential diagnoses
- assess disease severity
- provide baseline data for monitoring the progress of the disease

Which investigations are necessary depends on the findings of the clinical assessment and the suspected differential diagnosis. For example, a patient presenting with airways disease must have pulmonary function tests to identify any physiological defect and the degree of reversibility. In contrast, a patient presenting with suspected lung carcinoma requires radiological staging investigations (e.g. computerised tomography, CT, and positron emission tomography, PET) and a biopsy of abnormal tissue to confirm the suspected diagnosis. Many patients presenting with milder diseases do not need any investigations if the diagnosis is clear from the clinical presentation.

> **The clinical assessment is vital for an accurate interpretation of results of investigations.** For example, a chest X-ray showing consolidation in a patient with cough and fever probably represents pneumonia. However, the same radiographic changes in a patient with no fever and 3 months of coughing could be alveolar cell carcinoma or an unusual infection.

Various types of investigation are available for patients with suspected respiratory diseases.

- Tests of physiological function include pulmonary function tests, analysis of blood gases, sleep studies and PET scans
- Investigations of lung anatomy include chest X-ray, CT and magnetic resonance imaging (MRI) scans, ultrasound and bronchoscopy
- Cytological investigations include analysis of samples from bronchoscopy, percutaneous aspiration and surgery, as well as sputum
- Histological investigations include analysis of bronchoscopic, percutaneous and surgical biopsies
- Microbiological investigations include microscopy, cultures, serology, antigen testing, histology and nucleic acid amplification tests
- Immunological status include blood tests for inflammatory markers, autoantibodies and immunoglobulin (Ig) concentrations; and skin and blood allergen testing
- Blood tests to assess general health include full blood count and tests of liver and renal function

Useful investigations when assessing common respiratory presentations are listed in **Tables 2.20** and **2.21**.

Test sensitivity and specificity

The effectiveness of a particular investigation at confirming the presence or absence of a disease is measured using sensitivity and specificity.

- Sensitivity is the ability of the test to identify all cases of the disease, e.g. the proportion of people with a disease who will test positive
- Specificity is the likelihood that the test has accurately identified the disease, e.g. the proportion of positive results due to people with the disease

Both values are frequently expressed as percentages. The best test would clearly be 100% sensitive and 100% specific, but this is impossible to achieve. Many tests are either sensitive or specific; only a minority are both.

An important concept is that the pre-test probability of the presence of a disease has a major effect on the interpretation of a positive test result. For example, for a test that is 95% specific and 90% sensitive:

- when used as a screening test there will be one false positive result per 20 people tested. Therefore, for a disease with an prevalence of 1 per 10,000, there will be nearly 500 (9999 x 0.05) false positive results per true positive. This number of false positives would make the test very ineffective at identifying the single affected case
- when used as a diagnostic test for patients in which the clinical assessment suggests the patient has a 50% chance of the disease, then per every 200 patients the test will identify 100 x 0.90 cases accurately (90 cases) but will miss 10 cases. It will also identify 100 x 0.05 false positives (5 cases). So 1 result in every 18 will be a false positive, making the test clinically useful in these circumstances

This is another reason why the clinical assessment is essential for an accurate assessment of a positive test result.

Pulmonary function tests

Pulmonary function tests assess the physiological function of the lungs. These tests are most likely to be abnormal in diffuse lung diseases such as COPD and interstitial lung disease, and they are essential for both the diagnosis and monitoring of chronic lung disease.

The main difficulty with pulmonary function tests is that they depend on patient effort; the results are artificially low if a patient does not make a maximum effort. A core skill for technicians administering these tests is the ability to coax the best effort and technique from the patients doing them.

Pulmonary function tests are expressed as absolute values. However, the expected values vary markedly with sex, age and height, so results are also given as a percentage of expected for the individual patient. Values above 80% of expected are usually regarded as normal.

Investigations for acute respiratory presentations

Presentation	Investigation	Role
Acute dyspnoea	Chest X-ray	Identify pneumothorax, consolidation, effusion(s), left ventricular dilation, pulmonary oedema, pulmonary embolism, chronic lung disease
	PEFR	Identify and monitor airways disease
	ECG	Identify arrhythmias, pulmonary embolism, cardiac disease
	Echocardiogram	Identify left ventricular impairment (cardiac failure) or right heart strain (pulmonary embolism and pulmonary hypertension)
	Analysis of blood gases	Identify and assess severity of type 1 or type 2 respiratory failure
	Urea and electrolytes, liver function tests, full blood count	Identify kidney or liver impairment, abnormal white cell or platelet counts, anaemia, polycythaemia
	C-reactive protein and ESR	Markers of active inflammation
	Troponin	Increased in pulmonary embolism and cardiac disease
	D-dimer	Increased in pulmonary embolism
	CTPA	Identify pulmonary embolism
Major haemoptysis	Chest X-ray	Identify tuberculosis, lung cancer, aspergilloma, bronchiectasis
	CT scan	Identify tuberculosis, lung cancer, aspergilloma or bronchiectasis
	Full blood count and clotting screen	Identify thrombocytopenia or clotting disorders
	Sputum culture and acid-fast bacilli	Identify active tuberculosis or other bacterial infection
	Sputum cytology	Identify lung cancer or evidence of *Aspergillus* infection
	Bronchoscopy	Identify bleeding point and obtain diagnostic samples
	Pulmonary angiography	Identify bleeding vessel for embolisation or surgery
Cough and fever	Chest X-ray	Identify consolidation, lung nodules, cavities, pleural effusions
	Analysis of blood gases	Identify respiratory failure, acidosis or both; assess severity
	Urea and electrolytes, liver function tests, full blood count	Identify kidney or liver impairment, abnormal white cell or platelet counts, or anaemia or polycythaemia
	C-reactive protein and ESR	Markers of active inflammation
	Serological tests	Identify infection with atypical and viral pathogens
	Analysis of nasopharyngeal aspirate	Identify infection with viral pathogens
	Blood and sputum culture	Identify infection with bacterial pathogens
	Sputum and acid-fast bacilli test	Identify tuberculosis in high-risk patients
	Urine antigen testing	Identify infection with *Streptococcus pneumoniae* or *Legionella pneumophila*
Chest pain	Chest X-ray	Identify pneumothorax, consolidation, effusion(s) or the changes of pulmonary embolism or potential malignant disease
	CTPA	Identify pulmonary embolism, malignant and pleural disease
	ECG	Identify ischaemic heart disease, pericarditis or pulmonary embolism
	Urea and electrolytes, liver function tests, full blood count	Identify kidney or liver impairment, abnormal white cell or platelet counts, or anaemia or polycythaemia
	C-reactive protein and ESR	Markers of active inflammation
	Troponin	Increased in pulmonary embolism and cardiac disease
	D-dimer	Increased in pulmonary embolism

Table 2.20 Investigations used for common acute respiratory presentations

Investigations for chronic respiratory presentations		
Presentation	Investigation	Role
Dyspnoea	Spirometry with reversibility	Identify and assess severity and restrictive defects of airways disease
	Transfer factor	V decreases in transfer factor (in emphysema, interstitial lung disease, pulmonary embolism, anaemia and pulmonary hypertension)
	6-min walk test	Assess severity of exercise impairment
	Chest X-ray	Identify changes suggesting COPD, interstitial lung disease, cardiac failure, effusions, pneumoconiosis, etc.
	CT scan or CTPA	Further investigation of low transfer factor, suspected interstitial lung disease, emphysema, pulmonary embolism, pneumoconiosis
	Full blood count	Exclude anaemia as a cause of dyspnoea
	Serum angiotensin-converting enzyme, autoantibodies, avian precipitins, ANCA	If interstitial lung disease is suspected
	ECG, echocardiogram and other cardiac testing (e.g. nuclear scans and angiography)	Exclude active cardiac disease, diagnose chronic pulmonary emboli
Persistent cough with normal chest X-ray	Spirometry with reversibility test	Identify and assess the severity of airways disease (COPD and asthma)
	Home PEFR recordings	Identify asthma (variable PEFR)
	Skin allergen test	Identify atopic asthma
	Sputum eosinophilia	Identify cough variant asthma
	Sputum culture and acid-fast bacilli	Identify low-grade bacterial infection
	CT scan of sinuses	Identify chronic sinusitis
	CT scan of lungs	Identify bronchiectasis and endobronchial lesions
	Gastrointestinal tract tests (endoscopy and 24-h oesophageal manometry)	Identify gastro-oesophageal reflux
	Bronchoscopy	Identify endobronchial tumours or foreign body, obtain samples for culture
Lung mass on chest X-ray	CT scan of lungs and upper abdomen	Assess extent of lung mass and identify lung, pleural, liver, adrenal or lymph node (mediastinal, axillary, upper abdomen and cervical) metastases
	Urea and electrolytes, liver function tests, full blood count	Identify liver, bone or marrow involvement, or kidney impairment
	Biopsy: bronchoscopic or percutaneous (CT or ultrasound)	Obtain tissue for confirmed histological diagnosis
	Pulmonary function tests, ECG	Assess fitness for radical therapy with surgery or radiotherapy
	PET scan	Identify distal metastases before curative treatment
	CT scan of brain	If cerebral metastases suspected
	Bone scan	If bone metastases suspected
	MRI scan	Assess chest wall or mediastinal invasion
Minor haemoptysis	Chest X-ray	Identify lung masses, nodules, cavities, lobar collapse
	CT scan of lungs	Identify endobronchial tumours, bronchiectasis, aspergillomas or arteriovenous malformation, or to further assess chest X-ray abnormalities
	Bronchoscopy	Identify endobronchial tumours and obtain diagnostic samples
	Full blood count, clotting tests, ANCA	Identify thrombocytopenia, clotting disorders, vasculitis
	Sputum culture and acid-fast bacilli	Identify active tuberculosis, other bacterial infection
	Sputum cytology	Identify lung cancer

Table 2.21 Investigations used for common chronic respiratory presentations

Pulmonary function results may
be normal in patients with some
respiratory diseases, for example
intermittent diseases such as asthma.
Furthermore, localised diseases such
as lung cancer often affect too small a
volume to alter lung function.

The four main types of pulmonary function
test are:

- PEFR
- spirometry
- lung volumes
- transfer factor

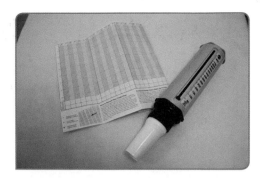

Figure 2.16 A peak expiratory flow rate meter.

Peak expiratory flow rate recording

This type of pulmonary function test measures the maximum expiratory flow in
L/ min. Values of PEFR are reduced in diseases causing airways obstruction.

To measure their PEFR, the patient blows
as hard and as fast as they can into the PEFR
meter. The best result of three blows is recorded. PEFR meters are small and portable (**Figure 2.16**), so can be used by patients at home.

Recordings of PEFR are used to identify
reversible airways obstruction and to assess
the severity of acute airways obstruction.

Identification of reversible airways obstruction

Repeated home recordings identify reversible
airways obstruction and confirm a diagnosis of
asthma. Patients record PEFR in the morning
and evening, as well as during periods when
they have respiratory symptoms. Diurnal variation (low PEFR in the morning, higher in the
evening) or a decrease in PEFR during symptoms of >15% confirms significant reversible
airways obstruction.

Assessment of severity of acute airways obstruction

The severity of acute airways obstruction is
assessed by comparing PEFR during an acute
attack to the patient's best recent PEFR. This
test is most useful for asthma; PEFR is less

useful in COPD, because values often do not
decrease greatly during exacerbations.

Spirometry

Spirometry is the single most useful test for
the diagnosis and monitoring of chronic lung
disease. It is also convenient. Spirometry can
be measured in outpatient units (**Figure 2.17**),
general practice surgeries, on home visits or
on the wards using handheld portable spi-
rometers, as well as in the respiratory physiology laboratory.

Results are produced by a forced prolonged expiration. As with PEFR recordings,
the best of three results is noted. Two components are measured (**Figure 2.19a**).

- Forced expiratory volume in 1 s (FEV_1) is a
  flow rate, but unlike PEFR, it is measured
  over 1 s and recorded as L/s
- Forced vital capacity (FVC) is the
  maximum ventilatory capacity of the lung
  and is measured in L.

FEV_1 can therefore never be greater than
FVC, and the FEV_1/FVC ratio is usually
around 0.80 (**Figure 2.18a**), although this
falls slightly with increasing age. Both FEV_1
and FVC are decreased by any lung disease
that reduces lung capacity. However, in airways obstruction the expiratory flow is particularly impaired and FEV_1 decreases to a
greater extent than the decrease in FVC. In
contrast, expiratory airflow tends to be preserved in chronic lung diseases not affecting
the airways, and there is a larger fall in FVC
than in FEV_1. This divides abnormal spirometry results into two main groups, obstructive

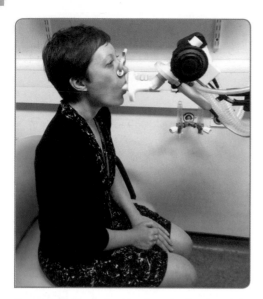

Figure 2.17 Measuring lung function in a hospital lung function laboratory.

and restrictive. Less commonly there can be a mixed obstructive and restrictive defect.

Obstructive lung function

A larger decrease in FEV_1 than that of FVC, with a FEV_1/FVC ratio < 0.70, shows obstructive lung function (**Figure 2.18b**). If a patient has obstructive spirometry results, then it is essential to test reversibility by recording the spirometry before and after inhaled or nebulised bronchodilator (usually a β2-agonist). If the treatment causes a significant increase in the spirometric values, defined as $> 15\%$ of precited values but of at least 200 mL, then the patient has reversible airways disease.

Obstructive lung function can be partially or fully reversible. Diseases are partially reversible if the spirometric values improve with treatment or between exacerbations but remain abnormal. Diseases are fully reversible if the spirometric values improve sufficiently to return to normal. Reversibility can also be tested in response to treatment with oral or inhaled corticosteroids over a period of days or weeks (usually 3 weeks).

Restrictive lung disease

The definition of restrictive lung function is a decrease in total lung capacity. However, in practice it is usually first identified by spirometric values (**Figure 2.18c**). Both FVC and FEV_1 decrease equally, or the decrease in FVC is greater, therefore the FEV_1/FVC ratio remains > 0.70. In fact, the FEV_1 is often almost equal to FVC. Some diseases, or the coexistence of two diseases (e.g. COPD and pulmonary fibrosis), cause mixed obstructive-restrictive lung function. Causes of obstructive and restrictive spirometric values are listed in **Table 2.22**.

Lung volumes

Spirometric values represent the usable lung volumes. The total volume of the lungs is measured by using specialist equipment in the lung function laboratory. The two main measures are residual volume and total lung capacity.

- Residual volume is the volume of air remaining in the lungs after a full expiration, and is increased in airways obstruction (e.g. COPD and acute asthma, called air trapping)
- Total lung capacity is the residual volume plus the spirometric values (FEV_1 and FVC); it is increased in airways obstruction because air-trapping causes the residual volume to increase. Due to loss of lung volume total lung capacity is reduced in interstitial lung disease and chest wall diseases (Figure 1.22).

Transfer factor

Transfer factor is a measure of potential oxygen uptake by the lungs. As oxygen uptake is dependent on diffusion across the alveolar membrane, transfer factor is measured using a readily diffusible gas, carbon monoxide, and specialist equipment in the respiratory physiology laboratory. Two values are given:

- T_{LCO} is the absolute value of the transfer factor, measured in mL/min/mmHg; any lung disease that reduces lung volume also reduces T_{LCO}
- K_{CO} is the transfer coefficient, the absolute transfer factor adjusted for lung size (T_{LCO} divided by alveolar volume VA, calculated from other lung variables);

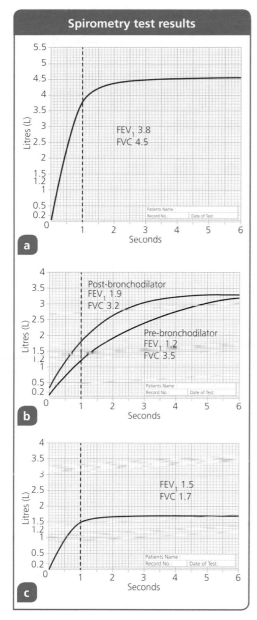

Spirometry test results

a FEV₁ 3.8
FVC 4.5

Patients Name
Record No. | Date of Test:

b Post-bronchodilator
FEV₁ 1.9
FVC 3.2

Pre-bronchodilator
FEV₁ 1.2
FVC 3.5

Patients Name :
Record No. | Date of Test:

c FEV₁ 1.5
FVC 1.7

Patients Name :
Record No.: | Date of Test:

Figure 2.18 Results of spirometry tests: (a) normal, (b) obstructive with partial reversibility and (c) restrictive. The forced expiratory volume (in 1 s) (FEV₁) value is where the curve meets the dotted line. The forced vital capacity (FVC) is the value where the curve crosses the y-axis on the right-hand side.

K_{CO} is a measure of the efficiency of oxygen diffusion per unit of lung, and is more useful than T_{LCO} for identifying lung diseases that affect oxygen uptake.

Causes of obstructive and restrictive spirometry results

Obstructive	Restrictive
Chronic obstructive pulmonary disease	Poor effort during test
Asthma	Extrathoracic or pleural causes, e.g. obesity, neuromuscular disease, chest wall deformities, diaphragmatic paralysis, large pleural effusions, pleural thickening
Other chronic airways diseases (e.g. bronchiolitis obliterans)	
Large airways obstruction	
	Interstitial lung disease
	Sarcoid or hypersensitivity pneumonitis*
	Extensive lung scarring due to previous infection, e.g. tuberculosis

*Often mixed obstructive–restrictive changes.

Table 2.22 Causes of obstructive and restrictive spirometry results

For example, after a pneumonectomy (surgical removal of a lung) the absolute value of transfer factor (T_{LCO}) will fall whereas K_{CO} will not as the remaining lung has normal efficiency at transferring oxygen to the blood. In contrast, in patients with interstitial lung disease oxygen diffusion into the blood is inhibited by the increase in alveolar wall thickness and both T_{LCO} and K_{CO} will be reduced.

Transfer factor is affected by lung disease, abnormalities of the pulmonary circulation and cardiac disease. It is also reduced by anaemia, and the result should be adjusted for the haemoglobin concentration. Causes of chronic reductions in transfer factor are shown in **Table 2.23**. Transfer factor is increased by pulmonary haemorrhage, polycythaemia and left-to-right cardiac shunts or pneumonectomy (because of increased haemoglobin or blood flow through the lungs).

Additional lung function tests

Additional lung function tests that are used for assessing respiratory diseases include

Causes of chronically reduced K_{CO}	
Category	Cause(s)
Pulmonary	Interstitial lung disease
	Emphysema
Pulmonary vascular	Pulmonary embolism
	Pulmonary hypertension
	Right-to-left shunts
Cardiac	Mitral valve disease
	Pulmonary oedema
Blood	Anaemia

Table 2.23 Causes of a chronically reduced transfer coefficient K_{CO}

flow volume loops, the 6-min walk, pulmonary challenge tests and respiratory muscle function tests.

Flow volume loops

Plots of flow rate (*y*-axis) against lung volume (*x*-axis) to obtain a flow volume loop during expiration and inspiration show characteristic patterns indicating the diagnosis. For example, rapid falls in expiratory flow in early expiration suggest dynamic airways collapse caused by emphysema, and large airways obstruction flattens the inspiratory flow volume loop (**Figure 2.19**).

The 6-min walk

The total distance a patient walks in 6 min is measured using a circuit of known distance, such as a long corridor. This provides a reproducible measure of the patient's exercise capacity that is used to judge response to treatment and disease progression. The patient's oxygen saturation is also recorded to identify exercise-induced desaturation and any response to portable oxygen therapy.

Pulmonary challenge tests

Although rarely necessary, a diagnosis of asthma can be confirmed by measuring spirometry responses to inhaled methacholine. The methacholine challenge causes a >20% decrease in FEV_1 in patients with asthma but not in healthy subjects.

Tests of respiratory muscle function

Measurements of the maximum airway pressure on inspiration or expiration (mouth pressures) and falls in spirometry when lying compared with when standing are used to

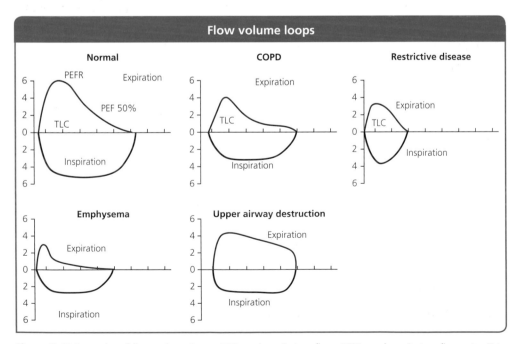

Figure 2.19 Examples of flow volume loops. PEF, peak expiratory flow; PEFR, peak expiratory flow rate; RV, residual volume; TLC, total lung capacity.

identify the rare patient who has respiratory muscle weakness.

Oxygen saturation and arterial blood gases

The ultimate role of the lungs is to oxygenate the blood and excrete carbon dioxide. Severe lung diseases result in changes in blood oxygen and carbon dioxide concentrations. Carbon dioxide concentration also affects acid–base balance, therefore severe lung disease affects blood pH and bicarbonate concentration.

Blood gases

Respiratory investigations commonly include some key analyses of blood gases. The normal values for these blood gas parameters are as follows:

- Oxygen saturation: >94%
- Pao_2: 11.3–14 kPa
- $Paco_2$: 4.7–6.0 kPa
- pH: 7.36–7.47
- HCO_3^-: 23–26 mmol/L
- Base excess: +/– 2 mmol/L

Blood oxygen levels

In the circulation, oxygen is either dissolved in the blood or bound to haemoglobin. The dissolved component, the partial pressure of oxygen (the Pao_2 for arterial blood) is measured using electrodes and an arterial blood gas analyser using a small amount of arterial blood. The result reflects how effectively oxygen is reaching the blood from the lungs.

The normal range of Pao_2 is 11.3–14 kPa (80–100 mmHg). A low Pao_2 is called arterial hypoxaemia and is the result of one of five broad mechanisms (**Table 2.24**). In practice, ventilation-perfusion mismatch is the dominant mechanism for most lung diseases.

> Blood gases are used to assess the severity of hypoxaemia, identify suspected hypercapnoea and assess acid-base imbalance. They provide diagnostic information (e.g. identifying type 2 respiratory failure) and are also valuable for assessing the severity of severe respiratory and systemic illnesses.

Mechanisms of arterial hypoxaemia*		
Broad mechanism	$P_{A-a}O_2$	Examples of causes
Reduced inspired Fio_2	Normal	High altitude
Alveolar hypoventilation	Normal	Sedative drugs
Impaired oxygen diffusion across alveoli	Increased	Interstitial lung disease
		Pneumocystis pneumonia
		Oedema
Ventilation–perfusion mismatch	Increased	Asthma
		COPD
		Most other lung diseases
Right-to-left shunts[†]	Increased	Pulmonary arteriovenous malformations
		Congenital cardiac diseases
		Lobar pneumonia

$P_{A-a}O_2$, alveolar–arterial oxygen partial pressure gradient; Pao_2, arterial partial pressure of oxygen; Fio_2, fractional concentration of oxygen in inspired air.

*Low Pao_2.

[†]Corrects poorly with oxygen therapy.

Table 2.24 Mechanisms causing arterial hypoxaemia

An accurate interpretation of a blood gas result requires knowing the F_{IO_2}, the percentage of oxygen in the air the patient is breathing. The F_{IO_2} is 21% (0.21) in air but with supplemental oxygen can increase to over 60%.

An important concept is the alveolar arterial oxygen gradient; this is a measure of the difference between the partial pressure of oxygen in the alveoli (P_{AO_2}) and the P_{aO_2}. A large difference occurs if the patient has a high F_{IO_2} but a low P_{aO_2}, which suggests a major problem with pulmonary gas exchange.

P_{IO_2} is the partial pressure of inspired oxygen reaching the lungs. The oxygen content of air (F_{IO_2}) is 21%, but when air enters the upper airway it becomes humidified and more saturated with water the further it moves down the trachea. This will dilute the proportion of oxygen in inspired air, and the P_{IO_2} is calculated using a dilution factor of 0.95 as follows:

$$P_{IO_2} = F_{IO_2} \times PB \times 0.95$$
$$= 0.21 \times 101.3 \times 0.95$$
$$= 20\,kPa$$

In this equation, PB is barometric pressure (101.3 kPa at sea level).

The partial pressure of oxygen in alveolar gas is P_{AO_2}, and the partial pressure of carbon dioxide in alveolar gas is P_{ACO_2}. The P_{AO_2} is calculated using the alveolar gas equation:

$$P_{AO_2} = P_{IO_2} - \left(\frac{P_{aCO_2}}{R}\right)$$

In this equation, R is the respiratory quotient (0.8) which is used to adjust the P_{aCO_2} (the arterial value) to provide an estimate of P_{ACO_2} (the alveolar value).

The alveolar–arterial partial pressure gradient ($P_{A-a}O_2$) is the difference between the P_{AO_2} and the P_{aO_2} (measured using arterial blood gas analysis). The following equation is used to calculate the $P_{A-a}O_2$:

$$P_{A-a}O_2 = P_{IO_2} - \left(\frac{P_{aCO_2}}{0.8}\right) - P_{aO_2}$$

The units in this calculation are kPa or mmHg (1 kPa = 7.5 mmHg).

For example, to calculate $P_{A-a}O_2$ for a patient breathing air with a P_{aO_2} of 6 kPa and a P_{aCO_2} of 4 kPa:

$$P_{A-a}O_2 = 20 - \left(\frac{4}{0.8}\right) - 6$$
$$= 9\,kPa$$

The normal alveolar–arterial partial pressure gradient is about 1 kPa, but it increases with age to about 3 kPa. The $P_{A-a}O_2$ is less accurate at high F_{IO_2}.

■ Hypoxaemia with a high $P_{A-a}O_2$ suggests problems with gas exchange or oxygen transfer: alveolar membrane disorders, interstitial lung diseases or ventilation–perfusion mismatch
■ Hypoxaemia with a normal $P_{A-a}O_2$ suggests hypoventilation

Respiratory failure is defined as P_{aO_2} < 8.0 kPa. Type 1 respiratory failure has a normal or low P_{aCO_2}, type 2 a high P_{aCO_2}. The causes of type 1 and 2 respiratory failure are listed in **Table 2.25**.

Carbon dioxide

The transport of carbon dioxide in the blood occurs in three ways: as dissolved gas (P_{aCO_2}), after chemical conversion to bicarbonate, or combined with haemoglobin (**Figure 1.26**). P_{aCO_2} is measured by arterial blood gas analysis. Finger probes that measure P_{aCO_2} are available but expensive and not very accurate; they are mainly used for continuous monitoring of P_{aCO_2} in sleep studies and in intensive care.

The normal range of P_{aCO_2} is 4.7–6.0 kPa (34–45 mmHg). Increased P_{aCO_2} is called hypercapnoea and occurs when reduced ventilation of the lung prevents adequate excretion of blood carbon dioxide.

Oxygen saturation

Most oxygen is transported in the blood bound to haemoglobin. Haemoglobin that is not associated with oxygen has a characteristic blue tinge, which is why patients with low P_{aO_2} have central cyanosis.

The proportion of haemoglobin that is bound to oxygen (the oxygen saturation) depends on P_{aO_2} (Figure 1.29) and can be measured by finger probes called oxygen saturation monitors. These devices are portable and give an instant result, providing a practical way to rapidly assess whether a patient has hypoxaemia.

Oxygen saturation is normally over 94%; a value of 93% suggests that the patient is hypoxic. A steep fall in haemoglobin oxygen saturation occurs with lower P_{aO_2}. When oxygen

Causes of respiratory failure	
Type	Causes
Type 1	Alveolar infiltrates:
	Pneumonia
	Pulmonary oedema
	Acute respiratory distress syndrome
	Interstitial lung diseases:
	Pulmonary fibrosis
	Sarcoidosis
	Airways disease:
	Some COPD patients ('pink puffers', Figure 3.10)
	Moderately severe asthma
	Pulmonary vascular disease:
	Pulmonary embolism
	Pulmonary hypertension
	Right-to-left shunts
Type 2	Central hypoventilation:
	Sedative drugs
	Brain diseases
	Obesity hypoventilation syndrome
	Respiratory neuromuscular dysfunction:
	Guillain–Barré syndrome
	Phrenic nerve palsies
	Cervical cord damage
	Motor neurone disease
	Muscular dystrophies and post-polio
	Chest wall disorders:
	Previous thoracoplasty
	Obesity
	Severe pleural disease
	Kyphoscoliosis
	Ankylosing spondylitis
	Airways disease:
	Some COPD patients ('blue bloaters', Figure 3.10)
	Severe asthma
	Large airways obstruction
	Obstructive sleep apnoea
	End stage of the causes of chronic type 1 respiratory failure

COPD, chronic obstructive pulmonary disease.

Table 2.25 Causes of type 1 and type 2 respiratory failure

saturation decreases to <90%, it often fluctuates rapidly over a range of 3–4%.

Oxygen saturation probes are placed over finger- or toenails. They provide inaccurate readings if the patient has nail varnish on or has poor peripheral perfusion.

Acid–base balance

Analysis of arterial or venous blood gases is also used to assess the acid–base balance by measuring $Paco_2$, pH, bicarbonate concentration, base excess (a measure of excess acid or base present) and sometimes lactate concentration.

Acid–base disorders are divided into respiratory and metabolic causes, and into acidosis (reduced pH) or alkalosis (increased pH). They can be uncompensated, partially compensated or totally compensated. The patterns and causes of acid–base disorders are summarised in **Table 2.26**.

Respiratory acidosis

This type of acid–base disorder is caused by an increased $Paco_2$ resulting from under-ventilation, therefore it occurs in type 2 respiratory failure. Respiratory acidosis is the most serious respiratory acid–base disorder. Acute respiratory acidosis causes a low pH, a high $Paco_2$ and an increase in bicarbonate of <1 mmol for each 0.1 decrease in pH. Metabolic compensation of the acidosis increases the bicarbonate (>1 mmol for each 0.1 decrease in pH) resulting in a base excess >2 mmol/L with a less acidotic pH.

Respiratory alkalosis

Hyperventilation results in the acid–base disorder called respiratory alkalosis. It does so by causing $Paco_2$ and bicarbonate to decrease and pH to increase.

Metabolic acidosis

When the body produces excess acid, this causes a decrease in pH, a negative base excess, and a low bicarbonate concentration. The resulting metabolic acidosis stimulates a compensatory hyperventilation that increases

Acid–base imbalances and causes		
Imbalance	Findings	Cause
Respiratory acidosis	Low pH High P_{ACO_2} High HCO_3^- (if compensated) Positive base excess (if compensated)	Type 2 respiratory failure (see Table 2.24)
Respiratory alkalosis	High pH Low P_{ACO_2} Low HCO_3^- Normal base excess	Hyperventilation Type 1 respiratory failure Excessive mechanical ventilation Increased respiratory rate caused by brain injury, shock, sepsis or aspirin overdose
Metabolic acidosis	Low pH Normal or low P_{ACO_2} Low HCO_3^- Negative base excess	Lactic acidosis resulting from shock, excessive exercise, convulsions or hypoxia Ketoacidosis Renal failure Excess bicarbonate loss (e.g. because of renal tubule defects or diarrhoea*)
Metabolic alkalosis	High pH Normal or slightly high P_{ACO_2} High HCO_3^- Positive base excess	Excess loss of stomach secretions (e.g. because of vomiting or nasogastric suction) Bicarbonate retention caused by diuretics

*Normal anion gap. Serum $[Na^+] - [Cl^-] - [HCO_3^-]$; should be 8 – 16 mmol /L

Table 2.26 Patterns and causes of acid–base imbalance

pH by removing CO_2 (and therefore HCO_3^-). This is sometimes mistaken for a primary lung problem.

Metabolic alkalosis

Rarely relevant for respiratory diseases, metabolic alkalosis leads to a high pH, a high bicarbonate concentration and a positive base excess. The patient may have a degree of hypoventilation to compensate for the increase in pH.

Mixed acid–base disorders

Mixed acid–base disorders are common. For example, patients with severe exacerbations of COPD commonly have a respiratory acidosis as a result of type 2 respiratory failure and a degree of metabolic acidosis caused by tissue hypoxaemia and low blood pressure.

Blood tests

The results of blood tests are rarely diagnostic for respiratory diseases. However, they provide information that can increase the likelihood of some respiratory diseases or help exclude a particular diagnosis. Blood tests that are frequently requested in patients presenting with acute or chronic lung disease include:

- full blood count
- urea and electrolytes, glucose, calcium and liver function tests
- inflammatory markers (CRP and ESR)
- blood tests for specific inflammatory, autoimmune and infectious diseases
- blood tests of cardiac and pulmonary circulation function

Full blood count

This blood test is essential for patients presenting with chronic dyspnoea to exclude anaemia as a cause. In addition, anaemia and thrombocythaemia (a high platelet count) sometimes indicate chronic inflammatory or neoplastic disease. An increased white cell count with neutrophilia suggests infection.

Eosinophilia is common in allergic disease (e.g. asthma and ABPA) and vasculitis.

Urea and electrolytes, glucose, calcium and liver function tests

Renal failure, liver disease, diabetes, bone disease, hypercalcaemia and hyponatraemia are all causes or complications of lung disease.

Inflammatory markers

The inflammatory markers C-reactive protein and erythrocyte sedimentation rate are useful markers of systemic inflammation. If their values are significantly increased, an explanation must be found. Both are increased by infectious, inflammatory and neoplastic diseases. For infections and inflammatory diseases, they are used to monitor the patient's response to treatment.

Blood tests for specific inflammatory, autoimmune and infectious diseases

A wide range of blood tests are available that, if positive, suggest that the patient has a specific inflammatory disease (Table 2.27) or infection (**Table 2.28**).

Blood tests of cardiac and pulmonary circulation function

Cardiac failure increases B-type natriuretic peptide concentration. Troponin T is increased by ischaemic heart disease but also during an acute pulmonary embolism. D-dimer is raised in pulmonary embolism but the test is non-specific; D-dimer is increased in almost any inflammatory condition.

Sputum tests

The collection of sputum samples provides material from the lower respiratory tract without invasive testing, and sputum tests can be diagnostic. The main problem is ensuring that an adequate non-salivary sample is obtained; the first sputum produced in the morning is usually the best quality sample. Inhalation of nebulised normal or hypertonic saline is sometimes used to induce sputum in patients with suspected infections who are otherwise unable to provide a sample. Sputum can be sent for cytology, microscopy and culture.

Sputum cytology

Cytological examination of the sputum occasionally identifies malignant cells in

Blood tests for inflammatory and autoimmune lung diseases	
Blood test	Associated inflammatory or autoimmune disease(s)
Serum angiotensin-converting enzyme	Increased in sarcoidosis (but non-specific)
Rheumatoid factor	Positive in rheumatoid arthritis
Autoantibody screen	Antinuclear antibody, anti-Jo-1 and other antibodies positive in autoimmune diseases causing interstitial lung disease
Avian precipitins	Positive in bird fancier's lung (a hypersensitivity pneumonitis)
Total IgG	Low in immunodeficiency
	Often polyclonal increases in inflammatory diseases
	Monoclonal increase in multiple myeloma
Total IgE	Mildly increased in asthma and allergic disease (up to 500 iu/L)
	Very high in ABPA (> 500 iu/L)
ANCA	Positive in vasculitis
ANCA, anti–neutrophil cytoplasmic antibody; Ig, immunoglobulin.	

Table 2.27 Blood tests for common inflammatory and autoimmune diseases of the lungs

Blood tests for infectious diseases	
Blood test	Function
Interferon-Y release assay	Latent tuberculosis infection (does not distinguish latent from active disease)
Serology for *Mycoplasma pneumoniae*	*M. pneumoniae* as potential cause of acute lung infection
Serology for *Chlamydophila pneumoniae*	*C. pneumoniae* as potential cause of acute lung infection
Serology for respiratory viruses	Potential viral cause of acute lung infection
HIV tests (serology, CD4 count and viral load)	HIV-positive patients and severity of their immunosuppression
CMV tests (serology and viral load)	Risk of CMV reactivation if immunocompromised and viral load once CMV infection is reactivated
Serology for parasites	Previous exposure to parasites (e.g. hydatid)
Serology for endemic fungi	Previous exposure to geographically restricted fungal pathogens (e.g. *Histoplasma*)
Serology for *Bordetella pertussis*	Recent whooping cough infection
CMV, cytomegalovirus.	

Table 2.28 Examples of blood tests for specific infectious diseases

patients with lung cancer, sputum eosinophilia in some patients with asthma, and *Aspergillus* in patients with allergic bronchopulmonary aspergillosis. Cytological examination of induced sputum is used in immunocompromised patients to identify *Pneumocystis* infection. The presence of haemosiderin-containing macrophages suggests pulmonary haemorrhage.

Sputum microscopy and culture

In patients with suspected lung infection, the sputum is used for microscopy and culture to identify bacteria, mycobacteria and fungi; it is not a good source for viral cultures. The standard test for pulmonary tuberculosis is microscopy with auramine or acid-fast staining and prolonged culture of three early morning sputum samples.

Pleural fluid

For patients with pleural effusions biochemical, cytological and microbiological testing of samples of pleural fluid are essential for identifying the cause (see Chapter 6).

Bronchoscopy

The tracheobronchial tree is directly accessed and visualised by bronchoscopy. In rigid bronchoscopy, a metal tube is passed through the vocal cords to reach the carina and proximal main bronchi. This procedure requires a general anaesthetic and is used for therapeutic bronchoscopic interventions and during thoracic surgery.

The majority of bronchoscopic procedures (95%) use flexible bronchoscopy, which requires only light sedation with topical anaesthesia. A fibre-optic bronchoscope is passed through the nose or mouth, past the vocal cords and into the trachea; it then easily reaches segmental bronchi. Bronchoscopy directly visualises bronchial lesions (e.g. tumours, bronchial stenosis, foreign bodies and sputum plugs) (**Figure 2.20**). A side channel allows suction of secretions and is used to obtain bronchial aspirates, bronchoalveolar lavage and bronchial brushings, as well as biopsies.

Bronchial aspirate

Small amounts of saline (5–20 mL) are injected down the bronchoscope and recovered by suction into a sterile sample tube to obtain a

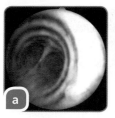 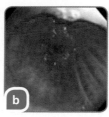 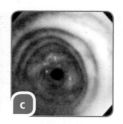

Figure 2.20 Bronchoscopy findings: (a) normal, (b) lung cancer and (c) tracheal stenosis.

sample of fluid from the bronchial tree. The fluid is sent for cytological and microbiological tests.

Bronchoalveolar lavage fluid

Samples from the alveoli are obtained by bronchoalveolar lavage. In this procedure, the end of the bronchoscope is wedged into a subsegmental bronchus and large volumes of saline are injected (100–200 mL). Suction is used to recover as much of the saline as possible into sterile sample tubes. The injected fluid reaches the alveoli, so bronchoalveolar lavage provides a sample of alveolar fluid for cytological investigation, a differential cell count to identify the relative proportions of different white cells (useful when investigating suspected interstitial lung disease) and microbiological tests.

Bronchial brushings

Visible bronchial abnormalities, especially suspected tumours, are sampled by rubbing with a bronchial brush. The material obtained this way is sent for cytological investigation.

Biopsies

Bronchoscopy is used during endobronchial, transbronchial and endobronchial ultrasound-guided biopsy procedures (see page 122). In the last of these, bronchoscopes fitted with bronchial ultrasound probes are used to visualise and biopsy peribronchial lesions, mainly mediastinal lymph nodes.

Indications for bronchoscopy

The main indications for bronchoscopy are as follows.

- A new lung shadow suspected to be a cancer
- Lobar collapse: to identify the cause and possibly treat the collapse by removing a foreign body or sputum plug
- Haemoptysis
- Suspected large airways obstruction
- Suspected interstitial lung disease (to obtain biopsies and a bronchoalveolar lavage cell differential)
- Difficult lung infection: examples are suspected tuberculosis without sputum production, pneumonia in the immunocompromised and lung abscess (to exclude proximal bronchial obstruction)
- Chronic cough (rarely)

Complications of bronchoscopy

Complications of bronchoscopy include:

- over-sedation
- increased hypoxia (especially after bronchoalveolar lavage)
- mild self-limiting pyrexia (after bronchoalveolar lavage)
- bleeding, mainly from biopsy sites, with post-procedure haemoptysis
- cough during and shortly after the procedure
- sore throat and hoarse voice

Allergen tests

Skin tests are used to identify allergies to specific allergens, such as house dust mite faeces, pollen, fungal spores and animal dander. The results are often positive in atopic patients and patients with asthma. Patients with ABPA are usually skin prick test–positive for *Aspergillus*. More complex allergen testing is needed for patients with suspected occupational asthma (e.g. assessing lung function after pulmonary challenge with the suspected cause) (**Figure 2.21a** and **b**).

Blood tests are used to identify hypersensitivity pneumonitis, for example avian precipitins in patients with bird fancier's lung. *Aspergillus*-specific IgE and IgG tests are used to identify sensitisation to *Aspergillus* in cases of ABPA.

Sleep studies

Patients with a suspected sleep disorder require a sleep study (see chapter 5). The simplest sleep study is an overnight recording of oxygen saturation. Oxygen saturation is measured by using a recording saturation probe lent to the patient overnight.

A simple sleep study suffices to exclude significant obstructive sleep apnoea in many patients. However, more complex tests are necessary for some patients and include assessment of chest wall and abdominal movement, heart rate, degree of snoring, sleep status (awake, REM or non-REM sleep), $Paco_2$, respiratory rate, electromyogram, electroencephalogram and airflow.

Chest X-ray

The posteroanterior chest X-ray is the standard radiological test used to visualise the anatomy of the lungs and thoracic cavity. It is an essential part of the diagnostic work-up for most patients presenting with suspected respiratory disease, and for monitoring changes in the disease over time. Lung tissue is not very visible on chest X-ray, showing up as grey or black areas traversed by lines representing bronchial walls and blood vessels. As most diseases cause an increase in cellular material or fluid, they are visible as different patterns of white patches in the lungs (chest X-ray opacities).

To ensure that no abnormalities are missed, assess each chest X-ray systematically as follows.

1. Is the film of adequate quality? Are the whole lungs visible, including both costophrenic angles? Is the patient rotated to the film? The ends of the clavicle should be evenly distanced from the vertebral bodies; if they are not, then the patient may have been rotated, which makes the chest X-ray more difficult to interpret.
2. Are the ribs normal, or are there fractures, lucencies or areas of increased density? Are the vertebrae straight, or is there a kyphosis or scoliosis? Do the ribs have the normal angle to the vertebrae?
3. Do the heart and mediastinum have a normal outline and size? Are mediastinal nodes present, and is there any density behind the left heart?
4. Is there evidence of changes in lung size? Is the trachea central? Is the horizontal fissure visible and in the correct place (horizontally at the level of the upper right hilum)? Are the diaphragms at the correct height, with the right diaphragm up to 2 cm higher than the left (because of the liver)?
5. Is there loss of the costophrenic angle, or evidence of pleural thickening or plaques?

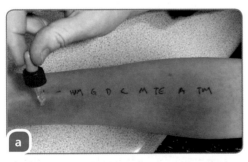

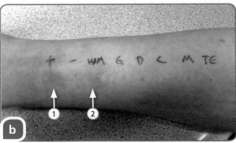

Figure 2.21 (a) Skin prick testing (b) and the results. +, positive control, −, negative control, letters represent different antigens (e.g. WM, house dust mite) (1) Reaction to positive control. (2) Reaction to house dust mite.

Does the diaphragm have its usual smooth curvature?

6. Are the lung zones normal? Each side should be compared with the other, looking at specifically at the apices, then the midzones and then the lower zones.

The structures visible on a normal chest X-ray are shown in **Figure 2.22**. The common potential abnormalities affecting the lungs, mediastinum and pleurae are:

- air space shadowing
- lobar collapse and atelectasis
- nodules and masses
- micronodules
- increased translucency
- diffuse lung diseases
- airways disease
- pleural abnormalities
- hilar abnormalities
- mediastinal abnormalities
- a so called 'white-out'

Air space shadowing

White or grey patches that obscure the underlying vascular markings represent parts of the lung where the alveoli have been filled with fluid or cellular material, and is called airspace shadowing or (when dense) consolidation. Their causes are listed in **Table 2.29**. Consolidation of an entire lobe or segment is called lobar consolidation (**Figure 2.23**).

Lobar collapse and atelectasis

Lobar collapse results in a shrunken white density representing the affected lobe, with volume loss on that side. Collapse of each lobe has a specific pattern (**Figure 2.24**). Small areas of collapsed alveoli only affecting part of a segment are called atelectasis and cause short lines of increased density on a chest X-ray.

Nodules and masses

Nodules and masses are visible as white opacities that are often roughly round. Common causes are listed in **Table 2.30**. Lung masses have a diameter > 3 cm; they are usually single.

Smaller opacities are called nodules and are often multiple.

Lung cancer must be considered if a chest X-ray shows a single large mass or nodule. Consider lung metastases if multiple nodules are present. Important considerations are:

- Has the mass or nodule increased in size since the last chest X-ray? A new or growing mass means that there is an active process that requires rapid investigation; if the patient has a large mass, is a smoker or has a history of extrathoracic malignancy then cancer is likely.
- Is there cavitation? Cavitation occurs when central necrosis of the lesion creates an air-filled cavity (**Figure 2.25**). Cavities that contain fluid have an air–fluid level: a straight line in the mass with opacity below and translucency above (**Figure 2.26**).
- What does the edge of the lesion look like? Smooth, defined edges are more likely to be caused by a benign process than indistinct edges or edges with short lines extending into surrounding lung (spiculation).
- What is the density? Very dense patches similar in density to bone represent calcification; this process occurs mainly during healing from an inflammatory process such as tuberculosis, which suggests a benign process is causing the shadow.
- Does the mass join with or erode into adjacent structures? For example, a lung tumour can invade the chest wall and destroy the adjacent rib (**Figure 2.25**).

Overlying skin or chest wall lesions can resemble a lung nodule on chest X-ray. For example, a lower zone mid-clavicular line shadow may be a nipple shadow.

Micronodules

Very small nodules (< 5 mm) are usually widespread through both lungs. They are more commonly caused by a diffuse process than by malignancy (**Figure 2.27**). The common causes are listed in **Table 2.31**. The speed of change over time is a key factor in identifying the potential cause; rapid changes occur in serious diseases and the cause must be identified immediately.

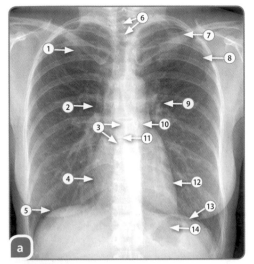

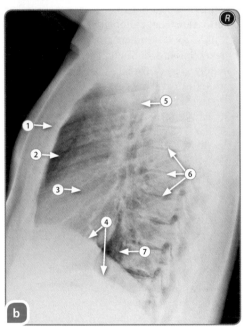

Figure 2.22 (a) Posteroanterior chest X-ray showing visible normal anatomical structures. ①, Anterior end of the right first rib. Count down from here to assess expansion of the chest. The diaphragm is crossed by the 5th and 7th ribs. ②, Right hilar point, formed by the meeting of the horizontal fissure and vessels from the upper and lower zones. ③, Pedicles of thoracic spine. ④, Right heart border, formed mainly from the border of the right atrium. ⑤, Dome of the right hemidiaphragm, crossed by the anterior end of the right 6th rib. ⑥, Spinous processes of the thoracic spine seen through the lucency of the trachea. ⑦, Left clavicle. ⑧, Border of the left scapula. ⑨, Left hilar point, slightly higher than the right and formed by the crossing of vessels from the upper and lower zones. ⑩, Edge of descending thoracic aorta. ⑪, Disc space of thoracic spine, which should be just visible on well-exposed film. ⑫, Left heart border, formed by the edge of the left and right ventricles. ⑬, Dome of the left hemidiaphragm, usually slightly lower than the right. ⑭, Gas in stomach lumen.
(b) Lateral chest X-ray. ①, Sternum. ②, Restrosternal space, hidden on a posteroanterior chest X-ray. ③, Heart. ④, Right and left hemidiaphragms. The stomach is below the left hemidiaphragm, which merges with the heart border. The right hemidiaphragm is usually higher than the left. ⑤, Lucency of the trachea. ⑥, Intervertebral thoracic disc spaces. The spine should appear gradually more lucent from the top down to the bottom because less tissue overlies the lower parts. ⑦, Retrocardiac space, hidden on posteroanterior chest X-ray.

Increased translucency

Increased translucency (blacker than usual parts of the lung) represents areas containing air or with reduced or absent tissue structures. Such areas are found in the:

- pleural space (pneumothorax, **Figure 2.28a**)
- muscles (subcutaneous emphysema, **Figure 2.28b**)
- mediastinum
- oesophagus (e.g. hiatus hernia and achalasia)

- diffusely throughout the lung(s), e.g. COPD and emphysema, or compensatory hyperinflation for lung collapse
- localised in a lung cavity, cyst or bullae
- under the diaphragm due to air in the peritoneum (e.g. due to a perforated ulcer) (**Figure 2.28c**)

Differences in chest wall density also affect the radiolucency of the underlying lung. For example, a previous mastectomy makes the lung look blacker on one side (**Figure 2.28d**).

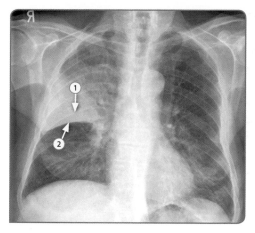

Figure 2.23 Chest X-ray showing lobar consolidation of the right upper lobe: ①, alveolar shadowing, and ②, bounded inferiorly by the horizontal fissure.

Diffuse lung diseases

Extensive diffuse lung shadowing has multiple causes and is difficult to define accurately using a chest X-ray. In the absence of an obvious clinical cause, a CT scan is necessary to define the anatomical pattern accurately. Diffuse lung shadowing can be described as:

■ reticular (multiple short irregular linear densities, often overlapping)

■ micronodular
■ reticulonodular (combinations of reticular and nodular shadowing)
■ ground glass shadowing (a generalised increase in density with still visible underlying vascular markings)

The distribution (apical versus basal, medial versus lateral) and speed of onset are important clues to the diagnosis. Causes are listed in **Table 2.30**.

Airways diseases

Tracheal narrowing is sometimes detected on chest X-ray. COPD, bronchitis and bronchiectasis all cause bronchial wall thickening, which produces parallel linear opacities arising from the hilar and a general increase in bronchial markings on chest X-ray. Dilated, thick-walled bronchi as a result of bronchiectasis can cause ring shadows (when seen end on) and tramline shadows (when seen side-on) (**Figure 2.29** and 9.3).

Pleural abnormalities

Pneumothoraces cause a contiguous area of radiolucency with no vascular markings between the lung and the chest wall. A pleural line should be visible (**Figure 2.28a**); a small

Causes of air space shadowing	
Cause(s)	Appearance on chest X-ray or CT scan
Common	
Pneumonia	Lobar: asymmetrical in a segmental or lobar distribution
	Bronchopneumonia: widespread small patches
Pulmonary embolism with pulmonary infarct	Wedge-shaped and peripheral
Pulmonary oedema	Bilateral, extensive, symmetrical ('bat's wing'), with upper lobe blood diversion and Kerley B lines*
Acute respiratory distress syndrome	Bilateral, extensive and symmetrical
Rarer	
Organising pneumonias	Bilateral and patchy peripheral
Pulmonary eosinophilia	Bilateral and patchy peripheral ('reverse bat's wing')
Alveolar cell carcinoma	Slowly progressive and asymmetrical
Lymphoma	
Pulmonary haemorrhage	
*Short horizontal linear opacities arising close to the pleurae basally.	

Table 2.29 Causes of air space shadowing on chest X-ray or CT scan

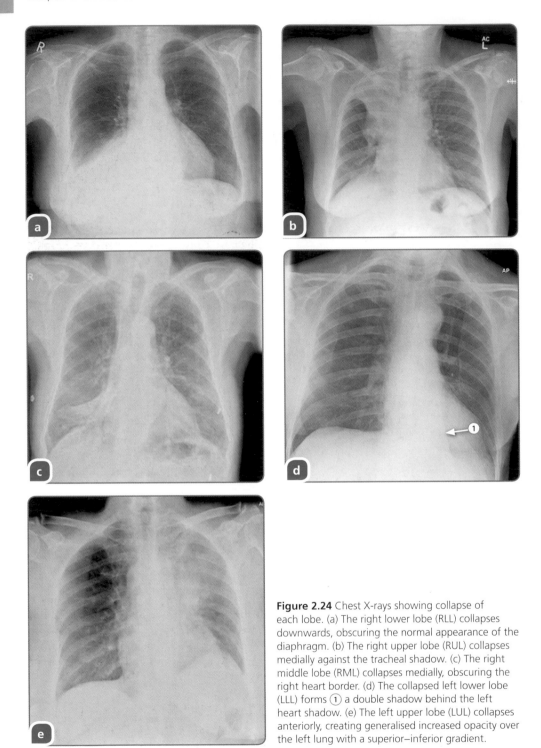

Figure 2.24 Chest X-rays showing collapse of each lobe. (a) The right lower lobe (RLL) collapses downwards, obscuring the normal appearance of the diaphragm. (b) The right upper lobe (RUL) collapses medially against the tracheal shadow. (c) The right middle lobe (RML) collapses medially, obscuring the right heart border. (d) The collapsed left lower lobe (LLL) forms ① a double shadow behind the left heart shadow. (e) The left upper lobe (LUL) collapses anteriorly, creating generalised increased opacity over the left lung with a superior–inferior gradient.

Causes of lung masses and nodules

No. of lung masses or nodules	Causes
Single or limited	Tumours:
	Lung cancer*
	Rarer lung tumours (carcinoid or hamartomas)
	Lung metastases
	Lymphoma
	Infective:
	Active tuberculosis*
	Previous tuberculosis (tuberculoma)
	Lung abscess*
	Aspergilloma (in a cavity with an air crescent)
	Fungal or parasitic infection*
	Other:
	Pulmonary infarcts (pulmonary embolism)*
	Enfolded lung (Blesovsky's syndrome)
	Pulmonary sequestration
	Rheumatoid nodules*
	Vasculitis*
	Encysted pleural fluid
Multiple	Tumours:
	Lung metastases
	Lymphoma
	Infective:
	Metastatic infection*
	Fungal or parasitic infection*
	Other:
	Rheumatoid nodules*
	Vasculitis*
	Arteriovenous malformations

*Frequently cavitate.

Table 2.30 Causes of lung masses and nodules on chest X-ray or CT scan

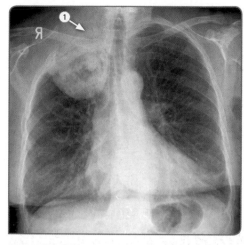

Figure 2.25 Chest X-ray of a right apical cavitating lung lesion with ① associated rib erosion: Pancoast's tumour.

pneumothorax is only visible at the apex of the lung. In contrast, pleural fluid causes a dense peripheral opacity that is basal, forming a curved meniscus unless there is loculation of the pleural space. Pleural thickening can be patchy and associated with calcification; the costophrenic angle may be blunted, with a squared-off appearance

Hilar abnormalities

Enlargement or focal lesions of the hilar occurs with pulmonary hypertension (most commonly secondary to COPD), hilar lymph node enlargement and tumours. The causes of enlarged hilar and mediastinal lymph nodes are:

- lung cancer
- extrathoracic tumour metastases
- sarcoidosis
- tuberculosis
- lymphoma

In pulmonary hypertension, blood vessels can usually be traced back to the enlarged vessel, whereas enlarged nodes or tumours have a lobulated appearance with defined lateral and inferior borders. A CT scan is often necessary to define suspected hilar abnormalities.

Mediastinal abnormalities

The mediastinal contours are abnormal if there are enlarged mediastinal nodes, aortic aneurysms and mediastinal tumours (**Figures 2.30** and **31**). However, even substantially enlarged mediastinal lymph nodes often

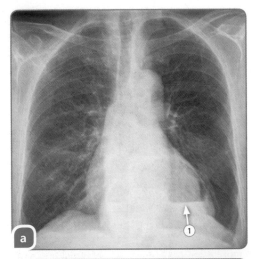

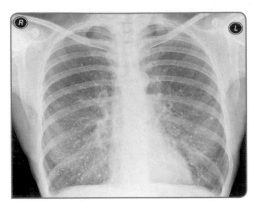

Figure 2.27 Chest X-ray showing a micronodular infiltrate, in this case caused by previous chickenpox pneumonia.

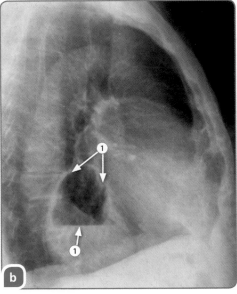

Figure 2.26 Chest X-rays showing an air–fluid level ① caused by a hiatus hernia. (a) Posteroanterior view showing the hiatus hernia as a retrocardiac opacity. (b) Lateral view showing ① the hiatus hernia in the middle mediastinum.

Causes of diffuse lung disease on chest X-ray	
Category	Disease
Interstitial lung disease and similar diseases	Sarcoidosis
	Pulmonary fibrosis
	Drug reactions
	Hypersensitivity pneumonitis
	Rare interstitial lung diseases
Pneumoconiosis	Asbestosis
	Berylliosis
	Silicosis
Malignancy	Extensive metastases (e.g. adenocarcinoma)
	Lymphangitis carcinomatosis
Infective	Miliary tuberculosis
	Pneumocystis
	Active viral lung infections
	Previous varicella pneumonia

Table 2.31 Causes of diffuse or micronodular lung disease on chest X-ray

remain undetected on chest X-ray. Again, CT is necessary if a mediastinal abnormality is suspected. Common causes of mediastinal masses are:

- enlarged mediastinal lymph nodes
- aortic aneurysms
- hiatus hernias
- thymomas and lymphomas
- retrosternal thyroid goitres (**Figure 2.32**)
- oesophageal lesions (e.g. tumours and pouches)
- teratomas and germ cell tumours
- paravertebral lesions (e.g. abscess and tuberculosis)
- neurogenic tumours
- congenital cysts

Pneumomediastinum is identified by lines of increased translucency between the lungs and the mediastinum and within mediastinal structures.

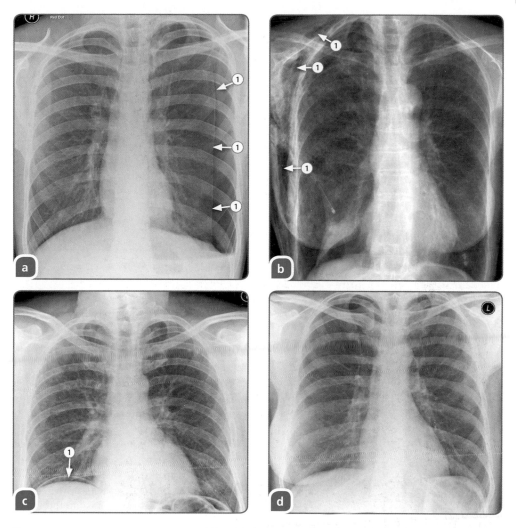

Figure 2.28 Chest X-rays showing different causes of increased translucency. (a) Pneumothorax ① Pleural line. (b) ① Subcutaneous emphysema. (c) ① Air under the diaphragm. (d) Previous left mastectomy.

'White out'

Complete white-out of a hemithorax has a limited number of causes.

- If the trachea is central, the causes include extensive unilateral or bilateral consolidation (**Figure 2.33a**) or air space shadowing, e.g. acute respiratory distress syndrome (**Figure 2.33b**), pleural mass (e.g. mesothelioma) and chest wall mass (e.g. Ewing's sarcoma)
- If the trachea is pulled towards the side of the opacification, the causes include pneumonectomy (**Figure 2.33c**) and total lung collapse

- If the trachea is pushed away from the side of opacification, the causes include pleural effusion (**Figure 2.33d**) and diaphragmatic hernia

A lateral chest X-ray (e.g. **Figure 2.26b**) helps when locating the exact position within the lungs of an abnormality detected on the posteroanterior film. Patients who are acutely ill may be unable to have a posteroanterior chest X-ray so instead have an anteroposterior chest X-ray. However, the anteroposterior view artificially enlarges the cardiac shadow and reduces the quality of the film.

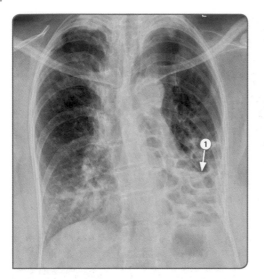

Figure 2.29 Plain chest X-ray of a patient with saccular bronchiectasis mainly affecting the left lower lobe. ① Ring shadows due to thin walled cysts. Some with fluid level representing dilated bronchi some with visible fluid levels due to mucous secretions.

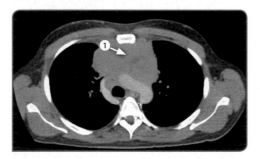

Figure 2.30 CT scan showing an anterior mediastinal mass ① due to lymphoma.

If the chest X-ray looks normal, check specifically for the following.

- Small apical pneumothorax
- An apical opacity produced by a Pancoast's tumour or pleural thickening from previous tuberculosis ('apical capping')
- Tracheal narrowing
- Absent breast shadowing
- Rib or vertebral fractures, sclerosis or erosions
- Air under the diaphragm as a result of perforation (**Figure 2.28c**)
- Density behind the heart (a left lower collapse or tumour)
- A central density with a fluid level behind the heart caused by a hiatus hernia (**Figure 2.26**)

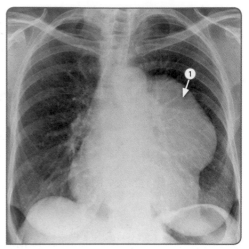

Figure 2.31 Chest X-ray showing a massive mediastinal mass ① due to a thymoma.

Computerised tomography

The chest X-ray remains the mainstay of lung radiology. However, it is a two-dimensional representation of thoracic anatomy and does not accurately define many lesions. CT scans of the thorax provide a three-dimensional assessment of the thoracic and lung anatomy, as well as much more detailed images of lung abnormalities. Consequently, CT is frequently used in the further investigation of the more severe lung diseases.

The density of CT images is altered to assess different anatomical areas. For CT scans of the thorax, the three main settings used assess the lungs, the soft tissues (mediastinum and pleura) and the bones. In addition scans vary in the depth of lung tissue displayed:

- Thin section CT scans show 1- to 2-mm transverse sections of lungs every 5–10 mm, providing detailed images of lung structure when investigating for interstitial lung disease or bronchiectasis
- Thicker sections are necessary to ensure that the whole lung is visualised during assessment for malignant disease

Intravenous contrast injections are required to separate vascular structures from mediastinal masses. Examples of the normal appearance of the thorax on CT are shown in **Figure 2.34**.

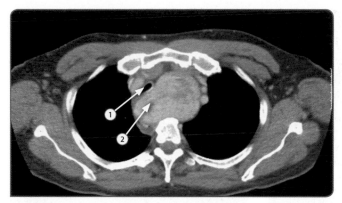

Figure 2.32 CT scan showing ① the trachea is displaced and compressed due to ② a superior mediastinal mass which is causing large airway obstruction.

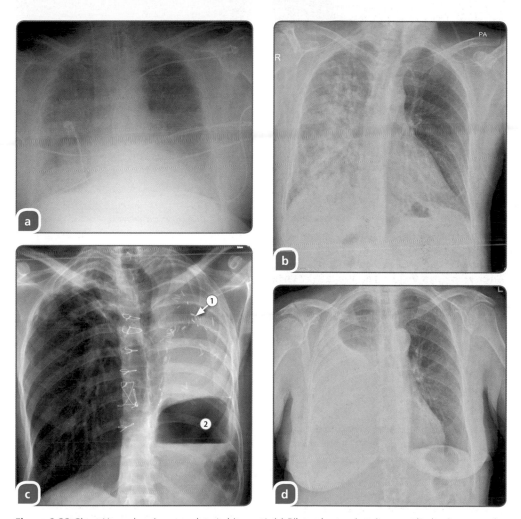

Figure 2.33 Chest X-ray showing complete 'white-out'. (a) Bilateral extensive air space shadowing caused by acute respiratory distress syndrome. (b) Extensive right-sided unilateral air space shadowing caused by consolidation (in this case, resulting from aspiration). (c) Left pneumonectomy: similar to total lung collapse, with mediastinal shift and raised left hemidiaphragm (identified by the high position of the gastric bubble ②)), but also with surgical clips ① visible in the left hemithorax. (d) Large right effusion: dense shadowing with a clear upper meniscus marking the top of the effusion.

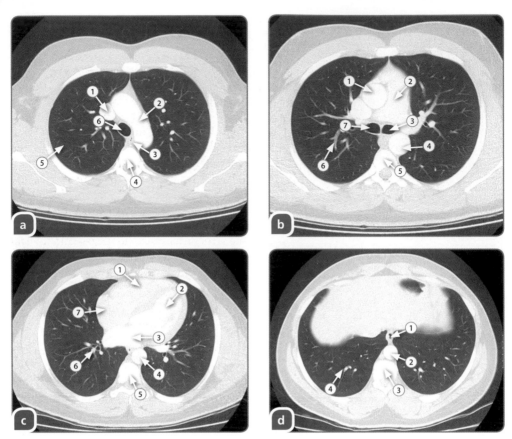

Figure 2.34 Normal appearance of the thorax on computerised tomography. (a) At the level of the of the arch of the aorta. ① Superior vena cava. ② Arch of the aorta. ③ Oesophagus. ④ Thoracic spine vertebra. ⑤ Lung parenchyma. ⑥ Trachea. (b) At the level of the carina. ① Ascending aorta. ② Pulmonary trunk. ③ Left main bronchus. ④ Descending aorta. ⑤ Thoracic spine vertebra. ⑥ Normal blood vessels. ⑦ Right main bronchus. (c) At the level of the heart. ① Right ventricle. ② Left ventricle. ③ Left atrium. ④ Descending aorta. ⑤ Thoracic spine vertebra. ⑥ Pulmonary blood vessels. ⑦ Right atrium. (d) At the level of the diaphragm. ① Oesophagus. ② Descending aorta. ③ Thoracic spine vertebra. ④ Pulmonary blood vessels.

Common indications

Computerised tomography is used in the following cases.

- Possible lung tumours: to define the anatomical site; identify pleural, chest wall or mediastinal invasion; and look for metastases (to the mediastinal, cervical or axillary nodes; lungs; liver; adrenal gland; thoracic spine; or ribs)
- Diffuse lung disease: CT appearances suggest the cause of an interstitial lung disease (see Chapter 4)
- Potential mediastinal, hilar and pleural abnormalities

- Lobar collapse or cavitating lung lesions
- Haemoptysis
- Suspected pulmonary embolism: a computerised tomography pulmonary angiogram (CTPA) is used (**Figure 2.35**); in CTPA, a large bolus of intravenous contrast is injected to identify opacities (clots) in pulmonary arteries
- Suspected bronchiectasis
- Suspected emphysema or bullae in patients with COPD
- Screening for lung metastases in patients with extrathoracic malignancies, or for lung cancer in high-risk patients

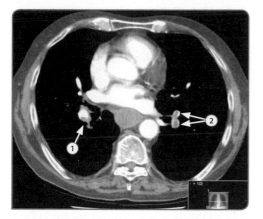

Figure 2.35 CT pulmonary angiogram showing large bilateral pulmonary emboli. ① Pulmonary embolus in right main pulmonary artery. ② Pulmonary emboli in left pulmonary arteries.

- Upper airways obstruction: sites are defined and potential causes identified
- Complex infection (e.g. pneumonia in the immunocompromised patient)

Disadvantages of computerised tomography

Computerised tomography has disadvantages: scans are very expensive, deliver a high dose of radiation and require a significant amount of time to complete. Furthermore, intravenous contrast can cause allergic reactions, nephrotoxicity and occasionally exacerbations of asthma; the use of contrast should generally be avoided in patients with unstable asthma or poor renal function.

The patient may not tolerate having a CT scan. They must be able to lie flat and hold their breath for the duration of the scan. This is only about 20 s with modern scanners but still too long for some patients with severe dyspnoea.

> **Some patients are unable to tolerate a CT scan because of severe claustrophobia.** Patients are more able to tolerate a scan if warned of these potential problems in advance.

Ultrasound

Ultrasound works best for identifying liquid or solid material, and so is not effective at assessing lung parenchyma, due to the air content. However, ultrasound is immensely helpful for assessing pleural effusions; it quantifies the amount of fluid present, identifies any loculations or pleural thickening, and guides safe pleural aspiration or pleural tube insertion. Ultrasound is used to assess potential phrenic nerve palsy by looking for movement of the diaphragm during sharp inspiration. Ultrasound is also used to assess the structure and guide biopsies of cervical or axillary lymph nodes and, via endobronchial ultrasound, mediastinal lymph nodes.

Magnetic resonance imaging

Magnetic resonance imaging scans provide poor assessments of the lung. However, they are useful for identifying the extent of tumour invasion of structures adjacent to the lung, such as major blood vessels, the chest wall and nerves. MRI is also used to assess pulmonary vascular abnormalities and pulmonary embolism.

Nuclear medicine scans

Nuclear medicine scans show the distribution pattern of a radionuclide tracer injected into patients. The nuclear medicine scans used in investigations of respiratory disease are:

- ventilation–perfusion scans (VQ scans)
- bone scans
- PET scans

Ventilation perfusion scans

Ventilation–perfusion scans are used mainly for the diagnosis of pulmonary emboli.

- Lung perfusion is shown by the pattern of distribution of injected technetium-99m–labelled macroaggregated albumin

- Lung ventilation is shown by the pattern of distribution of an inhaled radioactive gas (krypton-81 or xenon-133)

In a patient with a pulmonary embolus, the VQ scan shows areas of absent perfusion but with continued ventilation (mismatched defects). In chronic lung disease, the VQ scan shows matched defects in both perfusion and ventilation, which makes VQ scan assessment for a pulmonary embolus difficult. CTPA is generally used instead (**Figure 2.35**).

Bone scans

Bone scans are used to assess lung malignancies that may have spread to the bones. The patient is injected with technetium-99m–labelled diphosphonates, which concentrate in areas of bone metastases and are visible as hot spots.

Positron emission tomography

In the most common PET scan used in respiratory medicine, the patient is injected with radiolabelled glucose. The radiolabelled glucose concentrates at sites of high metabolic activity, such as malignancy and active infection or inflammation.

Because PET scans scan the whole body, they identify unsuspected metastases in either distal organs or mediastinal nodes in patients with lung cancer. Therefore PET is used before potentially curative therapy for lung cancer to ensure that the patient has localised disease.

Biopsy procedures

Histological confirmation of the diagnosis is essential for neoplastic disease. It is also used to confirm the diagnosis of some infiltrative, inflammatory and infectious diseases.

Focal lung disease is usually readily biopsied; the technique used depends on the anatomical location of the lesion. Diffuse lung disease cannot be biopsied using radiologically guided techniques, because of high complication rates and poor samples. Therefore

either a transbronchial biopsy, cryobiopsy or video-assisted thoracoscopic surgery biopsy is necessary.

Procedures to obtain biopsy material include:

- radiologically guided percutaneous lung biopsy
- extrathoracic radiologically guided biopsies
- biopsies during bronchoscopy
- surgical biopsies

Radiologically guided percutaneous lung biopsy

Focal abnormalities, including pleural, lung, chest wall and mediastinal lesions, can be biopsied under CT or ultrasound guidance. The main potential complications are haemorrhage or a pneumothorax.

In lung biopsy, the deeper the lesion to be biopsied, the greater the risk of a pneumothorax. The risk is also increased by underlying chronic lung disease. A pneumothorax in a patient with very poor lung function can cause respiratory failure and may be fatal. Therefore biopsy of deeper lesions is often contraindicated.

Extrathoracic radiologically guided biopsies

Extrathoracic involvement by a lung disease often provides the safest method to obtain a diagnostic biopsy. Examples include ultrasound-guided biopsy of cervical lymph node involvement in lung cancer, and skin biopsies of patients with cutaneous sarcoid.

Biopsies during bronchoscopy

Bronchoscopy allows direct access to the lower airways. Therefore endobronchial biopsies during bronchoscopy can be used to obtain material from the bronchial mucosa or endobronchial lesions (e.g. visible lung cancers).

Transbronchial biopsies are blind biopsies of distal airways, which can include lung interstitium, and are used in the investigation of diffuse lung disease. However, transbronchial biopsies are small and often not diagnostic, and the procedure can be complicated by pneumothorax. A newer technique called cryobiopsy may safely provide better samples than transbronchial biopsies.

Mediastinal lymph nodes can be visualised and biopsied using endobronchial ultrasound with excellent results. Endobronchial ultrasound-guided procedures can also be used to biopsy peribronchial masses.

Surgical biopsies

Enlarged mediastinal nodes or masses can be biopsied surgically through the suprasternal notch (mediastinoscopy) or a parasternal (mediastonotomy) approach. Pleural lesions can be biopsied using medical or surgical thorascopy, and lung lesions using video-assisted thoracoscopic surgery.

Surgical biopsies have a low but significant mortality and require a hospital stay of about 3 days. Therefore these procedures are reserved for when a histological diagnosis is essential and non-surgical biopsies are not possible.

Cardiac and pulmonary circulation tests

The differential diagnosis for many lung diseases is often heart disease, so tests of cardiac function are often required when investigating lung diseases. Cardiac tests are also needed to assess right heart circulation function in suspected cases of pulmonary vascular disease.

The most relevant tests are:

- electrocardiogram
- echocardiogram
- angiogram

Electrocardiogram

Electrocardiography provides evidence of left or right ventricular strain, ischaemic heart disease and pulmonary hypertension.

Echocardiogram

Echocardiography is used to identify valvular heart disease, left ventricular or diastolic impairment, right ventricular disease and pulmonary hypertension.

Echocardiograms are often unable to measure pulmonary artery pressure, because this requires Doppler assessment of regurgitant flow through the tricuspid valve. In addition, exacerbations of lung disease often cause temporary increases in pulmonary artery pressure that decrease when the patient recovers.

Angiogram

Coronary angiogram may be necessary to exclude coronary artery disease. Pulmonary angiogram is an important test for confirming pulmonary hypertension and identifying its cause. In patients with major haemoptysis, bronchial artery angiogram is used to identify bleeding points and to treat them by embolization.

Management options

Starter questions

Answers to the following questions are on page 140–141.

13. What are the common treatments used in respiratory medicine?
14. How should respiratory failure be treated?
15. What are the roles for surgery in respiratory disease?

The aims of therapeutic interventions for respiratory diseases are to:

■ alleviate symptoms
■ reverse or cure the respiratory condition
■ prevent progression
■ reduce mortality

Which of these aims is (or are) dominant depends on the disease process. For example, with infective disease cure and prevention of death are the main aims. In contrast, for most chronic lung diseases a cure is not possible, so the main aims are to minimise symptoms and preserve lung function, thereby delaying any associated disability and mortality. Therapeutic interventions include:

■ non-pharmacological interventions
■ pharmacological interventions
■ medical procedures
■ ventilatory support
■ surgical procedures

Patients usually require a mixed approach combining different therapeutic modalities. Of great importance is patient support and education, especially for patients with diseases for which no cure is possible. Patients who understand their condition are better able to cope with their illness as well as to manage their medication appropriately.

> **One of the major roles of a clinician is to explain disease and its prognosis to the patient**. Use terms that the average person readily understands and avoid medical jargon. Develop your own stock phrases to describe the common conditions; observe interactions between clinicians and patients to identify effective phrases.

Non-pharmacological interventions

Smoking cessation

Cigarette smoking is the leading cause of preventable mortality. It is responsible for nearly 6 million deaths annually worldwide. Smoking is extremely addictive. Most smokers want to stop smoking, but the long-term success rate of a single attempt to stop smoking without support is very low: 95% start smoking again within a year.

Helping a smoker stop smoking is one of the most cost-effective health interventions. Therefore physicians should have a good knowledge of the available smoking cessation interventions. The most effective strategy is a combination of behavioural (non-pharmacological) and pharmacological interventions.

Non-pharmacological interventions

Several approaches are used.

■ Identification of smokers is a prerequisite before smoking cessation interventions are used; any contact with health care services is an opportunity to identify smokers and educate them about the health benefits of quitting.
■ Behavioural interventions to address barriers to smoking cessation and help patients avoid triggers and remain motivated; options are one-to-one counselling, group therapy and support delivered by telephone or other media.
■ Alternative therapies such as hypnosis and acupuncture have been used but lack evidence for their efficacy.

Pharmacological

Various pharmacological treatments improve rates of smoking cessation. These include:

■ Nicotine replacement therapy to reduce the intensity of withdrawal symptoms (depression, difficulty sleeping, irritability, anxiety, poor concentration and restlessness) increases the chance of quitting by 1.5–2 times; the therapy is available without prescription and is available in a range of formats, including nicotine gum, lozenges, skin patches, nasal spray, electronic cigarettes and inhaler.
■ Bupropion acts on dopamine and noradrenaline (norepinephrine) pathways in the brain and increases the chance of quitting by 1.5–2 times when used for 7–12 weeks.
■ Varenicline is a partial agonist of the nicotinic acetylcholine receptor and improves the chance of quitting by

2–3 times; it is taken as a tablet twice a day for 12–24 weeks, but common adverse effects are nausea and odd dreams.

Active weight loss

Obesity (body mass index $>30\,\text{kg/m}^2$) adversely affects the respiratory system by increasing abdominal pressure on the diaphragm, residual volume, chest wall impedance and ventilation–perfusion mismatch. Therefore patients with any respiratory disease will experience greater dyspnoea if they are also obese. In addition, obstructive sleep apnoea and obesity hypoventilation syndrome are direct consequences of obesity, and obesity is strongly associated with increased risk of death from all causes.

Treatment options to help patients lose weight are as follows:

- Behavioural counselling, including one-to-one and group therapy, aims to identify and modify triggers, change eating patterns and reduce portion sizes
- Exercise to increase energy expenditure
- Pharmacological therapies include orlistat, which prevents fat absorption by inhibiting pancreatic lipase, and the appetite suppressants lorcaserin and phentermine; the use of these drugs is limited by adverse effects and safety concerns
- Surgical interventions such as gastric banding and gastric bypass are highly effective and should be considered for those with morbid obesity (body mass index $>40\,\text{kg/m}^2$)

Nutritional support

Emphysema, lung cancer, cystic fibrosis, bronchiectasis and chronic infection cause malnutrition and weight loss. Also, low body mass index increases the susceptibility of patients with cystic fibrosis or bronchiectasis to infective exacerbations. Nutritional support is essential to achieve normal growth in children and adolescents with cystic fibrosis, and to support optimal lung function and prolong life in all patients.

Methods of offering nutritional support include the following:

- Behavioural counselling and dietary education
- Oral nutritional support with high-calorie or high-protein supplements, usually in the form of drinks such as milkshakes
- Enteral support through nasogastric tubes (in the short term) or percutaneous endoscopic gastrostomy or jejunostomy (in the long term) is used if oral intake remains inadequate or is contraindicated (e.g. if there is a risk of aspiration)
- Parenteral nutrition through long-term central venous access is rarely necessary (e.g. after transplant in patients with cystic fibrosis), and it has a high frequency of adverse effects such as infections and venous thromboembolism.

Pulmonary rehabilitation

Pulmonary rehabilitation is a multidisciplinary, comprehensive intervention with proven benefits for patients with COPD. Rehabilitation probably also benefits patients with other chronic respiratory diseases, such as pulmonary fibrosis and bronchiectasis.

The aims are to provide education, reduce symptom burden and optimise functional status, thus enhancing quality of life and reducing hospital admissions. Components of pulmonary rehabilitation programmes include:

- upper and lower limb exercise conditioning to increase exercise endurance
- breathing retraining to increase tidal volume and reduce dyspnoea
- disease and treatment education to improve the patient's adherence to treatment and their ability to manage their own condition
- psychological support to identify and to target the treatment of depression
- smoking cessation advice and support
- nutritional support
- advance care planning, including discussion of the patient's preferences regarding use of cardiopulmonary resuscitation and invasive ventilation

Physiotherapy

As well as delivering pulmonary rehabilitation, physiotherapists can teach patients:

- lung clearance exercises to facilitate sputum expectoration (e.g. for patients with bronchiectasis)
- control of breathing patterns (for patients with chronic dyspnoea or with dysfunctional breathing such as hyperventilation)

Physiotherapists also actively clear sputum and tenacious secretions for acutely unwell patients and those with lobar collapse caused by a sputum plug.

Occupational therapy

Occupational therapists are key members of the multidisciplinary team who work closely with physiotherapists and social services to enable patients with respiratory disease to function at the highest level possible despite their physical impairment. Occupational therapists assess the patient's home environment and care needs. They then suggest modifications and care packages, and provide mobility aids and bathroom and self-care aids.

Pharmacological interventions

The main drug therapies used for respiratory disease are bronchodilators, anti-inflammatory and antimicrobial agents, and oxygen.

Routes of administration

Drug therapies are given through a wide range of routes. For respiratory diseases, drug therapies are usually oral, intravenous or inhaled.

Oral therapies

Most patients find the oral route the easiest way to take a drug. Oral therapies are appropriate for chronic diseases and acute treatments, unless a rapid onset of drug effects is required.

Intravenous therapies

Drugs are delivered intravenously to treat cases of acute disease in which any delay could have adverse effects. Intravenous administration is also necessary for drugs without an oral formulation, for example many chemotherapy agents and monoclonal antibody therapies.

Inhaled therapies

For respiratory diseases, inhaled therapies are attractive alternatives to oral and intravenous administration. Inhaled therapies deliver the drug directly to the lungs, which potentially gives a faster onset of its effects. Furthermore, lower doses may be used, which minimises systemic availability and consequent adverse effects.

Inhaled therapies include oxygen, bronchodilators, glucocorticoids and antimicrobials. Delivery devices for drug therapies (excluding oxygen) are divided into two broad categories: inhaler devices and nebulisers.

- A wide range of inhaler devices are available (**Figure 2.36**). The most widely used is the standard metred dose inhaler. Metred dose inhalers are quick to use, small and convenient to carry, but require good coordination to effectively deliver a dose to the airways. They are used with spacer devices to improve drug delivery to the lungs. Breath-actuated inhalers (e.g. accuhalers, easyhalers and turbohalers) require less coordination than standard metred dose inhalers, because the dose is triggered by taking a breath. Assessing adherence with and ensuring the effective use of inhaler therapies is a major cornerstone of respiratory medicine. Respiratory nurses have a vital role in helping patients select an inhaler device they can use effectively and are comfortable with.
- Nebulisers aerosolise the medication to create a fine mist that is then inhaled through a face mask. Nebulisers deliver a larger dose of the medication than inhalers do, and they are used by patients who are very breathless and would struggle to use an inhaler successfully. They are frequently used in hospital to treat acute asthma and COPD exacerbations. Methods for delivering oxygen are discussed below (page 149).

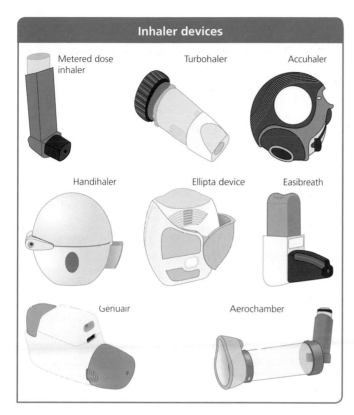

Inhaler devices

Metered dose inhaler

Turbohaler

Accuhaler

Handihaler

Ellipta device

Easibreath

Genuair

Aerochamber

Figure 2.36 Inhaler devices.

Bronchodilators

Bronchodilators are used for all types of airways disease to reduce the degree of airways obstruction and thus reduce dyspnoea and cough. They include β-agonists (e.g. salbutamol), anticholinergics (e.g. ipratropium bromide), magnesium and theophyllines (**Table 2.32**).

■ For most airways diseases, β-agonists are the first-line treatment and are given in inhaled, oral and intravenous forms. These drugs stimulate bronchial smooth muscle β_2 receptors to cause muscle relaxation and bronchodilation (**Figure 2.37**). There is evidence that they also interact with receptors on other cells implicated in asthma, such as mast cells, neutrophils, eosinophils and lymphocytes, and therefore have more long-term effects. Terbutaline and salbutamol have a rapid onset but are short-acting, with effects lasting < 4 h. Salmeterol has long lipophilic side chains

that increase the duration of its binding to the receptor, and is effective for up to 12 h. Although the β-agonists used for lung disease are relatively selective for β_2 receptors, they still cause significant β_1 receptor-related effects of tachycardia and tremor, which can limit their use. They also stimulate potassium shifts into muscle cells and in high doses sometimes cause hypokalaemia.

■ Anticholinergic drugs are antagonists of M_3 muscarinic receptors on airway smooth muscle cells, and are given as inhaled therapy. Activation of M_3 receptors by acetylcholine reduces intracellular cyclic AMP, causing contraction of airway smooth muscle and bronchoconstriction (**Figure 2.38**). Anticholinergics have a slower time of onset than that of β-agonists but act synergistically with them. They are used as second-line treatment of asthma and are first-line drugs for COPD. Ipratropium

Anti-inflammatory medications for asthma

Type	Example(s)	Mechanism of action	Indication(s) for use
Inhaled corticosteroids	Beclomethasone Fluticasone Budesonide	Broad inhibition of airways inflammation (**Figure 2.39**)	Mainstay of long-term asthma control
Systemic corticosteroids	Prednisilone (oral) Hydrocortisone (intravenous)	Broad inhibition of airways inflammation (**Figure 2.39**)	Treatment of severe acute exacerbations Continuous therapy in severe asthma (rarely necessary)
Chromones (rarely used in adults)	Nedocromil	Stabilisation of airway mast cells, preventing histamine release	Prevention of acute bronchoconstriction before anticipated exposure to a trigger Improved long-term asthma control
Leukotriene receptor antagonists	Montelukast	Blocking of action of leukotriene D4 and reduction of bronchoconstriction	Prevention of exercise-induced bronchoconstriction Improved long-term asthma control
Methlyxanthines (also are effective bronchodilators)	Theophylline Aminophylline	Inhibition of NF-κB transcription factor–mediated activation of inflammation	Improved long-term asthma control Acute treatment of asthma resistant to bronchodilators and glucocorticoids (bronchodilator effects)
Anti-IgE antibody	Omalizumab	Monoclonal antibody that binds IgE with high affinity	Improved long-term control of severe, inadequately controlled asthma associated with a raised IgE

Ig, immunoglobulin.

Table 2.32 Anti-inflammatory medications used to treat asthma

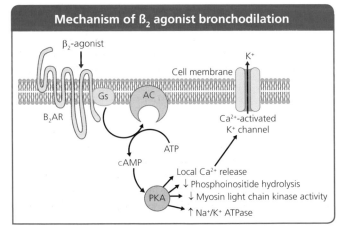

Mechanism of ß$_2$ agonist bronchodilation

Figure 2.37 Mechanism of bronchodilation by β$_2$-agonists. Activation of β$_2$ adrenergic receptor (B$_2$AR) by salbutamol, leads to activation of adenylyl cyclase (AC) through a stimulatory G protein (G$_s$), which in turn leads to an increase in cyclic AMP (cAMP). cAMP activates protein kinase A (PKA), which phosphorylates various proteins. This results in opening of calcium-activated potassium channels, increased Na$^+$/K$^+$ ATPase, decreased myosin light chain kinase activity and decreased phosphoinositide hydrolysis. These actions relax airway smooth muscle and thus bronchodilation.

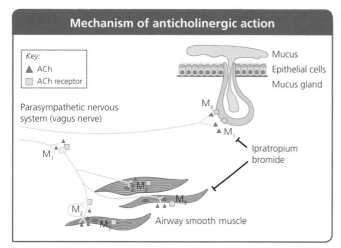

Mechanism of anticholinergic action

Key:
▲ ACh
☐ ACh receptor

Parasympathetic nervous
system (vagus nerve)

Mucus
Epithelial cells
Mucus gland

M_3
M_1
M_1
M_2
M_3
M_3

Ipratropium
bromide

Airway smooth muscle

Figure 2.38 Mechanism of anticholinergic action. Acetylcholine release from postganglionic parasympathetic nerve fibres stimulates muscarinic receptors on airway smooth muscle cells and mucus gland cells. This stimulation leads to smooth muscle contraction and mucus secretion. Anticholinergics such as ipratropium bromide block muscarinic receptors, leading to airway smooth muscle relaxation (and hence bronchodilation) and decreased mucus secretion. ACh, acetylcholine; M_1, M_2, M_3, muscarinic receptors.

bromide is a short-acting and tiotropium a long-acting anticholinergic agent. Anticholinergics have few adverse effects other than a bad taste, but they can cause paradoxical bronchoconstriction, and nebulised ipratropium can rarely precipitate glaucoma.

- Intravenous magnesium sulphate has bronchodilator activity in acute asthma. The mechanism of action is unclear, but it may inhibit calcium entry to smooth muscle cells in the airways. Evidence for the efficacy of magnesium is poor. However, it is a safe medication, and systematic reviews suggest that intravenous magnesium benefits patients with a severe asthma attack.

- Theophyllines are non-selective phosphodiesterase inhibitors that increase intracellular cyclic AMP, thereby causing smooth muscle relaxation and bronchodilation. Minor adverse effects include nausea, tremor and sleep disturbance; more seriously, theophyllines can precipitate arrhythmias (usually supraventricular). Theophylline and aminophylline are given orally or intravenously but have a narrow therapeutic index, therefore blood concentrations must be measured to avoid toxicity. These drugs also have some anti-inflammatory activity.

Common shorthand terms are used for inhaled therapies containing bronchodilators.

- SABA: short-acting β_2-agonist (e.g. salbutamol or terbutaline)
- LABA: long-acting β_2-agonist (e.g. salmeterol or formoterol)
- SAMA: short-acting muscarinic antagonist (e.g. ipratropium)
- LAMA: long-acting muscarinic antagonist (e.g. tiotropium)

Anti-inflammatory medications

Many respiratory diseases are associated with excessive inflammation at the site of disease, and consequently require treatment with anti-inflammatory medications. The mainstay of anti-inflammatory medication in respiratory disease is corticosteroids, but several other anti-inflammatory agents are also used in specific circumstances.

Corticosteroids

These anti-inflammatory drugs are available in inhaled, oral and intravenous formulations. Inhaled glucocorticoids suppress airways inflammation in various ways: they activate anti-inflammatory genes and suppress proinflammatory genes, including those that encode cytokines and chemokines (**Figure 2.39**). They have other effects on both structural and inflammatory cells (**Table 2.33**). Inhaled steroids cause mild local immunosuppression, allowing oral candidiasis to develop and increasing the risk of pneumonia in COPD patients. They also cause a reversible laryngeal myopathy that causes a hoarse and weak voice. Good inhaler technique and gargling to remove locally deposited drug help prevent upper airways adverse effects.

Systemic steroids are powerful anti-inflammatory agents. However, they cause significant immunosuppression and have several other major adverse effects that restrict their use to severe or life-threatening conditions:

- infection with conventional pathogens
- infection with opportunistic pathogens (e.g. *Aspergillus* and *Pneumocystis*)
- increased appetite and weight gain
- osteoporosis (vertebral collapse and fractures)
- thinning of the skin, with easy bruising
- 'moon facies': facial swelling affecting the cheeks

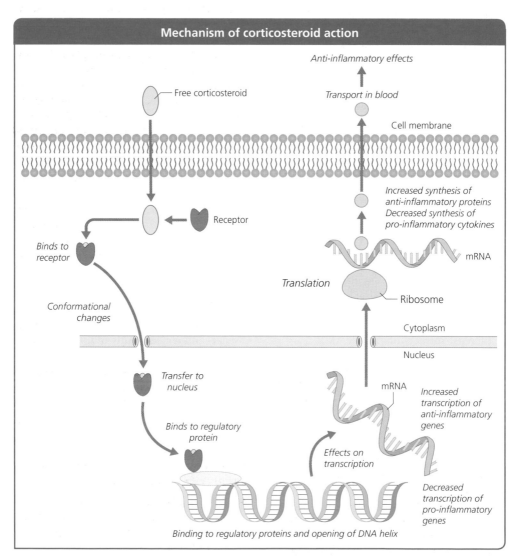

Figure 2.39 Mechanism of corticosteroid action. mRNA, messenger RNA.

Corticosteroid effects on cells	
Cell type	Action of steroid on cell
Inflammatory	
Eosinophil	Decreased eosinophil numbers
Lymphocyte	Decreased lymphocyte numbers
	Decreased cytokine production
Macrophage	Decreased cytokine production
	Impaired host defence
Dendritic cells	Decreased numbers and cytokine responses
Structural	
Epithelial	Decreased production of cytokines and other mediators
Endothelial	Decreased leak across endothelium
Airway smooth muscle	Decreased β_2 receptor expression
	Decreased cytokine production
Mucus glands	Decreased mucus secretion

Table 2.33 Effect of corticosteroid on other cells

- central obesity
- cataracts
- psychosis
- diabetes
- proximal myopathy
- avascular necrosis, e.g. of the hip
- Addisonian collapse on withdrawal or during acute illness (hypotension, prostration, vomiting)
- growth retardation in children

Long-term oral corticosteroids must be withdrawn slowly to prevent Addisonian-type symptoms. Patients on high-dose inhaled corticosteroids have a degree of systemic absorption, which rarely causes milder versions of the adverse effects seen with oral therapy.

Other anti-inflammatory agents

A number of other anti-inflammatory agents are used to treat asthma (**Table 2.32**). These include leukotriene antagonists and possibly theophylline. Non-steroidal anti-inflammatory drugs are useful anti-inflammatory agents and analgesics for the treatment of pleurisy and

musculoskeletal disorders. Cytotoxic agents such as methotrexate, cyclophosphamide and cyclosporine are used in the treatment of severe inflammatory lung disease such as progressive sarcodiosis or vasculitis.

Specific monoclonal antibody therapies have been developed to target specific elements of the inflammatory response. Examples include the inhibition of tumour necrosis factor by infliximab as treatment for sarcoidosis, and anti-IgE therapy with omalizumab for allergic asthma.

Antimicrobial agents

Antimicrobial agents are used to treat active infections and also as prophylactic therapy for patients at high risk for specific infections. Antimicrobial agents can be given by oral, intravenous or nebulised routes.

Which antimicrobial to use, and the duration and route of therapy, depend on the infecting pathogen or the clinical presentation (see Chapter 8). Generally, nebulised antimicrobials are reserved for prophylactic therapy, because they are not sufficiently efficacious for treatment of active infections.

A major issue is microbial drug resistance, because this prevents effective treatment. However, it is difficult to identify drug resistance without a positive culture for the infecting organism.

Oxygen

Oxygen is one of the most common drugs given in hospital practice. For any patient on oxygen, the route of administration, delivery device and flow rate should be prescribed on the drug chart. Various devices are used to administer oxygen (**Table 2.34**). The correct device for oxygen delivery depends on the indication.

Oxygen therapy is potentially life-saving for hypoxaemic patients but has significant adverse effects, including:

- Drying and crusting of the nasal and oral mucosa, especially with high flow rates: humidified oxygen is used to help prevent these effects.

Routes of oxygen administration			
Device	Flow rate (L/min)	F_{IO_2} (%)	Indications
Nasal cannula	1–6	Depends on flow rate (1–6 L/min) and respiratory rate 24–28 (at 2 L/min)	Minimal acute respiratory distress or oxygenation problem Patients with stable long-term oxygen requirements (e.g. long-term oxygen therapy) Allows patient to talk, eat and drink comfortably
Simple (Hudson) face mask	5–8	40–60	Similar indications to nasal cannula but requires higher oxygen concentrations Some patients prefer facemasks to nasal cannula
Venturi mask	2–12	24, 28, 35, 40 and 60	When exact F_{IO_2} is important (i.e. in patients at risk of hypercapnia or severe hypoxaemia)
Non-rebreathe mask (with reservoir bag)	6–15	50–80	Any spontaneously breathing patient who requires the highest possible F_{IO_2} (e.g. in cases of severe pneumonia or pulmonary oedema, shock, trauma or carbon monoxide poisoning)
Non-invasive ventilation or CPAP	Variable	Up to 80	Non-invasive ventilation used mainly for type 2 respiratory failure with lower levels of F_{IO_2} CPAP mainly used for severe type 1 respiratory failure with high F_{IO_2}
Mechanical ventilation	Variable	Up to 99	Invasive and only available on the intensive care unit or in theatres. Not appropriate for all patients with chronic respiratory disease
Hyperbaric oxygen chamber	n/a	High atmospheric pressure Increases amount of oxygen dissolved in blood	Treatment for carbon monoxide poisoning

CPAP, continuous positive airway pressure; F_{IO_2}, fractional concentration of oxygen in inspired air; n/a, not applicable.

Table 2.34 Routes of administration of oxygen

- Hypercapnia and respiratory acidosis: the respiratory drive of patients with type 2 respiratory failure depends on hypoxaemia, because their response to increased $Paco_2$ is blunted. If these patients receive a high F_{IO_2}, they frequently develop worsening hypoventilation and consequently an increase in $Paco_2$. Therefore patients with type 2 respiratory failure should initially receive lower oxygen concentration, increasing the F_{IO_2} if there is persisting hypoxaemia with no rise in $Paco_2$ identified on repeated arterial blood gas analyses.
- Pulmonary oxygen toxicity: breathing oxygen at increased partial pressures (> 50 kPa) causes release of oxygen free radicals, resulting in diffuse alveolar damage.
- Alveolar collapse (atelectasis): preterm neonates and patients who are mechanically ventilated are at risk of atelectasis if they spend prolonged periods breathing high concentrations of oxygen.
- Cerebral oxygen toxicity: breathing hyperbaric oxygen at pressures > 160 kPa (e.g. by deep sea divers) can cause severe cerebral vasoconstriction and seizures.
- Fire: oxygen promotes combustion. Patients who smoke while using inhaled oxygen therapy are at high risk of facial burns.

In some patients who are not hypoxaemic, oxygen is harmful. For example, oxygen therapy increases mortality in non-hypoxaemic patients with myocardial infarction or stroke.

> **Oxygen should not be given to patients who are not hypoxaemic and have myocardial infarction, stroke, anaemia, or an obstetric emergency.** However, it should be given in all cases of hypoxaemia, shock, cardiac arrest, anaphylaxis and carbon monoxide poisoning.

Long-term oxygen therapy

Long-term oxygen therapy used at home for at least 15h daily increases survival and improves quality of life in hypoxaemic patients with severe COPD and other chronic lung diseases. The therapy is delivered using oxygen concentrators and nasal cannula.

Indications for long-term oxygen therapy in chronic lung disease are:

- Pao_2 of $< 7.3\,kPa$
- Pao_2 of $< 8.0\,kPa$ in the presence of cor pulmonale
- OSA with nocturnal hypoxaemia not corrected by CPAP

Long-term oxygen therapy helps control secondary pulmonary hypertension and cor pulmonale. It may also improve cognitive function and exercise capacity, and reduce the frequency of hospital admissions. Ambulatory oxygen cylinders are also used for some patients with chronic hypoxic lung disease to improve the distances they can mobilise when out of their home.

Other general pharmacological therapies used in respiratory disease

Other drug therapies that are frequently used for patients with respiratory disease are listed in **Table 2.35**.

Other respiratory disease therapies	
Therapy	Indication(s)
Chemotherapy	Various chemotherapy agents are used to treat lung cancers
Paracetamol (acetominophen)	Used to treat pain and reduce pyrexia
NSAIDs (e.g. ibuprofen)	Used to treat pain, particularly pain caused by inflammation and pleuritic chest pain
Opiates Weaker: codeine, dihydrocodeine and co-codamol Strong: diamorphine, fentanyl and morphine	Analgesics for severe pain, particularly pain associated with malignancy and severe pleurisy, post-operative or post-procedure pain, and pain from fractured ribs or vertebrae Used to alleviate dyspnoea and cough in patients with advanced malignancy or terminal chronic lung disease
Benzodiazepines	For anxiety caused by severe dyspnoea in severe respiratory disease (e.g. sublingual lorazepam) Temporary sedation for procedures (e.g. intravenous midazolam)
Nebulised saline	To improve clearance of tenacious sputum
Carbocysteine	To improve clearance of tenacious sputum
N-acetyl cysteine	Antioxidant therapy for pulmonary fibrosis
Hyoscine butylbromide	An anticholinergic used in palliative care to decrease distressing airway secretions
NSAID, non-steroidal anti-inflammatory drug.	

Table 2.35 Examples of other therapies used in respiratory disease

Medical procedures

Some pleural and bronchial diseases are treated by physical procedures.

Pleural procedures

Air or fluid is removed from the pleural space by pleural aspiration (thoracocentesis) to give immediate relief from dyspnoea or life-threatening haemodynamic effects. A cannula or needle is advanced into the pleural space through a rib space, and air or fluid is drawn off with a syringe. The cannula or needle is then removed.

Continuous drainage of a pneumothorax or pleural effusion air or fluid requires insertion of a chest drain, usually within the 'safe triangle' (**Figure 2.40**). Chest drains may be inserted with the Seldinger technique: a guide wire is inserted into the pleural space before the tract is dilated, and a drain is advanced over the guide wire. Alternatively, a 'surgical chest drain' is inserted, creating access to the pleural space by blunt dissection of the subcutaneous tissues and the external and internal intercostal muscles; the drain is then inserted down this dissected tract.

Pleural effusions are prevented by obliterating the pleural space by a medical pleurodesis. In this procedure, a proinflammatory agent (e.g. talc or tetracycline) is introduced into the pleural space through a chest drain to cause inflammation and fusion of the visceral and parietal pleurae.

The main complications of pleural procedures are pain, syncope, local infection of the insertion site, empyema (**Figure 2.41**), haemorrhage and puncture of underlying organs. These procedures are safest when done using ultrasound guidance. The course of the intercostal bundle (Figure 1.15) should be avoided; this runs just under the inferior aspect of the ribs.

> **Draining very large effusions too rapidly causes marked cardiovascular effects, resulting in pain, dyspnoea and syncope.** When doing a pleural tap, remove a maximum of 1 L of fluid at one go. If a chest drain is inserted, the three-way tap may need to be closed or the drain clamped for 1–2 h after each 500–1000 mL is drained.

Bronchoscopic interventions

Bronchoscopy can be used to remove mucus plugs or foreign bodies that are occluding large airways. An airway that is narrowed by a benign or malignant process can be treated with balloon dilatation, laser or cryotherapy ablation, or stenting under bronchoscopic guidance. Radiotherapy can be given to bronchial tumours through a bronchoscope (brachytherapy).

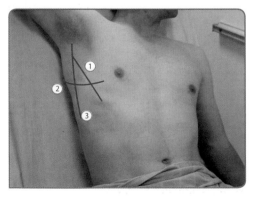

Figure 2.40 The safe triangle for insertion of chest drains: ① lateral border of pectoralis major; ② 5th intercostal space; and ③ mid-axillary line.

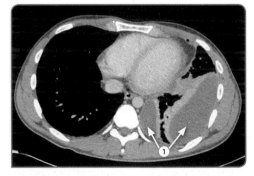

Figure 2.41 CT scan of empyema. ① Loculated pocket of fluid with thick surrounding rind, indicating empyema.

Ventilatory support

As well as oxygen therapy, patients with respiratory failure can be given additional positive pressure on inspiration to increase ventilation. Ventilator support can be given by non-invasive ventilators administered through tight-fitting face or nasal masks. Non-invasive ventilation does not require insertion of an endotracheal tube and can be administered on a normal ward without sedation. Alternatively, patients are sedated, paralysed and ventilated through an endotracheal tube inserted into the trachea using mechanical ventilation in an intensive care ward.

Bilevel non-invasive ventilation

This type of ventilatory support is used to reduce increased $Paco_2$ as well as improve oxygenation. Bilevel non-invasive ventilation cycles between higher inspiratory support (usually 10–20 cm of water) and lower expiratory pressure support (usually 0-4 cm of water).

- The inspiratory positive airway pressure decreases the work of breathing and improves tidal volume
- The expiratory positive airway pressure increases the functional residual capacity, splinting open the airways and preventing alveolar collapse

Bilevel non-invasive ventilation is an acute treatment of type 2 (hypercapnoeic) respiratory failure with acidosis (e.g. pH < 7.35) mainly as a result of COPD. It is also used as a chronic treatment nocturnally for chronic type 2 respiratory failure caused by chest wall, neuromuscular and chronic lung diseases.

Long-term non-invasive ventilation may reset the respiratory control centre to increase responsiveness to a rising $Paco_2$.

Continuous positive airway pressure

Continuous positive airway pressure provides single-level pressure support throughout the respiratory cycle, usually set at 5–10 cm of water. When combined with high-flow oxygen, it improves oxygenation and so is used to treat severe type 1 respiratory failure. However, it may increase $Paco_2$. Nocturnal CPAP without oxygen is also an effective treatment for OSA.

Mechanical ventilation

All modern ventilators use positive pressure ventilation. Patients must have an endotracheal tube inserted and are then connected through this to the ventilator. Mechanical ventilation allows precise control of the entire ventilator cycle, including pressure, volume, respiratory rate and Fio_2 at all points in the cycle.

Different modes of ventilation are available, but the following are most commonly used.

- Volume-controlled: a fixed volume is delivered and the airway pressures are variable
- Pressure support: a fixed positive pressure is delivered every time the patient triggers a breath, and the tidal volume is variable
- Synchronised intermittent mandatory ventilation: this allows the patient to breathe spontaneously between machine delivered breaths

Mechanical ventilation is used for severe respiratory failure not responding to supplemental oxygen, treatment of the underlying disease or (if used) non invasive ventilation. However, mechanical ventilation is inappropriate if the patient's underlying disease does not have a significant potentially reversible element.

Many potential complications are associated with mechanical ventilation, including:

- over-ventilation with respiratory alkalosis
- gastric distension
- barotrauma with pneumothorax, pneumomediastinum or air embolism
- tissue injury during endotracheal tube placement
- post-intubation tracheal stenosis
- ventilator lung injury
- ventilator-acquired pneumonia
- impaired cardiac output

- fluid retention and oedema
- inability to communicate
- post-ventilation psychological effects

> **Non-invasive ventilation is contraindicated in uncooperative patients or those with severe unstable disease that would be more safely treated by intubation and mechanical ventilation.** However, mechanical intubation is inappropriate for many patients with exacerbations of severe chronic lung disease; non-invasive ventilation provides a life-saving alternative.

Surgical interventions

Several surgical procedures are potentially curative for specific lung diseases. Thoracic surgery requires a general anaesthetic, and the patient is intubated with a double-lumen tube for individual ventilation of the unaffected lung.

The surgery can be done using minimally invasive video-assisted thoracoscopic surgery techniques. In these techniques, small incisions are used to allow surgical instruments into the thoracic cavity. The other option is open surgery, which requires a large incision running parallel to the rib called a thoracotomy (**Figure 2.4**). Post-operative complications and recovery times are much better for video-assisted thoracoscopic surgery than for open surgery. However, more complex operations, such as large lung resections and chest wall surgery, usually require an open procedure.

Lung resection

In diseases causing focal lung pathology, the lung can be resected by:

- wedge resection (removing the affected tissue only)
- lobectomy (removing the affected lobe)
- pneumonectomy (removing the whole lung)

The commonest disease treated by resection is lung cancer. However, resection is also used to treat other tumours, sites of major uncontrolled haemoptysis, and severe focal infections unresponsive to antimicrobial agents (e.g. aspergillosis, lung abscess and pulmonary gangrene).

Bullectomy and lung volume reduction surgery

Excision of large bullae (bullectomy) and emphysematous upper lobes (lung volume reduction surgery) sometimes improves lung function in patients with COPD. However, the results are difficult to predict, and the procedures have significant morbidity and mortality. Newer techniques use bronchoscopes to place coils in the bronchi of emphysematous patients. This has a similar effect to lung volume reduction surgery and may be a safer alternative.

Pleural surgery

Recurrent pneumothorax is treated by surgical pleurectomy (removal of pleura) or pleurodesis; continuing air leaks can be stopped by over-sewing the leak at the same time. Recurrent pleural effusions are prevented by surgical pleurodesis. Surgical pleural drainage and decortication (removal of thickened pleura) is used for patients with poorly controlled or extensive empyema.

Lung transplant

Progressive chronic lung diseases resulting in respiratory failure are cured by lung transplant with a size-, human leucocyte antigen– and blood group–matched donor organ. Common indications are cystic fibrosis, idiopathic pulmonary fibrosis, COPD and primary pulmonary hypertension.

The shortage of donor organs and the high morbidity and mortality generally restrict transplant to patients younger than 65 years.

Depending on the condition needing treatment, the transplant may be one lobe, a single lung, a double lung or a combined heart and lung procedure.

Perioperative mortality is about 10%. A further 40% of patients die of complications, mainly infection and progressive small airways obstruction caused by chronic host-versus-graft disease (bronchiolitis obliterans) within 5–10 years. Patients need lifelong immunosuppression to prevent organ rejection.

Judging when a patient with chronic lung disease is suitable for lung transplant is difficult. Predicted survival should be <5 years, but they should not be so debilitated that the surgery has unacceptable mortality.

Answers to starter questions

1. The type of chest pain does not necessarily indicate its cause, but certain features ring alarm bells. Dull, persistent, progressive pain that wakes the patient at night suggests malignancy. Pleuritic chest pain often has a serious cause, such as infection or pulmonary embolism. Of course, chest pain of cardiac origin is serious: it is more central, feels crushing and is usually worse on exertion.

2. Non-respiratory symptoms, such as weight loss, fever, bone density loss and joint inflammation, are significant in respiratory diseases for several reasons. They:
   - help identify extra-thoracic sites affected by the underlying disease, particularly in cases of malignancy
   - indicate disease severity, e.g. weight loss in patients with COPD
   - help determine prognosis
   - are part of the disease's negative effects on patients' quality of life
   - indicate the presence of an infective or inflammatory condition (e.g. fever)

3. This question has no single answer; it depends on the individual patient. An occupational history and general social history, including social support and housing arrangements, are likely to be necessary for all patients. Occupational history is essential for diagnosis in patients with possible pneumoconiosis or asbestos-related disease. For those with severe dyspnoea, the presence of stairs at home is one factor to consider. Part of the holistic care of a patient is to facilitate the provision of social support when needed. Therefore the social history will identify patients with specific needs and to refer them to the social services and community respiratory teams.

4. The most relevant aspects of the past history depend on the presenting complaint and the individual patient. However, a thorough history of respiratory and cardiac disease is likely to be useful. For some conditions, the history must include a childhood history. For example, whooping cough or recurrent infections as a child are sometimes a cause of bronchiectasis in adulthood.

Answers *continued*

5. Various ways are used to assess the severity of a chronic respiratory disease.

   ■ Exercise capacity should be assessed by asking the patient how far they can walk, and whether they can climb stairs.
   ■ Rate of deterioration can be assessed by comparing current exercise capacity with baseline exercise capacity.
   ■ For conditions that have exacerbations, exacerbation frequency can be a strong indicator of severity (particularly true of COPD)

   An objective measurement of severity should be made alongside the patient's subjective assessment of severity. Some patients adapt to a given severity of lung disease (as measured by FEV_1) much better than others, and have less of a subjective feeling of breathlessness. Therefore quality of life varies significantly between patients with the similar physiological severity of disease.

6. Examining all patients presenting with respiratory symptoms is essential. It can identify serious and life-threatening problems such as acute severe asthma or tension pneumothorax, in which waiting for imaging tests before starting treatment could be fatal. Examination also helps determine which investigations will be most useful for the patient, preventing them from receiving unnecessary tests.

7. The requirement for investigations depends on the severity of the haemoptysis and other associated symptoms. Reasons to investigate extensively include:

   ■ risk factors for malignancy (e.g. smoking)
   ■ 'red flag' symptoms (e.g. weight loss)
   ■ severe and persistent haemoptysis
   ■ lack of any other explanation for the haemoptysis (e.g. recent severe chest infection)

8. Dullness to percussion may indicate solid material or fluid under the area percussed. Causes include consolidation of the lung, a large mass in the lung parenchyma and a thickened pleura, haemothorax or chylothorax (which are rare) or a pleural effusion (which is common and has many possible causes).

9. The A–a gradient is a measure of the difference between the alveolar concentration of oxygen (A) and the arterial concentration of oxygen (a). The A–a gradient helps determine the cause of hypoxaemia, because an abnormally high A–a gradient suggests a defect in diffusion, ventilation–perfusion mismatch or right-to-left shunt.

10. Dyspnoea is usually caused by anaemia, cardiac disease or lung disease. A full blood count will identify a patient with anaemia. An ECG and echocardiogram assess ventricular function and will exclude cardiac causes in most patients. Exertional dyspnoea due to atypical and painless angina is an exception and an exercise test, nuclear scans or coronary artery angiography are needed to diagnose it.

    Chronic airways diseases cause an obstructive pattern reduction in spirometry values and an increase in residual and total lung volumes. Interstitial lung disease causes a restrictive pattern on spirometry and a reduction in total lung capacity and transfer factor (both T_{LCO} and K_{CO}). Chest wall or neuromuscular disease causes a restrictive pattern on spirometry and a fall in total lung capacity. However, patients present with a normal transfer factor when adjusted for lung size (the K_{CO}). Pulmonary vascular disease does not affect spirometry or lung volumes, but it does cause a fall in transfer factor.

Answers *continued*

In some patients it leads to right heart strain and pulmonary hypertension which are identified using an ECG or echocardiogram. Asthma will often give normal lung function results but the patient should have variable PEFR results over time, especially when feeling short of breath.

Sometimes, after multiple investigations, if no obvious cause is found it is necessary to decide whether the symptoms are due to the patient being unfit or deconditioned, or whether further specialist investigations are likely to help with diagnosis.

11. The nature and site of the lesion, and the patient's underlying lung function and general condition, dictate the biopsy method used. The best sample should be obtained at the lowest discomfort and risk to the patient. Needle biopsies are excellent ways of obtaining histology of focal lung lesions such as nodules and dense patches of consolidation. Radiologists perform percutaneous needle biopsies with ultrasound or CT guidance which are best for peripheral lung or pleural lesions. The safest percutaneous needle biopsies are when the lesion is in the pleura. If a patient has COPD or interstitial lung disease, there is significant risk of pneumothorax if the needle traverses lung tissue. A needle biopsy can only be done if the patient has adequate lung function to cope with a pneumothorax without serious risk of respiratory failure.

Lesions inside a bronchus are best biopsied during bronchoscopy. Lesions adjacent to a major bronchus (e.g. mediastinal lymph nodes or a central tumour) can be biopsied during bronchoscopy using endobronchial ultrasound guidance. These are performed by respiratory physicians or thoracic surgeons.

If percutaneous or bronchoscopic biopsies are not possible, surgical biopsies of solid lesions are performed. Needle biopsies are not appropriate for diffuse alveolar infiltrations or interstitial lung disease as there is a high risk of bleeding and pneumothorax; in addition the quantity of tissue obtained is limited. Diffuse alveolar infiltrations and interstitial lung disease need a surgical biopsy, usually by video-assisted thoracoscopic surgery. Transbronchial biopsy samples are possible but they are often too small to be diagnostic.

Newer methods such as cryobiopsy via a bronchoscope may improve sample size without increasing the risk of complication. All patients undergoing a lung biopsy need to be assessed for potential bleeding risk, i.e. is the platelet count >50, is blood coagulation normal, is the patient taking any anticoagulant or antiplatelet therapies such as low molecular weight heparin, warfarin, aspirin or clopidogrel?

12. Advantages for using CT scans are:

- They provide a three dimensional view of the lungs
- They give excellent resolution of pulmonary and intrathoracic anatomy
- They are essential for the accurate, non-invasive assessment of lung diseases including interstitial lung disease, pulmonary artery abnormalities, pulmonary emboli, lung masses and mediastinal lesions

However, they do have disadvantages compared to chest X–rays:

- They are expensive
- They require a higher radiation dose (100 times greater than a X-ray, depending on the CT technique), so can be only used intermittently

Answers *continued*

Frequent monitoring of radiological abnormalities is, therefore, done using chest X-rays, as they sometimes provide a better indication of disease progression as all of the lungs are visible in one picture whereas CT scans give an image of only one cross section of lung. Most patients are able to have a chest X-ray, but those with orthopnoea or severe claustrophobia cannot easily tolerate a CT scan. Patients are given intravenous contrast when pulmonary vessels and mediastinal abnormalities are being assessed using CT. This can cause renal failure in patients with pre-existing renal impairment or exacerbate asthma.

13. The most common treatments are antibiotics, bronchodilators (e.g. anticholinergics and β-agonists) and anti-inflammatories (e.g. steroids). Other pharmacological agents are available; details are provided under the individual conditions in Chapters 3–12. Non-pharmacological therapies, such as smoking cessation, improved nutrition, exercise and physiotherapy, are helpful in many conditions.

14. Principles of treating respiratory failure:

    1. Identify and treat the cause

    2. Correct Pao_2 and $Paco_2$ abnormalities

    Some causes of respiratory failure can be rapidly reversed by a physical procedure, e.g. pleural drainage for a patient with pre-existing lung disease presenting with sudden onset deterioration due to a pneumothorax. Many causes of respiratory failure will respond to treatment in minutes to hours (e.g. bronchodilators for airways obstruction) or days (e.g. antibiotics for pneumonia). However, some causes of respiratory failure require several days or weeks to respond to treatment (e.g. systemic corticosteroids for exacerbations of COPD). Sometimes there are no effective therapies for example in ARDS. The time taken for a response to treatment dictates how long the patient will require respiratory support to correct Pao_2 and $Paco_2$.

    Type 1 respiratory failure is treated with supplemental inhaled oxygen to increase oxygen saturation >92% (preferably >95%). The method of oxygen delivery depends on the severity of hypoxia:

    - Mild hypoxia: nasal specula, 24–28% Fio_2
    - Severe hypoxia: face mask, 24–60% Fio_2
    - Severe hypoxia with no response to face mask alone: face mask and CPAP

    Type 2 respiratory failure is caused by under ventilation of the lungs and cannot be corrected by supplemental inhaled oxygen alone. In patients with raised $Paco_2$, if Fio_2 is too high it often reduces the hypoxic respiratory drive and causes a further increase in $Paco_2$ and worsening respiratory acidosis. Type 2 respiratory failure is treated with low levels of supplemental oxygen, e.g. Fio_2 24–28%, aiming for oxygen saturation > 88%. If the patient also has respiratory acidosis, then they may be given bilevel non-invasive ventilation to increase alveolar ventilation; however, this is sometimes poorly tolerated.

    For type 1 and 2 respiratory failure, intubation and mechanical ventilation can be used if non-invasive therapies fail to adequately correct the blood gas abnormalities.

Answers *continued*

15. Although most respiratory diseases do not require surgery, it is a vital component for diagnosis and treatment of a small proportion of patients. Surgical biopsies, performed using VATs, are necessary for the accurate diagnosis of interstitial lung diseases, mediastinal or intrapulmonary nodules, or pleural effusions in some patients. Benign or malignant thoracic tumours and unresolved lung infections (e.g. lung abscesses or pulmonary gangrene) can be eradicated with surgical resection. Surgery is a commonly required treatment for patients with pleural infection, and persisting or recurrent pneumothorax. Bullectomy or lung volume reduction surgery is used in very select patients with COPD. Lung transplants are a potential cure for patients with chronic lung disease.

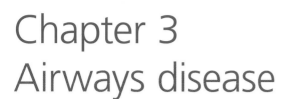

Chapter 3
Airways disease

Starter questions

Answers to the following questions are on pages 165–166.

1. Is chronic asthma the same as chronic obstructive pulmonary disease (COPD)?
2. What are the risk factors for developing asthma?
3. Why do only some smokers develop COPD? And can non-smokers develop the disease?
4. Is COPD ever reversible?
5. Do corticosteroids increase the risk of infection in patients with COPD?
6. Why is large airways obstruction often misdiagnosed as asthma?

Introduction

Airways diseases are lung diseases that cause obstruction of the bronchial tree, the small airways or both. This group of diseases includes asthma and COPD.

Asthma and COPD both affect the small and medium airways, and are the most common chronic respiratory diseases. In the UK, more than 5 million people have asthma, and 900,000 have a diagnosis of COPD (a further 2 million are thought to be undiagnosed). COPD is predicted to be the third leading cause of death by 2030.

Diseases of the trachea and large airways are rare. However, they can be life-threatening.

Case 1 Recurrent cough and wheeze

Presentation

Mr Lewis, aged 28 years, has been referred to the respiratory outpatient department by his general practitioner (GP). He has had a cough on and off for 6 months, following a chest infection over the winter.

Initial interpretation

Persistent cough (lasting >8 weeks) has various possible causes, including infection, smoking, postnasal drip, gastro-oesophageal reflux disease, and the use of certain medications (e.g. angiotensin-converting enzyme inhibitors). A more serious cause is cancer. However, asthma is a common cause of persistent cough in younger patients.

There is no standard test for asthma, and there are often few signs. The diagnosis is based primarily on identifying features in the history that suggest reversible airways obstruction.

History

Mr Lewis notices the cough particularly in the morning, after exercise and during periods of cold weather. When the cough is severe, it wakes him at night. It is associated with a whistling sound on breathing in and a feeling that his chest is 'tight'. He is usually a keen cyclist but has found it increasingly difficult to cycle his normal distances. The cough is usually dry but occasionally produces small amounts of yellow phlegm. His GP prescribed a salbutamol inhaler, which eased the cough a little.

Interpretation of history

The variability of the symptoms suggests reversible airways disease. Breathlessness, cough and wheeze that are worse with exercise, at night or on waking in the morning are typical of asthma. The symptoms are clearly not controlled, despite the use of the salbutamol inhaler.

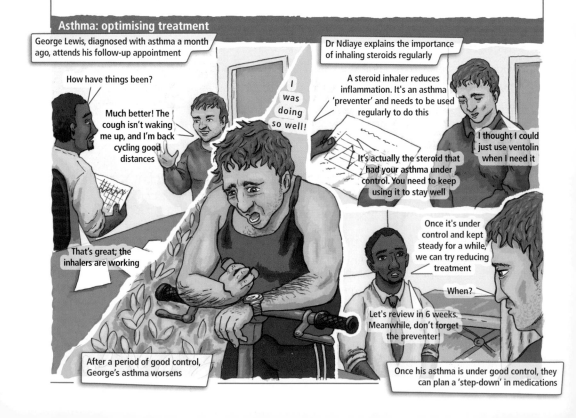

Asthma: optimising treatment

George Lewis, diagnosed with asthma a month ago, attends his follow-up appointment

How have things been?

Much better! The cough isn't waking me up, and I'm back cycling good distances

That's great; the inhalers are working

I was doing so well!

Dr Ndiaye explains the importance of inhaling steroids regularly

A steroid inhaler reduces inflammation. It's an asthma 'preventer' and needs to be used regularly to do this

It's actually the steroid that had your asthma under control. You need to keep using it to stay well

I thought I could just use ventolin when I need it

Once it's under control and kept steady for a while, we can try reducing treatment

When?

Let's review in 6 weeks. Meanwhile, don't forget the preventer!

After a period of good control, George's asthma worsens

Once his asthma is under good control, they can plan a 'step-down' in medications

Case 1 *continued*

Further history

Mr Lewis had no respiratory problems during childhood. He has hay fever every spring, and there is a strong family history of asthma. He is otherwise well and on no regular medications. He smokes 10 cigarettes a week.

Examination

He looks well and has a normal body mass index. Cardiovascular and respiratory examinations are normal. Peak expiratory flow rate (PEFR) is 610 L/min. Oxygen saturation is 99% on room air.

Interpretation of findings

Unless someone is having an asthma exacerbation or has poorly controlled asthma, the examination and pulmonary function test results are often normal. It is important to remember that the absence of wheeze, a normal single PEFR reading, and normal spirometry results do not exclude a diagnosis of asthma.

Investigations

Chest X-ray and spirometry results in clinic are normal. Blood tests show no eosinophilia and a normal total immunoglobin (Ig) E. Home PEFR recordings show significant variability, decreasing from >600 L/min in the evening to 380 L/min in the morning or during exercise.

Diagnosis

The history strongly suggests asthma. This diagnosis is confirmed by the variation in PEFR recordings. The symptoms are frequent, so regular treatment with inhaled steroids is warranted. The aim is to achieve day-to-day freedom from symptoms. Mr Lewis must stop smoking.

Post-viral hyperactivity syndrome is a possible differential diagnosis. It is treated similarly to asthma but the symptoms settle and do not require long-term treatment.

Case 2 Worsening breathlessness in a 70-year-old smoker

Presentation

Mr Williams is referred to the respiratory outpatient clinic with worsening breathlessness over the past year. He now finds it difficult to climb the stairs at home.

Initial interpretation

In older patients, COPD, pulmonary fibrosis and heart failure are possibilities. It is crucial to elicit any other symptoms and to find out more about the duration and time course of the deterioration of the breathlessness.

History

Mr Williams first noticed he was getting breathless about 5 years ago. Since then, the problem has worsened; he now has an exercise tolerance of about 50 m and can barely walk up hills or stairs. He does not get breathless on resting or when lying down at night. He has no chest pain or ankle swelling.

Interpretation of history

Gradually deteriorating breathlessness on exertion over years is a common

Case 2 *continued*

symptom in COPD. The lack of orthopnoea and peripheral oedema make cardiac causes less likely. Other symptoms suggesting COPD include frequent chest infections, wheeze, chronic cough and regular sputum production.

Further history

Mr Williams has noticed a wheeze (a whistling noise in his chest). He does not cough up sputum unless he has a chest infection. He needed a course of antibiotics for a chest infection 6 months ago.

He has smoked since the age of 15 and now smokes 10 cigarettes a day, having cut down from 40. He has a history of benign prostatic hypertrophy, hypertension and atrial fibrillation.

He lives with his wife and is a retired flooring contractor. He is taking atorvastatin, alfuzosin, salbutamol, omeprazole, perindopril, glucosamine, doxazosin and warfarin.

Examination

Mr Williams looks cachectic. He is not cyanosed, and there is no clubbing of his fingers or toes. However, he is breathless and using his accessory muscles when breathing. His fingers are nicotine-stained.

His heart rate is 76 beats/min and is irregularly irregular. However, his jugular venous pressure is not increased, and his heart sounds are normal. His chest is hyperexpanded, and there is bilaterally reduced expansion on inspiration. He has generally quiet breath sounds and a mild end expiratory wheeze on auscultation. Oxygen saturation is 92% on air.

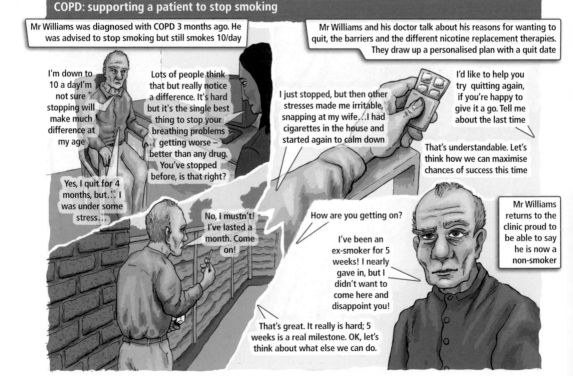

COPD: supporting a patient to stop smoking

Mr Williams was diagnosed with COPD 3 months ago. He was advised to stop smoking but still smokes 10/day

Mr Williams and his doctor talk about his reasons for wanting to quit, the barriers and the different nicotine replacement therapies. They draw up a personalised plan with a quit date

I'm down to 10 a day I'm not sure stopping will make much difference at my age

Lots of people think that but really notice a difference. It's hard but it's the single best thing to stop your breathing problems getting worse – better than any drug. You've stopped before, is that right?

I just stopped, but then other stresses made me irritable, snapping at my wife...I had cigarettes in the house and started again to calm down

I'd like to help you try quitting again, if you're happy to give it a go. Tell me about the last time

That's understandable. Let's think how we can maximise chances of success this time

Yes, I quit for 4 months, but... I was under some stress...

No, I mustn't! I've lasted a month. Come on!

How are you getting on?

I've been an ex-smoker for 5 weeks! I nearly gave in, but I didn't want to come here and disappoint you!

Mr Williams returns to the clinic proud to be able to say he is now a non-smoker

That's great. It really is hard; 5 weeks is a real milestone. OK, let's think about what else we can do.

Case 2 *continued*

Interpretation of findings

The hyperexpanded chest wall shape, reduced expansion on inspiration, quiet breath sounds and wheeze are in keeping with a diagnosis of COPD. There are no signs of cardiac failure. Mr Williams seems to be hypoxic, which suggests that he is developing respiratory failure. The fact that he appears cachectic does not necessarily mean he has cancer, because advanced COPD can also produce this appearance.

Investigations

Pulmonary function tests show a forced expiratory volume in 1s (FEV_1) of 0.9 L (38% of predicted) and a forced vital capacity (FVC) of 1.5L, giving a FEV_1/ FVC ratio of 58% (**Figure 3.1**). Chest X-ray shows hyperexpanded lung fields with flattened diaphragms (**Figure 3.2**).

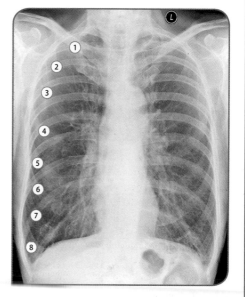

Figure 3.2 Chest X-ray showing hyperexpanded lung fields in chronic obstructive pulmonary disease. The diaphragm is depressed and flattened by hyperinflation (arrows). There are sparse coarse lung markings. ①–⑧ Visible anterior rib ends; normally, fewer than 6 are visible.

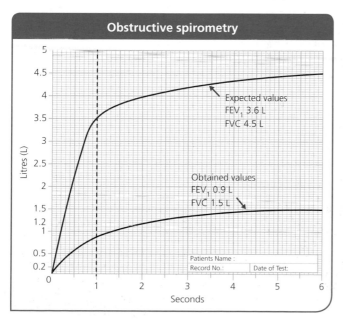

Obstructive spirometry

Expected values
FEV_1 3.6 L
FVC 4.5 L

Obtained values
FEV_1 0.9 L
FVC 1.5 L

Patients Name :
Record No.:   Date of Test:

Litres (L)

Seconds

Figure 3.1 Spirometry results for a 70-year-old man showing obstruction. The forced expiratory volume (in 1 s) (FEV_1) value is the point at which the curves meet the dashed line. The forced vital capacity (FVC) value is the point at which the curves cross the y-axis on the right-hand side.

Case 2 *continued*

Diagnosis

These history and examination findings in a patient with a significant smoking history strongly suggest COPD. The diagnosis is confirmed by the spirometry results, which show severe obstructive changes.

The diagnosis is explained to Mr Williams, and he is started on long-acting β agonist inhalers, used regularly. A referral is made for pulmonary rehabilitation and smoking cessation services.

> **Patients often ignore COPD symptoms, which start gradually and progress over years.** They may attribute breathlessness to ageing and modify their lifestyle to cope. Therefore they may not be diagnosed until they have severe disease or are admitted to hospital with an acute exacerbation.

Large airways obstruction

Large airways obstruction includes obstruction of the main bronchi, trachea, larynx or pharynx (**Figure 3.3**). The disease can be acute and life-threatening or occur gradually, depending on the cause. The management of an acute presentation of stridor (a harsh vibrating sound) and upper airways obstruction is discussed in Chapter 11.

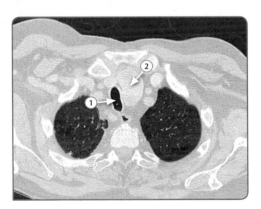

Figure 3.3 Computerised tomography showing major airways obstruction. ① Trachea displaced to the right and with a narrowed lateral diameter. ② Left paratracheal mass.

Epidemiology

About a fifth of lung cancer patients develop complications associated with large airways obstruction. Other causes of the condition are uncommon.

Aetiology

The causes of large airways obstruction are divided into acute, subacute or chronic (**Table 3.1**). Most cases are caused by malignancy or infectious disease.

Clinical features

The presentation of large airways obstruction is extremely varied and depends on the cause. Acute presentations are discussed in Chapter 11. Chronic large airways obstruction presents with gradually increasing breathlessness and cough, and can also cause bronchiectasis distal to the obstruction.

The speed of progression depends on the cause, and patients can be misdiagnosed as having asthma or COPD. The patient sometimes hears stridor, which often varies in intensity over

Large airways obstruction causes	
Speed of onset	Common causes
Sudden	Aspiration of a foreign body
	Mucus plug (especially if there is a pre-existing stricture)
Acute infective	Epiglottitis
	Diphtheria
	Tonsillar or pharyngeal abscess
Acute non-infective	Smoke or fire inhalation
	Chemical exposure burns
Subacute (often with acute deteriorations)	Primary malignancy (e.g. bronchogenic carcinoma, laryngeal carcinoma, thyroid carcinoma or mediastinal tumour)
	Secondary malignancy
	Massive lymphadenopathy (e.g. lymphoma or tuberculosis)
	Vocal cord paralysis
Chronic	Post-intubation tracheal stenosis
	Effects of radiotherapy or surgery
	Vasculitis (granulomatosis with polyangiitis)
	Tracheomalacia
	Goitre or retrosternal goitre
	Post-infective (e.g. after tuberculosis)

Table 3.1 Causes of large airways obstruction

time or with changes in position. For example, stridor may be increased by lying flat. Mild obstruction may cause no symptoms. Other symptoms of malignant obstruction include haemoptysis, hoarseness, chest pain and dysphagia (if the oesophagus is compressed). Breathlessness at rest is a sign of severe obstruction.

Diagnostic approach

The diagnosis is based on history, clinical examination, pulmonary function tests and imaging. Stridor is a very specific sign of large airways obstruction and must be investigated thoroughly.

Investigations

Useful investigations in upper airways obstruction include:

- X-ray of the chest and neck
- computerised tomography (CT)
- spirometry, PEFR and flow volume loop
- bronchoscopy

X-rays of the chest and soft tissue of the neck

Chest and neck X-rays sometimes show tracheal deviation, a large mass lesion, consolidation, bronchiectasis or lobar collapse distal to the obstructed airway. These findings are not usually diagnostic.

Computerised tomography of the neck and chest

A CT scan of the neck and chest identifies the site, potential cause and severity of large airways obstruction.

Pulmonary function tests

Spirometry shows obstruction, and the PEFR is reduced. The flow volume loop has a characteristic shape and provides information on whether the obstruction is dynamic or fixed, and extra- or intra-thoracic (Figure 2.18). The ratio of FEV_1 (mL):PEFR (L/min) (the Empey index) is helpful to distinguish large airways obstruction from lower airways disease; a ratio > 10 suggests large airways obstruction.

Bronchoscopy

Bronchoscopy is the most sensitive test for large airways obstruction. It provides information on the cause, location and degree of large airways compression.

The procedure also allows a biopsy of the lesion to be taken for histological investigation. However, in severe obstruction, biopsies are potentially dangerous; bleeding or swelling can further compromise the airway.

Specific tests are required to confirm the cause. For example, a biopsy can be examined to detect malignancy, and anti–neutrophil cytoplasmic antibody (ANCA) can be measured to help identify vasculitis.

Management

The cause should be treated. The obstruction is relieved by endobronchial therapies (stenting, balloon dilatation or laser ablation), surgery and tracheostomy (as a last resort).

The immediate management of severe large airways obstruction is:

- high-flow oxygen or heliox (an oxygen–helium mixture, the lower viscosity of which aids respiration)
- high-dose corticosteroids to reduce airway oedema
- nebulised bronchodilators and adrenaline (epinephrine)
- surgery (sometimes; see Chapter 11)

Prognosis

Acute stridor is life-threatening. The condition must be treated immediately. Infective causes have a good prognosis, but the prognosis for malignant causes is poor.

Asthma

Asthma is a common condition in which there is hyper-reactivity of the airways and chronic inflammation. These changes cause variable airflow obstruction that in the early stages is fully reversible. However, over time asthma can cause irreversible airways obstruction if not well-controlled.

Types

The following terms are used to describe asthma.

- Allergic: caused by inhalation of allergens (e.g. pollen).
- Chronic: asthma requiring long-term maintenance treatment (e.g. inhaled steroids) to control symptoms.
- Acute: a short-term exacerbation.
- Brittle: asthma in patients whose PEFR variability is significant despite considerable medical therapy, or in patients prone to sudden acute attacks without an obvious trigger on a background of good control. In both groups, the risk of death from asthma is higher than in other asthma patients.
- Difficult: asthma in a patient with a confirmed diagnosis and whose symptoms, lung function abnormalities, or both are poorly controlled despite treatment that would usually be effective. Mild, moderate or severe asthma can be classified as difficult. Further assessment is needed to determine whether the cause is related to the disease, the patient (poor adherence) or the physician (inappropriate therapies).
- Severe: asthma with severe symptoms or requiring hospital treatment. Any patient may have severe asthma at some point. Sometimes the term is used to describe brittle or steroid-resistant asthma.
- Steroid-resistant: some patients respond poorly to steroid therapy, with no significant increase in FEV_1 or PEFR after a 2-week trial of oral steroids. Others

need such high doses that adverse effects become a problem. All patients with steroid-resistant asthma require further assessment to ensure that the diagnosis is correct and that there are no unidentified precipitating factors.

■ Status asthmaticus: a prolonged and severe asthma attack that fails to respond to initial treatment and is life-threatening (see Chapter 11).

Epidemiology

Asthma is the most common chronic respiratory disease. An estimated 300 million people worldwide (5.4 million in the UK) have asthma. It is more prevalent in high-income countries. However, its incidence has been increasing in both high-income and low- to middle-income countries.

Asthma is a common childhood diagnosis, but occurs in all ages and there is a second peak in people older than 60 years. In adults, asthma is more common in women than in men. Also, adults who are obese are more likely to have the disease than those with normal body mass index.

Aetiology

The causes of asthma are complex and poorly understood. Risk factors for developing the disease include:

■ family history of asthma
■ history of other atopic conditions (e.g. hay fever and eczema)
■ bronchiolitis in childhood
■ childhood exposure to tobacco smoke
■ maternal vitamin D deficiency during pregnancy
■ premature birth (especially if neonatal ventilation was necessary)
■ low birth weight

Genetic factors also predispose individuals to airway hyper-responsiveness after exposure to environmental triggers. Some genetic associations have been identified, for example polymorphisms of *ADAM33*, a gene encoding a disintegrin and metalloproteinase domain 33 protein. However, many other genes are likely to be involved.

Triggers for asthma are listed in **Table 3.2**, and its pathogenesis is shown in **Figure 3.4**. Occupational exposure can cause asthma in paint sprayers, bakers, cleaners, chemical workers and solderers.

Prevention

If the patient is overweight, weight loss can improve symptoms. Smokers must stop smoking. If they continue to smoke, control of their asthma will be poor; tobacco smoke makes inhaled corticosteroids less effective.

Patients should avoid sources of known triggers, such as dust and pet cats. Sometimes this necessitates significant changes to the home environment. For example, carpets may need to be removed if regular vacuuming provides inadequate dust control.

Pathogenesis

Exposure to an environmental trigger or allergen causes the release of inflammatory mediators in the airways. These mediators activate more inflammatory cells, thus creating a cycle of airway inflammation involving eosinophils, CD4$^+$ T helper (Th) 2 lymphocytes, interleukins,

Asthma triggers	
Type of trigger	Examples
Allergens	House dust mite
	Pollen
	Animal dander and feathers
Airborne irritants	Pollution
	Tobacco smoke
	Fumes
	Cold air
	Thunderstorms
	Mould and damp
Drugs	Non-steroidal anti-inflammatory drugs
	Beta-blockers
Infections	Upper respiratory tract infection
	Acute bronchitis
Foods	Sulphites in preservatives and wine
Physical activity	Exercise

Table 3.2 Potential asthma triggers

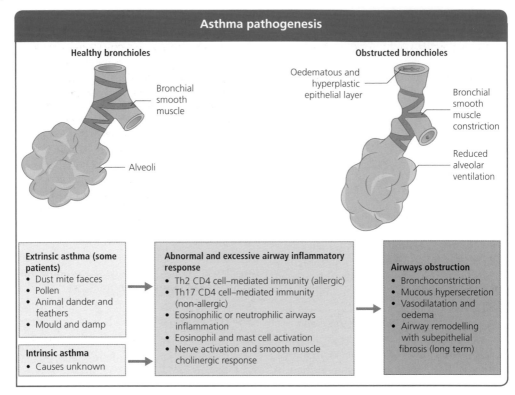

Asthma pathogenesis

Healthy bronchioles

Bronchial smooth muscle

Alveoli

Obstructed bronchioles

Oedematous and hyperplastic epithelial layer

Bronchial smooth muscle constriction

Reduced alveolar ventilation

Extrinsic asthma (some patients)
- Dust mite faeces
- Pollen
- Animal dander and feathers
- Mould and damp

Intrinsic asthma
- Causes unknown

Abnormal and excessive airway inflammatory response
- Th2 CD4 cell–mediated immunity (allergic)
- Th17 CD4 cell–mediated immunity (non-allergic)
- Eosinophilic or neutrophilic airways inflammation
- Eosinophil and mast cell activation
- Nerve activation and smooth muscle cholinergic response

Airways obstruction
- Bronchoconstriction
- Mucous hypersecretion
- Vasodilatation and oedema
- Airway remodelling with subepithelial fibrosis (long term)

Figure 3.4 Pathogenesis of asthma. Immunoglobulin (Ig) E, interleukin (IL)-4, IL-5, IL-13, IL-17, IL-33, histamine and leukotrienes are key mediators. Th, T-helper cells.

tumour necrosis factor α, leukotrienes and mast cell tryptase (**Figure 3.4**). In some cases, neutrophils play a role.

The inflammation narrows the small airways by increasing mucus secretion, constricting smooth muscle and causing oedema. These pathological changes make breathing more difficult.

Long-term airway remodelling occurs when subepithelial fibrosis prevents airways from returning to their normal diameter.

Clinical features

The most common symptoms of asthma are:

- episodic breathlessness
- wheeze
- dry cough

The dyspnoea and cough are worse on waking or during exercise, as well as after a viral upper respiratory tract infection or exposure to fumes or changes in weather.

Mild disease causes episodes of cough alone. During periods of worse asthma, patients are often woken by cough and dyspnoea in the middle of the night. Some patients produce small amounts of white or yellow sputum. In more severe episodes, dyspnoea is usually the dominant symptom and may necessitate emergency treatment in hospital (see page 303).

Between episodes of asthma, patients may have no symptoms. However, with very longstanding disease a degree of chronic airways obstruction can develop, which causes persistent dyspnoea on exertion.

Patients with asthma are often atopic. A history of eczema, hay fever and nasal polyps is common.

Chronic cough, sometimes producing yellow phlegm, with few other symptoms is a common presentation of asthma. The diagnosis is often not suspected. The cough varies in intensity over time but if severe can wake the patient at night. It is exacerbated by tobacco smoke or other fumes, and eased by bronchodilator treatment.

Between episodes, there are no signs. However, on examination during periods of poor control, a polyphonic expiratory wheeze may be audible.

During more severe exacerbations, the patient has:

- tachycardia
- an increased respiratory rate
- pulsus paradoxus (an exaggerated drop in blood pressure on inspiration)
- evidence of a hyperexpanded chest
- poor chest expansion on inspiration bilaterally
- a widespread expiratory polyphonic wheeze

Bilateral quiet breath sounds and central cyanosisare signs of a very severe attack (see Chapter 11).

Complications of asthma include:

- allergic bronchopulmonary aspergillosis (ABPA)
- lobar collapse (sputum plugs)
- pneumothorax and pneumomediastinum

- chronic respiratory failure (in severe, long-standing disease)
- complications of corticosteroid therapy

> **Asthma exacerbations requiring hospital treatment are frequently preceded by a period of increasingly poor disease control.** Worsening symptoms and increased use of bronchodilators suggest poor control.
>
> Hospital admissions can be prevented by educating patients to recognise poor control and accordingly increase their use of regular medications (e.g. inhaled corticosteroids). A course of oral prednisolone may also be beneficial.

Diagnostic approach

No simple diagnostic test is available for asthma. The diagnosis is made by identifying variable airflow obstruction. This is done either through a classic history combined with a good response to inhaled treatment, or through home PEFR recordings (**Figure 3.5**) or pulmonary function tests.

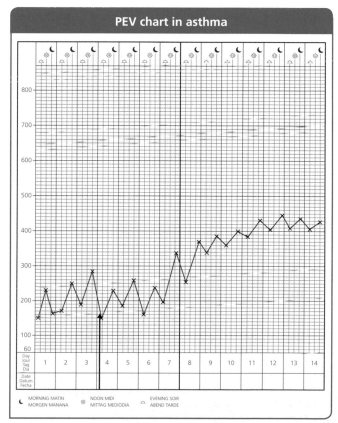

Figure 3.5 Peak expiratory flow chart showing diurnal variation in asthma and the response to preventer inhaler treatment starting on day 4 (arrow).

The following features increase the likelihood of a diagnosis of asthma.

- A cough that is worse early in the morning or at night or is associated with a trigger (e.g. exercise, medications, cold air or stress)
- A family history of asthma
- Peripheral blood eosinophilia
- Wheeze on auscultation
- Spirometry results showing partial or complete reversibility of airflow obstruction after salbutamol, or home PEFR recordings showing diurnal variation and decreases of $\geq 20\%$ during symptomatic periods
- A significant response to treatment (in terms of symptoms or the results of pulmonary function tests)

Differential diagnoses to be considered are:

- post-viral bronchial hyper-reactivity syndrome: temporary episode of mild reversible airways obstruction caused by a preceding viral URTI
- hyperventilation syndrome
- vocal cord dysfunction
- rhinitis or sinusitis
- gastro-oesophageal reflux
- heart failure
- COPD
- bronchiectasis
- interstitial lung disease
- inhaled foreign body
- bronchiolitis obliterans
- chronic large airways obstruction

> In middle and old age, long-standing asthma can change from an episodic illness characterised by full recovery with effective treatment to a disease with less day-to-day variation in symptoms but increasing chronic dyspnoea. Pulmonary function tests may not show full reversibility of an obstructive defect, even after intense treatment with oral prednisolone and nebulised bronchodilators.

Investigations

The following investigations are used in asthma:

- spirometry with reversibility
- home PEFR recordings
- chest X-ray
- skin prick allergen tests
- eosinophil count, total immunoglobulin (Ig) E, *Aspergillus* antibody and ANCA
- bronchial challenge testing (rarely necessary)
- vasculitis (very rare)

Spirometry

The results are usually normal between episodes. However, they show obstructive changes when the patient is symptomatic. FEV_1 improves by $\geq 15\%$ with bronchodilator treatment (Figure 2.16b).

Peak expiratory flow rate

The patient's PEFR is lower in the morning (diurnal variation), decreases during symptomatic episodes, and increases in response to inhaled or oral corticosteroids (**Figure 3.5**).

Chest X-ray

In asthma, the chest X-ray is usually normal. However, it can show hyperexpanded lungs if the patient has a severe attack or poorly controlled disease. The chest X-ray is more likely to be abnormal if the asthma is associated with another disease (e.g. ABPA and vasculitis) or if there is a complication (e.g. lobar collapse, pneumonia and pneumothorax).

Blood tests

Full blood count may show mild eosinophilia, and IgE may be mildly to moderately increased. In severe disease, measurements of ANCA and *Aspergillus* antibody help exclude vasculitis and ABPA, respectively.

Skin prick allergy testing

Many patients are allergic to one or more allergens. Sources of allergens include house dust mites, pet cats and dogs, and moulds (e.g. *Aspergillus*).

Bronchial challenge tests

Bronchial challenge is a spirometric test done before and after inhalation of histamine or methacholine. In patients with asthma, these agents decrease FEV_1.

Newer tests

Asthma is associated with an increase in exhaled nitric oxide, and cytological analysis of sputum shows eosinophils. These tests are usually available only in specialist clinics.

Management

The aim is to prevent symptoms and exacerbations. Ideally, treated patients will be largely symptom-free, with:

- minimal symptoms day and night
- minimal need for reliever medication
- no exacerbations
- no limitation of physical activity
- normal lung function (FEV_1, PEF, or both >80% of predicted or best value).

Asthma symptoms may be eased non-pharmacologically by:

- weight loss
- smoking cessation
- breathing exercises (e.g. Buteyko breathing)
- allergen reduction or removal (e.g. By regularly vacuuming or ridding the home of carpets)
- psychological help (e.g. for stress)

> **Buteyko breathing** is a set of breathing exercises used to help reduce dysfunctional breathing and develop a good breathing pattern.

Medication

Medical therapy for asthma is stepwise. As the disease worsens, the strength and variety of treatments used to control symptoms are increased. Thus, mild disease requires step 1 treatment (intermittent use of bronchodilators only), and severe disease that is difficult to control requires step 5 treatment (a range of anti-inflammatory and bronchodilator medications) (**Figure 3.6**).

Steroids and anti-inflammatory agents

The mainstay of treatment is regular use of inhaled corticosteroids. These drugs reduce inflammation of the airways, thus controlling chronic symptoms and preventing exacerbations. The dose of inhaled steroid is increased until symptoms are controlled. It is then reduced to a dose that maintains freedom from symptoms. Symptoms worsened by a trigger are treated by increasing the dose temporarily.

The choice of inhaled steroid largely depends on which inhaler the patient is best able to use effectively. The following are added to inhaled corticosteroids to treat patients whose asthma symptoms are not controlled by inhaled corticosteroids alone (**Figure 3.6**):

- long-acting bronchodilators (e.g. Salmeterol and tiotropium)
- leukotriene antagonists
- aminophylline or theophylline

Systemic corticosteroids are necessary for more severe exacerbations. They are sometimes used in the long term for patients with very severe asthma not controlled by high doses of inhaled therapies alone.

Bronchodilators (β-agonists or muscarinic antagonists, and theophyllines)

Inhaled short-acting bronchodilators (**Table 2.32**) are used when necessary to relieve residual symptoms and regularly during exacerbations. Examples are salbutamol, terbutaline and ipratropium bromide. The frequency of their use indicates the patient's level of asthma control.

During more severe exacerbations, salbutamol and ipratropium are given by nebuliser. Nebulisers deliver the drugs at a higher dose, and one that is not reliant on the patient's inhaler technique. Intravenous magnesium or infusions of salbutamol or aminophylline are used for very severe attacks.

Patients experiencing very severe attacks (status asthmaticus) may require intubation and mechanical ventilation to give the treatments time to reduce the degree of airways obstruction (see page 303).

Specialist therapies for severe poorly controlled asthma

Anti-IgE therapy with omalizumab benefits some patients with severe poorly controlled asthma and high IgE. Bronchial thermoplasty

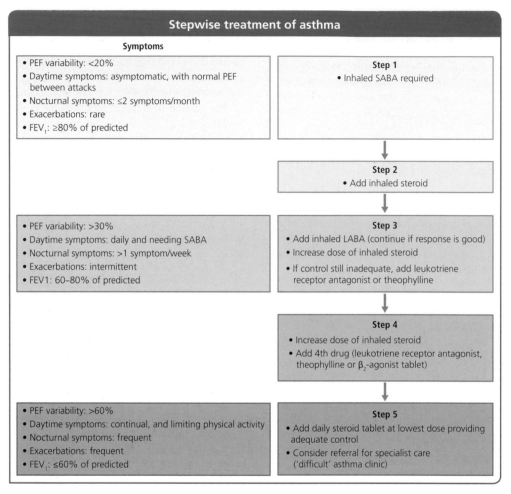

Figure 3.6 Stepwise treatment of asthma. FEV_1, forced expiratory volume (in 1 s); LABA, long-acting β_2 agonist; PEF, peak expiratory flow; SABA, short-acting β_2-agonist.

(radiofrequency heat treatment of bronchial walls to reduce smooth muscle content) can help patients with severe steroid-dependent asthma.

Prognosis

Asthma has a good prognosis if treated successfully. However, poorly controlled asthma is responsible for about 1100 deaths/year in the UK and 250,000 deaths/year worldwide. An estimated 75% of hospital admissions for asthma and 90% of deaths in the UK could be avoided with improved management of chronic disease. To achieve this goal, it is essential to ensure that patients have a good understanding of their treatment.

If a patient with asthma develops worsening symptoms, check the following:

- Adherence: are they using the inhaled steroids regularly?

- Inhaler technique: poor technique results in poor asthma control

- Trigger factors, e.g. a new pet, smoking, untreated oesophageal reflux, non-steroidal anti-inflammatory drugs, starting β blockers, and personal stress

- Allergic bronchopulmonary aspergillosis: the patient may have developed ABPA, so total IgE and *Aspergillus* precipitans are measured.

Chronic obstructive pulmonary disease

Chronic obstructive pulmonary disease (COPD) is characterised by largely irreversible airways obstruction caused by exposure to an environmental irritant. In high-income countries, the irritant is usually smoke from cigarettes.

The disease is common worldwide. COPD is an umbrella term for a heterogeneous mix of pathological changes ranging from chronic bronchitis to emphysema.

> **Exacerbations of COPD are a leading cause of hospital admission.** Some patients have recurrent admissions, often several a year. Others have largely stable disease with infrequent exacerbations. Reasons for the difference are unclear, but both pathological and psychosocial factors may be involved.

Types

There are various types of emphysema, including:

- Centriacinar emphysema, also known as centrilobular emphysema, usually involves the upper part of the lungs. Changes spread outwards, starting from the bronchioles
- Panacinar emphysema is commonly seen in the lower part of the lungs. The alveoli are completely destroyed. It is usually seen in people with alpha-1 antitrypsin deficiency.
- Paraseptal emphysema involves the distal airways and can be associated with apical bullae.

Epidemiology

COPD is a leading cause of morbidity and mortality worldwide. The World Health Organisation estimates that 65 million of the world's population have moderate to severe COPD. However, the prevalence of the disease varies enormously between countries; it is only 0.2% in Japan but 6.3% in the USA. In the UK, about 900,000 people have a diagnosis of COPD, and an estimated further 2 million have undiagnosed disease.

The prevalence of COPD is underestimated, because the disease is often diagnosed only at an advanced stage. The prevalence of COPD increases with age; the median age at diagnosis is 53 years.

Overall, COPD is more common in men. However, in the USA and Canada the prevalence of COPD in women has increased as more women take up smoking.

Aetiology

Smoking is the single most common risk factor for COPD; it accounts for almost all COPD cases in high-income countries. However, tobacco smoke is not the only cause. Exposure to smoke from solid fuel used for cooking is a major cause of COPD in low- and middle-income countries (**Table 3.3**).

> **Tobacco smoke includes smoke from pipes and cigars, as well as from water pipes (smoking shisha) and cannabis cigarettes. All these forms increase the risk of developing COPD.** Inhalation of recreational drugs (crack cocaine and heroin) can cause more severe COPD.

Lung function naturally decreases with age. However, lung function declines faster in people who smoke. In those who give up smoking, the rate of decline decreases to fall in line with that of people who have never smoked (**Figure 3.7**).

Other factors that accelerate lung function decline are smoke exposure during childhood, maternal vitamin D deficiency during pregnancy, low birthweight, low socioeconomic status and poor diet (low fruit and vegetable intake).

Prevention

The most effective way to prevent COPD is to stop smoking. Once COPD has developed, smoking cessation can slow the rate of decline in lung function (**Figure 3.7**). Therefore newly diagnosed patients must be supported in their efforts to stop smoking.

Risk factors for COPD	
Environmental factors	**Host factors**
Occupational exposures	Smoking
Indoor air pollution	Alpha-1 antitrypsin deficiency
Outdoor air pollution	Childhood respiratory infections
	Bronchial hyper-responsiveness
	Asthma
	Low socioeconomic status
	Low birthweight
	Genetic predisposition
	Low intake of vitamin C
	Pulmonary tuberculosis
	Poor lung growth and development

Table 3.3 Risk factors for the development of chronic obstructive pulmonary disease

Pathogenesis

Exposure to noxious particles, such as oxidants in tobacco smoke, causes an excessive inflammatory response in the airways (**Figure 3.8**) driven mainly by macrophages, CD8 lymphocytes and neutrophils. This inflammation causes scarring and thickening to the respiratory epithelium that narrows the airways, and increases the number of mucous-secreting cells. Noxious particles also increase the number of proteinases in the lungs. These are normally neutralised by antiproteinases, but this increase upsets the proteinase–antiproteinase balance allowing the proteinases to digest lung tissue. These processes result in the three main features of COPD:

- hypersecretion of mucus
- small airways obstruction
- alveolar destruction (emphysema)

The relative extent of each of these pathological features varies between patients. One may be dominant, or there may be a more equal mix of two or all three. These features of COPD cause the physiological changes of airflow limitation, hyperinflation, gas exchange abnormalities and secondary pulmonary hypertension.

Chronic obstructive pulmonary disease usually progresses slowly. However, its severity increases if the patient has frequent exacerbations and comorbidities. Chronic bacterial colonisation of the bronchi is common.

Figure 3.7 Lung function decline in smokers. FEV_1, forced expiratory volume (in 1 s).

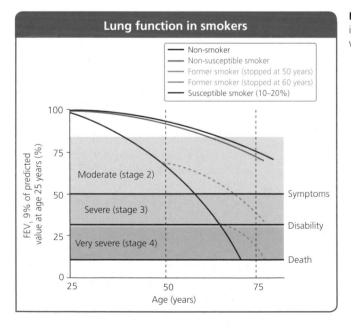

Lung function in smokers

- Non-smoker
- Non-susceptible smoker
- Former smoker (stopped at 50 years)
- Former smoker (stopped at 60 years)
- Susceptible smoker (10–20%)

FEV_1 9% of predicted value at age 25 years (%)

Moderate (stage 2)

Severe (stage 3)

Very severe (stage 4)

Symptoms

Disability

Death

Age (years)

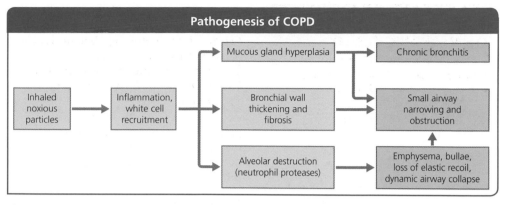

Figure 3.8 Pathogenesis of COPD.

Alpha-1 antitrypsin (A1AT) deficiency is a genetic condition that can lead to emphysema and liver cirrhosis. A1AT inhibits protease enzymes released by neutrophils. Therefore in A1AT deficiency there is uncontrolled lung damage in response to inflammation caused by smoking. About 1 in every 4000 people has A1AT deficiency in the UK, and 1 in 25 carry the faulty A1AT gene.

Clinical features

COPD is mainly diagnosed in the middle-aged and elderly. The disease is rare in people under 40 years of age, unless they have A1AT deficiency, HIV infection or a history of mis-using drugs (inhaled or injected).

Patients with COPD usually have a long history of gradually worsening exertional breathlessness over years. They also complain of a chronic cough, sputum production, wheeze and frequent attacks of acute bronchitis.

Many, but not all, patients with COPD experience exacerbations. These are defined as 'acute changes in a patient's baseline dyspnoea, cough and/or sputum beyond day-to-day variability sufficient to warrant a change in therapy'. Exacerbations are often caused by a viral upper respiratory tract infection or by a viral or bacterial bronchitis. However, they may also be brought on by changes in temperature or levels of pollution.

Exacerbations cause increased breathlessness, wheeze, cough and the production of sputum (which may be purulent). These symptoms may be preceded by coryzal symptoms (runny nose and sneezing) suggesting a viral upper respiratory tract infection.

Patients with severe exacerbations present to hospital. They may be confused and drowsy because of type 2 respiratory failure (Table 2.25). Exacerbations can be associated with a decrease in lung function; this can take patients up to 3 months to recover from, or it may become permanent. Patients with frequent exacerbations (two or more annually) have higher levels of lung inflammation, worse quality of life, a greater degree of chronic bacterial colonisation and higher mortality.

COPD is not just a disease of the lungs. General health status needs to be taken into account. Other factors to ask the patient about include comorbidities, psychological status and body mass index (**Table 3.4**).

Common complications of COPD are acute episodes of respiratory failure during exacerbations, chronic respiratory failure, cor pulmonale, pneumonia, a pneumothorax, bullae, slow weight loss with cachexia, lung cancer, pulmonary emboli, cardiovascular disease and depression.

Examination

Patients with mild to moderate disease may have few obvious signs. With more severe disease, many of the features of COPD can be identified from general inspection of the patient (see page 94).

The presentation of COPD can vary considerably between patients in:

Systemic consequences of COPD	
System	Consequence(s)
Psychological	Depression
	Anxiety
	Social isolation
Neurological	Cognitive impairment (caused by chronic hypoxia, inflammation or both)
Haematological	Polycythaemia
Cardiac	Ischaemic heart disease
	Left ventricular dysfunction
	Cor pulmonale
	Arrhythmias
Respiratory	Emphysema
	Chronic bronchitis
	Pulmonary hypertension
Musculoskeletal	Skeletal muscle atrophy and wasting
	Deconditioning
	Osteoporosis
	Fragility fractures

Table 3.4 Systemic consequences of chronic obstructive pulmonary disease

- the degree of airways obstruction versus the degree of emphysema
- the reversibility of the obstructive lung function changes
- the extent of associated bullous change
- the degree of associated systemic muscle wasting and weight loss
- the frequency of associated bacterial infection
- the frequency of exacerbations
- the severity of secondary pulmonary hypertension

'Pink puffers' and 'blue bloaters' are terms sometimes used to describe the two extremes of this phenotypic variation (**Figure 3.9**).

Diagnostic approach

Chronic presentations

In most patients, the history strongly suggests COPD. The main differential diagnoses to exclude are chronic asthma, pulmonary fibro-sis, chronic pulmonary emboli, cardiac failure and cardiac valvular disease. Examination helps exclude these diagnoses by assessing for:

- heart murmurs
- signs of cardiac failure (although these could also be caused by cor pulmonale)
- basal crepitations (suggesting pulmonary fibrosis)

Selected investigations are then necessary to confirm the presence of COPD and exclude other causes of chronic dyspnoea.

Acute presentations

The main differential diagnoses to consider for an acute exacerbation of COPD are left ventricular failure with pulmonary oedema, pneumonia, pulmonary embolism and a pneumothorax. These can largely be distinguished by chest X-ray, electrocardiography and blood tests. However, if pulmonary embolism is suspected computerised tomography pulmonary angiography (CTPA) is necessary.

Investigations

The following investigations are useful in diagnosing COPD:

- spirometry with reversibility, lung volumes, transfer factor and flow volume loop
- chest X-ray
- CT scan
- pulse oximetry and blood gases (in severe disease)
- electrocardiogram (ECG) and echocardiogram
- sputum microbiology

Pulmonary function tests

The diagnosis of COPD is confirmed by spirometry results showing irreversible airflow obstruction (**Figure 3.1**). FEV_1 is usually <80% of the patient's predicted values; if FEV_1 is ≥80% of predicted, a diagnosis of COPD is made only if respiratory symptoms are also present.

Disease severity is graded according to spirometry results or symptoms (**Table 3.5**).

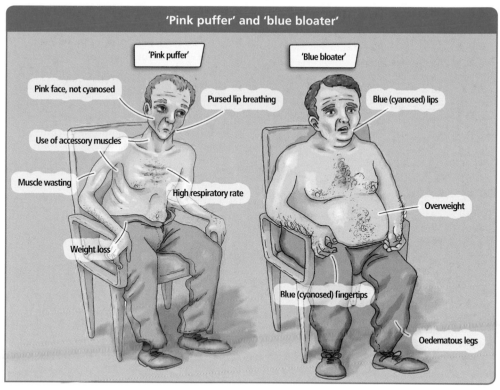

Figure 3.9 Classical presentations of chronic obstructive pulmonary disease: 'pink puffer' and 'blue bloater'.

Reversibility is assessed by spirometry before and after β agonist treatment or a 3-week course of oral prednisolone 30 mg/day. Many patients with COPD have a degree of reversibility in lung function, but some persistent obstructive changes will always remain.

Residual volume and total lung capacity are increased in COPD, reflecting air trapping and hyperexpansion of the lungs as a result of airways obstruction. COPD patients with emphysema have reduced gas transfer (transfer factor of the lung for carbon monoxide, T_{LCO} and transfer coefficient of the lung for carbon monoxide, K_{CO}). This decrease is caused by alveolar destruction reducing the surface area of the lung available for gas exchange. Emphysema results in loss of support of the bronchi. This loss of support causes a characteristic flow volume loop appearance resulting from dynamic collapse of the airways (Figure 2.19).

Pulse oximetry shows decreased oxygen saturation in patients with respiratory failure. If oxygen saturation is low, either acutely or chronically, a blood gases need to be done to measure $Paco_2$ as well as Pao_0, pH and HCO_3 to determine whether the patient has type 1 or type 2 respiratory failure (Chapter 2).

Radiology

Chest X-ray can show hyperexpanded lung fields, flattened diaphragm, and a paucity of lung markings. Bullae may be present (**Figure 3.10**), usually most obviously in the apices.

> **Care is needed to avoid mistaking a bulla for a pneumothorax.** This misdiagnosis and subsequent insertion of a chest drain could cause a bronchopleural fistula, which has a significant mortality and sometimes requires surgical intervention. The edge of a bulla curves out from the pleura at an acute angle, whereas the pleural edge in a pneumothorax curves away from the chest wall at a much shallower angle (Figure 3.10). A CT scan is sometimes necessary to help distinguish a bulla from a pneumothorax.

Classification of COPD severity

Grade	Definition
A Low risk and low symptom burden	Low symptom burden (mMRC 0–1 or CAT score < 10) **and** FEV$_1$ ≥ 50% (old GOLD 1–2) and low exacerbation rate (none or one annually)
B Low risk but higher symptom burden	Higher symptom burden (mMRC ≥ 2 or CAT ≥ 10) **and** FEV$_1$ ≥ 50% (old GOLD 1–2) and low exacerbation rate (none or one annually)
C High risk but low symptom burden	Low symptom burden (mMRC 0–1 or CAT score < 10) **and** FEV$_1$ < 50% (old GOLD 3–4) and/or high exacerbation rate (at least two annually)
D High risk and higher symptom burden	Higher symptom burden (mMRC ≥ 2 or CAT ≥ 10 **and** FEV$_1$ < 50% (old GOLD 3–4) and/or high exacerbation rate (at least two annually)

Table 3.5 Global initiative for chronic obstructive lung disease (GOLD) classification of chronic obstructive pulmonary

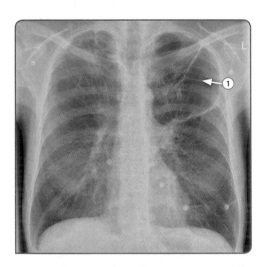

Figure 3.10 Chest X-ray of left upper lobe bullae ①.

A CT of the lungs or a CTPA is indicated:

- if transfer factor is reduced (to identify emphysema)
- if bullae are present (to define their extent, because surgery may be considered)
- if lung reduction surgery is being considered (see below)
- in COPD affecting younger patients or those with no obvious cause for their symptoms (to help clarify the diagnosis)
- if the clinical assessment or radiological findings suggest lung fibrosis, pulmonary emboli, cancer or bronchiectasis
- to investigate coincidental suspicious lesions on chest X-ray

The CT scan can show areas of emphysema (**Figure 3.11**), mild bronchiectasis (present in a quarter of patients with severe COPD) and an enlarged pulmonary artery trunk (if the patient has secondary cor pulmonale).

Blood tests

Stable COPD causes no major blood test abnormalities. However, COPD patients are often elderly and could have coexisting renal or liver disease. Serum A1AT levels are measured in younger patients with basal emphysema, or those with a family history of A1AT deficiency.

Additional blood tests may be required to exclude other diagnoses, for example B-type natriuretic peptide for cardiac failure or IgE for chronic asthma. C-reactive protein is not usually increased to >50 mg/L in acute exacerbations; a higher C-reactive protein concentration suggests a diagnosis of pneumonia or sepsis.

Cardiac investigations

An echocardiogram and ECG are often required to assess for cor pulmonale or cardiac causes of dyspnoea. Patients with severe COPD may have signs of right heart strain on ECG: right axis deviation and right ventricular hypertrophy. They can also develop multiple atrial ectopics (a 'wandering pacemaker'). Echocardiogram may show pulmonary hypertension before clinical cor pulmonale has developed.

Microbiology

Many patients with COPD are colonised with bacteria, usually *Haemophilus influenzae, Moraxella catarrhalis* or *Streptococcus pneumoniae.* Sputum culture helps exclude unusual pathogens that can complicate

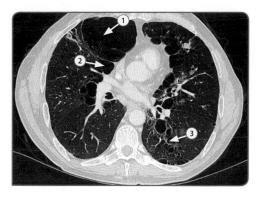

Figure 3.11 CT appearance of emphysema. ① Bulla. ② Paraseptal emphysema. ③ Centrilobular emphysema.

chronic COPD, for example *Pseudomonas* and non-tuberculous mycobacteria.

Exacerbations are often caused by bacterial bronchitis. Bacterial bronchitis normally causes purulent phlegm, which should be cultured to determine if resistant bacteria are present.

Management

The management of COPD requires a multi-disciplinary approach that includes educating the patient about:

- the background to their condition
- how to prevent and manage exacerbations
- breathing strategies (usually through a pulmonary rehabilitation course)
- smoking cessation
- the function of oral and inhaled medications
- oxygen use

For severe disease, patient education would also include consideration of home non-invasive ventilation, lung transplantation and eventually palliative care interventions.

Details of how the multidisciplinary approach is applied are in Chapter 12.

Non-pharmacological management

Various options are available for the non-pharmacological treatment of COPD patients.

- Smoking cessation. Patients with COPD must stop smoking. Smoking cessation leads to reduced symptoms, a small increase in lung function, and slowing of the rate of lung function decline.

- Pulmonary rehabilitation. Patients with a Medical Research Council breathlessness score of ≥ 3, those who have frequent exacerbations and those who have recently been admitted to hospital with an exacerbation are offered pulmonary rehabilitation (Chapter 2). Pulmonary rehabilitation improves exercise tolerance and quality of life.
- Non-invasive ventilation. Home non-invasive ventilation may help some patients with chronic type 2 respiratory failure.
- Palliative care. In severe disease with a poor prognosis, referral to the palliative care team can greatly help patients manage their symptoms (see Chapter 12).

Pharmacological treatments

The following drugs are prescribed to treat COPD:

- Inhalers. Inhaled therapies are the mainstay of the pharmacological treatment of COPD. Patients have varying responses to specific inhaler types, so different inhalers may need to be tried to identify which (if any) are most beneficial. An algorithm for the use of inhaled therapies to treat COPD is shown in **Figure 3.12**.
- Theophyllines. These may help control symptoms of dyspnoea and wheeze.
- Mucolytics. These may help loosen sputum to improve clearance.
- Oral steroids. Some patients with COPD feel that their symptoms improve when they are treated with long-term low-dose oral prednisolone. However, this treatment has serious adverse effects and should be avoided, if possible.
- Oxygen. Long-term oxygen therapy is offered to patients with $Pao_2 < 7.3$ on two blood gas samples 6 weeks apart when stable. This threshold for long-term oxygen therapy is lowered in some patients with cor pulmonale or high pulmonary artery pressures. Ambulatory oxygen therapy is offered to patients if it improves their exercise tolerance on a 6-min walk test or similar, and if they have significant desaturation on exercise.

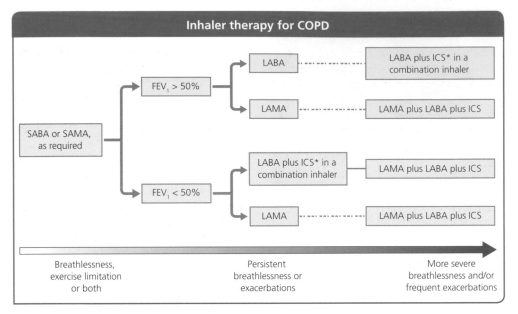

Figure 3.12 Inhaler therapy for chronic obstructive pulmonary disease. Dashed lines indicate when therapy should be considered. Solid lines indicate when therapy should be offered. FEV$_1$, forced expiratory volume (in 1 s); ICS, inhaled corticosteroid; LABA, long-acting β$_2$-agonist; LAMA, long-acting muscarinic antagonist; SABA, short-acting β$_2$ agonist; SAMA, short-acting muscarinic antagonist. *Consider LABA plus LAMA if ICS is declined or not tolerated.

Surgery

Surgical resection or closure of bullae can benefit selected patients. In lung volume reduction surgery, highly emphysematous parts of the lung are removed to allow less affected lobes to expand. Lung volume reduction surgery improves airflow, chest wall and diaphragm movements, and gas exchange in a small proportion of patients. However, it has a significant mortality and is suitable for only a small number of selected patients. Insertion of one-way valves via bronchoscopy is an alternative.

Lung transplantation is sometimes considered in patients with severe COPD who are under 65 years of age and who have responded poorly to treatment. They must have stopped smoking.

Management of exacerbations

Exacerbations are treated with oral corticosteroids (e.g. prednisolone 30 mg once daily for 5 days) and antibiotics (amoxicillin 500 mg three times daily for 7 days or doxycycline 100 mg once daily if the patient has an allergy to penicillin). More severe exacerbations may require the following.

- Hospital admission
- Regular nebulised bronchodilators
- Controlled oxygen therapy
- Non-invasive ventilation or possibly intubation and mechanical ventilation in cases of type 2 respiratory failure; however, mechanical ventilation is not appropriate for all patients, so this option must be considered carefully (see Chapter 11).

Prognosis

A significant proportion (14%) of patients admitted to hospital with an exacerbation of COPD die within 3 months.

Allergic bronchopulmonary aspergillosis

Asthma and cystic fibrosis can be complicated by allergic bronchopulmonary aspergillosis (ABPA). Patients with ABPA are allergic to *Aspergillus*. Inhaling of the fungal spores (ubiquitous in the environment) stimulates allergic airways inflammation causing:

- episodes of increased airways obstruction (manifesting as poorly controlled asthma)
- proximal bronchiectasis
- production of sputum cast and bronchial obstruction by tenacious sputum resulting in lobar collapse and bronchoceles (dilated fluid filled bronchi due to a proximal blockage by a sputum plug)

Diagnosis is made using blood tests that show very high levels of serum IgE (> 1000 IU/mL) and sensitisation to *Aspergillus* (raised *Aspergillus* specific IgG and IgE levels, *Aspergillus* skin prick test positive).

Treatment is the same as for asthma and for bronchiectasis, although many patients need oral corticosteroids to control their asthma symptoms. Patients are often treated with antifungal agents, e.g. itraconazole. Significant irreversible airways obstruction is common and a minority of patients develop progressive bronchiectasis and/or respiratory failure.

Other causes of irreversible airways obstruction

A proportion of patients with fixed airways obstruction have never smoked and do not have COPD. Causes of non-COPD fixed airways obstruction include:

- chronic asthma and ABPA
- bronchiectasis and cystic fibrosis
- post-tuberculosis
- bronchiolitis obliterans:
  - autoimmune disorders (e.g. rheumatoid arthritis and Sjögren's syndrome)
  - post-viral (usually after a childhood infection)
- graft-versus-host disease after stem cell transplantation
- graft-versus-host disease after lung transplantation
- use of certain medications (e.g. Penicillamine)
- chronic microaspiration
- exposure to toxic fumes

Treatment is similar to that for COPD. However, the response to corticosteroids and bronchodilators is usually minimal.

Answers to starter questions

1. No. Asthma and COPD are distinct entities. Asthma that is poorly controlled for a long time can lead to irreversible airways obstruction, which is clinically similar to COPD. However, the inflammatory processes underlying the two diseases are different.

2. Asthma is more common in people who:
   - have a parent or sibling with asthma
   - are overweight
   - smoke
   - have another allergic condition (e.g. hay fever or eczema)
   - have a mother who smoked during pregnancy
   - had a low birthweight

Answers *continued*

3. Only a small proportion (up to 50%) of smokers go on to develop COPD. This is largely because genetic factors determine the extent of the inflammatory reaction in response to exposure to tobacco smoke, as well as the lung tissue's susceptibility to damage. In the UK, the greatest risk factor for COPD is smoking (including passive smoking). Worldwide, other risk factors are significant; these include pollution and occupational exposure to triggers such as dust and fumes.

4. Some patients with COPD may have a partially reversible element to their airways obstruction, but most will not. Clinical trials have provided evidence for a small degree of reversibility in some COPD patients treated with certain inhaler combinations. In those with a more emphysematous COPD phenotype, significant reversibility is very unusual.

5. Results from large observational studies suggest that the risk of developing pneumonia is increased, possibly doubled, in COPD patients taking high doses of inhaled corticosteroids. The relationship is stronger with some types of inhaled corticosteroids than with others. The use of these drugs may also be associated with non-tuberculous mycobacteria infection. However, the evidence for a link between inhaled corticosteroids and infections is inconclusive, and inhaled steroids do reduce COPD exacerbations and still have a role in their management.

   Higher doses of oral prednisolone (>15 mg/day) are strongly immunosuppressive if taken for long periods, which increases the incidence of bacterial, fungal and viral infections. However, COPD patients rarely require prolonged high-dose oral corticosteroids.

6. Acute large airways obstruction causes acute stridor (wheeze on inspiration), which is a very specific sign for the disease. Therefore large airways obstruction is rarely confused with acute asthma. However, chronic large airways obstruction can present with cough or dyspnoea with obstructive lung function, and the chest X-ray can appear normal. These findings, and the fact that asthma is much commoner, mean that long-standing large airways obstruction is often mistakenly diagnosed as asthma.

   The actual diagnosis is suggested by the following.

   - A history including a possible cause of large airways obstruction (e.g. prolonged intubation, tracheostomy, foreign body inhalation, tuberculosis and vasculitis)
   - Lack of exacerbations caused by the usual triggers for asthma
   - Slow progression over many years
   - Fixed monophonic wheeze on examination

   The most crucial evidence that the patient does not have asthma is the absence of significant variation in lung function (either PEFR or FEV_1) and a positive Empey index (ratio of FEV_1, in mL, to PEFR, in L/min, > 10). A diagnosis of large airways obstruction is confirmed by a CT scan of the large airways and bronchoscopy.

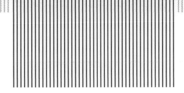

Chapter 4
Interstitial lung disease

Starter questions

Answers to the following questions are on page 183–184.

1. What investigations are needed for diffuse abnormalities on chest X-ray?
2. ILD, DPLD, HP, IPF, UIP, NSIP – why is it essential to become familiar with the meaning of so many abbreviations in this group of diseases?
3. How is disease severity judged in pulmonary fibrosis?
4. What tests are used to identify the underlying causes of a patient's interstitial lung disease?
5. Which patients with pneumoconiosis are entitled to compensation?

Introduction

Interstitial lung disease (ILD), also called diffuse diseases of the lung parenchyma or diffuse parenchymal lung disease (DPLD), is a heterogenous group of diseases featuring non-infective infiltrations of the interstitium and alveoli (**Figure 4.1**). ILD affects about 80/10,0000 men and 70/10,0000 women worldwide.

Interstitial lung diseases generally present with progressive breathlessness, restrictive lung function and reduced transfer factor. However, there are differences in the detail of their presentation. Diagnosis depends on the computerised tomography (CT) scan, and sometimes on lung biopsy.

The two most common ILDs are pulmonary fibrosis and sarcoidosis. These conditions are idiopathic or associated with a known cause (e.g. rheumatoid arthritis).

- Pulmonary fibrosis is often aggressive and progressive.
- Sarcoidosis is usually less aggressive, but it is persistent.

In all ILDs, long-standing disease produces changes similar to those seen in pulmonary fibrosis.

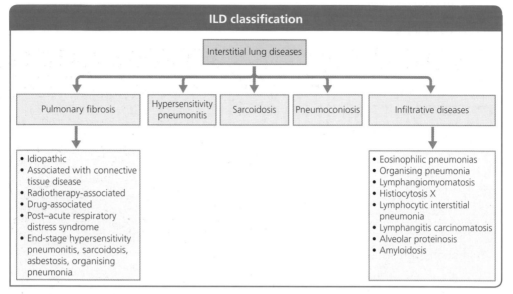

Figure 4.1 Classification of interstitial lung diseases.

Case 3 Progressive shortness of breath

Presentation

Mr Burrows, aged 70 years, is referred to the chest clinic with an 8-month history of progressive breathlessness and a non-productive cough.

Initial interpretation

In Mr Burrows's age group, common conditions causing slowly progressive dyspnoea are chronic obstructive pulmonary disease (COPD), heart failure and pulmonary fibrosis. The rate of progression and the variability and severity of the dyspnoea need to be assessed.

History

Over the past year, Mr Burrows has found it difficult to keep up with friends on outings with the local rambling association. His breathlessness has slowly worsened. He now finds himself breathless after climbing one flight of stairs and walks only slowly on level ground.

He is not breathless at rest or lying flat, so he does not have orthopnoea. He sometimes coughs but rarely produces sputum. He reports no swelling of his legs or systemic symptoms such as malaise, weight loss and fevers. He has never smoked cigarettes.

Interpretation of history

The lack of variation in the symptoms and the lack of both orthopnoea and ankle oedema point away from a cardiac cause of breathlessness. The history of slow progression suggests COPD or pulmonary fibrosis. However, Mr Burrows has never smoked, so COPD is unlikely.

Risk factors or exposure to possible aetiological agents must be identified. Therefore a thorough treatment and occupational history is required.

Further history

Mr Burrows has not had any rashes, skin thickening or muscle or joint pain.

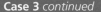
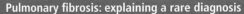

Case 3 *continued*

Pulmonary fibrosis: explaining a rare diagnosis

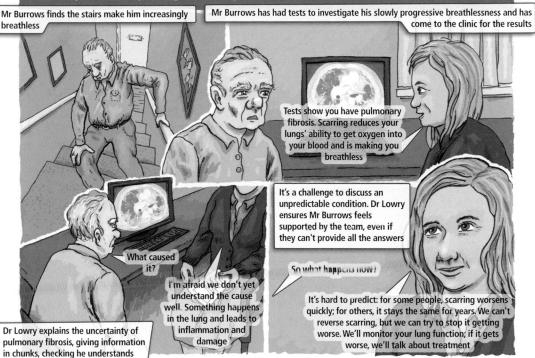

Mr Burrows finds the stairs make him increasingly breathless

Mr Burrows has had tests to investigate his slowly progressive breathlessness and has come to the clinic for the results

Tests show you have pulmonary fibrosis. Scarring reduces your lungs' ability to get oxygen into your blood and is making you breathless

It's a challenge to discuss an unpredictable condition. Dr Lowry ensures Mr Burrows feels supported by the team, even if they can't provide all the answers

What caused it?

So what happens now?

I'm afraid we don't yet understand the cause well. Something happens in the lung and leads to inflammation and damage

It's hard to predict: for some people, scarring worsens quickly; for others, it stays the same for years. We can't reverse scarring, but we can try to stop it getting worse. We'll monitor your lung function; if it gets worse, we'll talk about treatment

Dr Lowry explains the uncertainty of pulmonary fibrosis, giving information in chunks, checking he understands

He takes amlodipine for hypertension, but no other medication. He has no history of rheumatological diseases or cancer.

He worked as a salesman for many years and is not aware of any exposure to asbestos or other occupational dusts. He does not keep pigeons or other types of bird.

Examination

Mr Burrows is not breathless at rest. He has finger clubbing, but his joints are normal and he has no rashes or peripheral oedema. His jugular venous pressure is not increased, and his heart sounds are normal. The trachea is central. Lung expansion is equal but slightly reduced bilaterally, and percussion is normal. On auscultation there are bibasal fine inspiratory crepitations. Oxygen saturation is 95% on air but falls to 91% after walking 50 m.

Interpretation of findings

Mr Burrows has a typical presentation of pulmonary fibrosis: chronic progressive dyspnoea but few other symptoms, and characteristic fine basal crepitations. The latter are sometimes called Velcro crepitations, because they sound like Velcro being pulled apart.

In the early stages of pulmonary fibrosis, oxygen saturation is typically normal at rest but characteristically falls on exercise. The absence of rheumatological disease (e.g. rheumatoid arthritis and systemic sclerosis) or exposure to other causes of ILD (e.g. asbestos or pet birds, which cause hypersensitivity pneumonitis, HP) means that Mr Burrows probably has idiopathic pulmonary fibrosis (IPF). Further investigations are needed to confirm this diagnosis and assess its severity.

Case 3 *continued*

Investigations

Chest X-ray shows diffuse reticulonodular shadowing (**Figure 4.2a**), which was not visible on an X-ray taken 5 years ago. The results of routine blood tests including creatine kinase, erythrocyte sedimentation rate and C-reactive protein are normal. Tests for rheumatoid factor and antinuclear antibodies are negative.

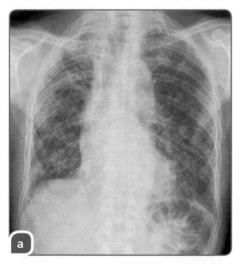

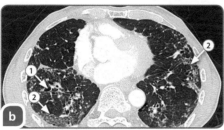

Figure 4.2 Idiopathic pulmonary fibrosis. (a) Chest X-ray showing diffuse reticulonodular infiltrates. (b) High-resolution computerised tomography shows pulmonary fibrosis in a pattern typical of usual interstitial pneumonia. ① Traction bronchiectasis. ② Septal thickening and possible honeycombing.

Electrocardiographic and echocardiographic findings are normal.

Spirometry shows a forced expiratory volume (in 1 s) of 2.25 L (69% of predicted) and a forced vital capacity of 2.74 L (65% of predicted). The ratio is 0.82, which indicates a restrictive lung defect. More detailed tests of pulmonary function show reduced lung volume (79% of predicted) and reduced transfer factor (transfer factor of the lung for carbon monoxide, T_{LCO}, 48% of predicted; transfer coefficient of the lung for carbon monoxide, K_{CO}, 61% of predicted).

High-resolution CT of the lungs shows subpleural and mainly basal fibrosis with areas of honeycombing (**Figure 4.2b**). The radiologist describes the subpleural and basal predominance and presence of honeycombing as typical of usual interstitial pneumonia (UIP).

Diagnosis

Investigations have confirmed that Mr Burrows has the changes in lung function and CT scan abnormalities of pulmonary fibrosis. The diagnosis is idiopathic pulmonary fibrosis, because the history, examination and blood tests have not identified a cause of ILD. Clubbing also strongly suggests idiopathic pulmonary fibrosis.

Because the clinical and radiological features are highly consistent with idiopathic pulmonary fibrosis, the respiratory consultant feels that a bronchoscopy or lung biopsy would provide no additional information.

Mr Burrows is given patient information leaflets on idiopathic pulmonary fibrosis. He also receives a follow-up appointment with repeat pulmonary function tests to help assess the rate at which his condition is deteriorating.

Case 4 Cough and painful shin rash

Presentation

Mrs O'Connor is 34 years old. She presents to her general practitioner with 3 weeks of dry cough, fatigue, and aching knees and ankles. Yesterday, she developed a rash on her legs.

Initial interpretation

Many diseases present with a dry cough. However, the rash is unusual and narrows the differential diagnosis considerably.

History

Mrs O'Connor was previously healthy. Her cough came on gradually and was not preceded by a respiratory infection. She describes the rash as painful and red, with tender lumps on both shins.

Interpretation of history

The history of painful rash on the shins suggests erythema nodosum, making the associated diseases sarcoidosis and tuberculosis possible diagnoses. A primary rheumatological problem should also be considered.

Sarcoidosis can affect many organs, not just the lungs. Therefore a full systemic enquiry is required (see **Table 4.6**).

Further history

Mrs O'Connor was born in the UK and does not smoke. She had a bacille Calmette–Guérin (BCG) vaccination in childhood and has never had tuberculosis or been in contact with anyone with tuberculosis.

Examination

Mrs O'Connor looks generally well. Her knees and ankles are swollen and red. However, they are not tender and no effusions are detected. Multiple raised, red, tender nodules are present on the anterior shins.

She has no finger clubbing or palpable lymph nodes. The results of cardiovascular, respiratory, abdominal and neurological examinations are all normal.

Interpretation of findings

The clinical examination suggests the rash is erythema nodosum. The history has established a low risk of tuberculosis, therefore sarcoidosis is likely. Other causes of erythema nodosum do not cause respiratory symptoms.

Investigations

Chest X-ray shows symmetrical and bilateral hilar lymphadenopathy (**Figure 4.3**). High-resolution CT of the chest confirms symmetrical smooth enlargement of multiple hilar and mediastinal nodes, with normal lung parenchyma. Bronchoscopy with endobronchial ultrasound-guided biopsy of the mediastinal lymph nodes identifies non-caseating granulomas.

Blood tests show high serum angiotensin-converting enzyme (ACE). The results of other blood tests, including full blood count, renal and liver function tests and

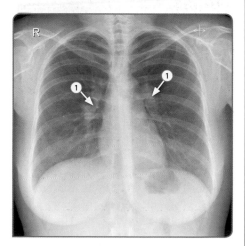

Figure 4.3 Chest X-ray showing bilateral hilar lymphadenopathy in sarcoidosis. ① The hilar nodes are enlarged.

Case 4 *continued*

calcium, are otherwise normal. Mantoux test and interferon-gamma release assay results are negative.

Diagnosis

The combination of bilateral mediastinal lymphadenopathy and erythema nodosum strongly suggests acute sarcoidosis. This type of sarcoidosis is known as Löfgren's syndrome. Non-caseating granulomas in the lymph node biopsy confirm the diagnosis, and the high serum ACE is supportive.

The negative Mantoux and interferon-gamma release assay results make tuberculosis unlikely. Löfgren's syndrome is usually mild and resolves spontaneously in 1–2 years.

Pulmonary fibrosis

In pulmonary fibrosis, the alveoli and lung interstitium are infiltrated by mesenchymal cells and increased amounts of extracellular matrix and collagen. The result is impaired lung function, progressive shortness of breath, and characteristic appearances on high-resolution CT.

Clinically, the term *pneumonia* describes alveolar infection; pathologically, it describes all infiltrations affecting the alveoli, whether infective or not. Many patients find the name organising pneumonia confusing, because they associate it with infection rather than non-infective consolidation of the lung.

Types and aetiology

Pulmonary fibrosis has multiple causes.

- Idiopathic pulmonary fibrosis, formerly cryptogenic fibrosing alveolitis (60% of patients with ILD). The most common histological pattern seen in idiopathic pulmonary fibrosis is that of usual interstitial pneumonia (see page 173).
- Connective tissue disease (10–20% of patients with ILD). Among patients with pulmonary fibrosis caused by connective tissue disease, 80% have rheumatoid arthritis, 14% have systemic sclerosis and 6% have other diseases (e.g. dermatomyositis). The histological pattern of a non-specific interstitial pneumonia (NSIP) (see page 173) is usually present.
- Drugs (**Table 4.1**). The drugs that most commonly cause pulmonary fibrosis are chemotherapy agents.
- Radiotherapy. Depending on the dose given and individual susceptibility, 5–15% of patients develop pneumonitis within 1–3 months of completing radiotherapy. This progresses to mature pulmonary

Drugs that cause pulmonary fibrosis	
Class	Example(s) known to cause pulmonary fibrosis
Chemotherapy agents	Bleomycin
	Busulfan
	Mitomycin
	Cyclophosphamide
	Methotrexate
	Melphalan
Antibiotics	Nitrofurantoin
Antiarrhythmic agents	Amiodarone
Disease-modifying antirheumatic drugs	Gold
	Leflunomide
	Penicillamine
	Sulfasalazine
	Etanercept

Table 4.1 Drugs that cause pulmonary fibrosis

fibrosis over 6–12 months.

- Acute respiratory distress syndrome.
- Other causes. Pulmonary fibrosis also occurs in hypersensitivity pneumonitis, sarcoidosis, pneumoconiosis and with chronic aspiration. It also occurs after heavy asbestos exposure (called asbestosis).

Epidemiology

The incidence of idiopathic pulmonary fibrosis (IPF) is 5/100,000 person years. In the UK, 2000 new cases are diagnosed annually. The incidence of IPF ranges from 14–43/100,000 worldwide

IPF is 1.5–2.0 times more common in men than in women. The disease is commoner in smokers and in persons whose occupations exposed them to dusts and fumes.

The median age for presentation of IPF is 70 years. Fibrosis associated with connective tissue disease typically occurs between the ages of 50 and 60 years.

Pathogenesis

Pulmonary fibrosis is characterised by an abnormal alveolar epithelium. Epithelial to mesenchymal transition leads to increased production of extracellular matrix proteins, destruction of lung tissue and scarring. The extent of associated inflammation varies.

There are two main patterns of pneumonia seen in people with IPF.

1. Usual interstitial pneumonia. The pattern is heterogeneous, with areas of normal lung, interstitial inflammation, fibroblasts and fibrotic cysts (honeycombing). The disease is resistant to treatment.
2. Non-specific interstitial pneumonia. The histological findings are thickening of the alveolar septum, variable inflammation and fibrosis. Non-specific interstitial pneumonia has a better prognosis than usual interstitial pneumonia.

These histological patterns correlate with radiological patterns (usual interstitial pneumonia, **Figure 4.4**, and non-specific interstitial pneumonia, **Figure 4.5**). The radiological

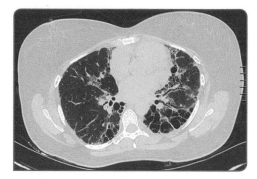

Figure 4.4 High-resolution computerised tomography shows pulmonary fibrosis of the usual interstitial pneumonia histological type. Subpleural basal fibrosis with extensive honeycombing is visible.

appearances of the end stage of many other ILDs are similar to those of usual interstitial pneumonia.

Clinical features

Pulmonary fibrosis presents with progressive dyspnoea over months and a dry cough. Pulmonary fibrosis caused by chemotherapy or radiotherapy presents more acutely, progressing over weeks.

On examination, patients have:

- finger clubbing (15–25%)
- reduced chest expansion bilaterally
- fine, late inspiratory Velcro crepitations, usually bibasal
- cyanosis and signs of cor pulmonale (in severe disease)

Signs of associated disease, for example rheumatoid arthritis, may also be present.

Diagnostic approach

Patients with suspected ILD need pulmonary function tests, chest X-ray and high-resolution CT. The diagnosis requires a multidisciplinary team approach. The joint American Thoracic Society–European Respiratory Society diagnostic criteria for idiopathic pulmonary fibrosis are shown in **Table 4.2.**

Blood tests

Abnormal blood tests can identify specific causes:

Diagnostic criteria for idiopathic pulmonary fibrosis	
Major criteria	**Minor criteria**
Exclusion of known causes of interstitial lung disease (e.g. drug toxicity, environmental exposures and connective tissue diseases)	Age > 50 years
	Bibasilar Velcro inspiratory crackles
Restrictive pulmonary function (reduced vital capacity with an increased FEV_1/FVC ratio) and impaired gas exchange (decreased Pao_2 or T_{LCO})	Insidious onset of breathlessness
	Duration of illness > 3 months
Bibasilar reticular abnormalities with minimal ground glass opacities on high-resolution computerised tomography	
Transbronchial lung biopsy or bronchoalveolar lavage showing no features to support a different diagnosis	

FEV_1, forced expiratory volume (in 1 s); FVC, forced vital capacity; T_{LCO}, transfer factor of the lung for carbon monoxide.

Table 4.2 American Thoracic Society–European Respiratory Society diagnostic criteria for diagnosis of idiopathic pulmonary fibrosis in the absence of a surgical lung biopsy

X-ray appearances in interstitial lung disease	
Disease	**Finding**
Idiopathic pulmonary fibrosis	Bibasal involvement, usually typical of disease with a usual interstitial pneumonia histological pattern
Associated with connective tissue disease	Bibasal, usually typical of disease with a non-specific interstitial pneumonia histological pattern
Radiotherapy-associated	Characteristic straight edge corresponding to field
Sarcoidosis	End-stage disease, predilection for upper lobes
Hypersensitivity pneumonitis	Predilection for upper lobes

Table 4.3 Characteristic X-ray appearances in interstitial lung diseases

- rheumatoid factor, antinuclear antibodies, creatine kinase, anti–neutrophil cytoplasmic antibody and extractable nuclear antigens (connective tissue diseases)
- avian precipitins (hypersensitivity pneumonitis)
- serum ACE (sarcoidosis)

Pulmonary function tests

Pulmonary fibrosis causes a restrictive lung defect. Lung volumes are small and transfer factor reduced. T_{LCO} <40% indicates severe disease. A 6-min walk test can be used to monitor progress and indicate prognosis.

Imaging

Chest X-ray shows diffuse, basal reticulo-nodular shadowing, but this investigation is insensitive (**Table 4.3**). High-resolution CT is essential and shows thickened intralobular septa, ground glass infiltration and honey-combing in a subpleural and basal distribution (**Table 4.4** and **Figure 4.5**). Pulmonary fibrosis caused by radiotherapy corresponds with the radiation field and has a straight edge.

Bronchoscopy and bronchoalveolar lavage

Bronchoscopy with bronchial/EBUS lymph node biopsies and bronchoalveolar lavage helps exclude other diagnoses, such as sarcoidosis, hypersensitivity pneumonitis, infection and rarer causes of lung infiltrations.

Lung biopsy

Histological findings usually suffice to confirm a diagnosis. Surgical biopsy (video-assist-

CT findings in interstitial lung disease	
Disease	**Finding(s)**
Common	
Pulmonary fibrosis	Basal subpleural arcading
	Honeycombing
	Some ground glass infiltrates
Sarcoidosis	Bilateral hilar lymphadenopathy
	Diffuse parenchymal nodules (especially along fissures and pleura)
	Upper lobe predominance
Hypersensitivity pneumonitis	Ground glass infiltrates
	Poorly formed centrilobular nodules
	Cysts
	Upper lobe predominance
Pneumoconiosis (asbestosis)	Identical to idiopathic pulmonary fibrosis but often with pleural plaques
Pneumoconiosis (other)	Simple: micronodular infiltrates
	Complicated: upper lobe nodular infiltrates that coalesce into masses and cavitate
Rarer	
Lymphangitis carcinomatosis	Localised thickening of interlobular septa
Langerhans cell histiocytosis	Irregular bizarre cysts
	Predilection for upper zones
Lymphangioleiomyomatosis	Scattered regular cysts
	Effusions
	Pneumothoraces
Alveolar proteinosis	Crazy paving thickened interlobular septa
	Ground glass infiltrates
Eosinophilic pneumonia	Patchy bilateral peripheral consolidation
Organising pneumonia	Patchy bilateral peripheral consolidation

Table 4.4 Characteristic high-resolution computerised tomography findings in interstitial lung diseases

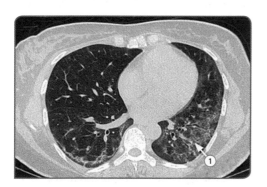

Figure 4.5 High-resolution computerised tomography showing pulmonary fibrosis of the non-specific interstitial pneumonia histological type. ① Ground glass shadowing and septal thickening.

ed thoracoscopic surgery or open procedure is warranted only if the diagnosis is unclear or if management depends on the results.

Management

The aims of management are to and treat underlying causes (e.g. drugs or gastro-oesophageal reflux), advise patients who smoke to stop and prevent progression with medical treatment if possible. However, clinical trial data on the efficacy of different treatments are limited. Options include:

- high-dose systemic corticosteroids (initially 0.5–1 mg/kg)
- *N*-acetylcysteine

- azathioprine, cyclophosphamide or both
- pirfenidone or nintedanib

The fibrosis component is considered largely irreversible. Non-specific interstitial pneumonia, and drug- and radiotherapy-induced pulmonary fibrosis, respond better.

Patients age <65 years with severe (T_{LCO} <40%) or progressive (reduction of >10% in forced vital capacity or >15% in T_{LCO} over 6 months) disease are suitable candidates for lung transplant. Pulmonary rehabilitation and oxygen therapy help relieve symptoms.

Prognosis

Idiopathic pulmonary fibrosis has a 5-year survival rate of 10–15%. Pulmonary fibrosis associated with connective tissue disease has a better prognosis. Drug- or radiotherapy-induced pulmonary fibrosis initially progresses rapidly and can be fatal. However, it then stops progressing and can even improve. Pulmonary fibrosis after acute respiratory distress syndrome improves over time.

> **Most patients will not have heard of intersititial pulmonary fibrosis, or know about its symptoms and course**. This lack of knowledge makes breaking the news of its incurable nature very challenging.

Hypersensitivity pneumonitis

Hypersensitivity pneumonitis (also called extrinsic allergic alveolitis) is an ILD caused by an immunological reaction to an inhaled antigen. Exposure to the antigen is usually related to the patient's occupation or a hobby. Examples are listed in **Table 4.5**.

Epidemiology

In the UK, bird fancier's lung is the most common form of hypersensitivity pneumonitis, and farmer's lung affects 0.4–7% of farm workers. Smoking decreases the risk of hypersensitivity pneumonitis.

Aetiology

Multiple exposures to the antigen cause a type 4 (cell-mediated delayed hypersensitivity) reaction. The reaction leads to pulmonary fibrosis predominantly in the upper lobes.

Clinical features

Acute and chronic hypersensitivity pneumonitis presents in different ways.

- Acute hypersensitivity pneumonitis presents with episodes of breathlessness, wheeze, cough, fever and crepitations

Specific hypersensitivity pneumonitis examples		
Disease	Antigen	Cause of exposure
Bird fancier's lung (caused by exposure to pet birds, pigeons and duck down duvets, for example)	Avian protein (from feathers, droppings or serum proteins)	Cleaning cages precipitates acute episodes
Farmer's lung	Thermophilic actinomycetes (e.g. *Micropolyspora faeni, Aspergillus* species)	Mouldy hay
Mushroom worker's lung	Thermophilic actinomycetes and mushroom spores	Picking mushrooms
Malt worker's lung	*Aspergillus clavatus*	Spreading barley
Winemaker's lung	*Botrytis cinerea*	Mould on grapes
Hot tub lung	*Mycobacterium avium*	Inhalation of aerosolised bacteria

Table 4.5 Examples of specific types of hypersensitivity pneumonitis

4–6 h after exposure. Symptoms settle within 48–72 h.

- Chronic hypersensitivity pneumonitis presents with progressive dyspnoea and cough. In this way, the presentation is similar to that of pulmonary fibrosis, but chronic hypersensitivity pneumonitis also causes the systemic symptoms of fatigue and weight loss. The patient may have no history of acute hypersensitivity pneumonitis.

Diagnostic approach

Diagnosis requires identification of exposure to a causative antigen (**Table 4.5**). The antigen may be cryptic (concealed or indirect), for example, in a case of bird fancier's lung caused by a new duck down duvet.

Pulmonary function tests

Hypersensitivity pneumonitis causes a restrictive or mixed restrictive–obstructive defect with reduced transfer factor.

Evidence of immunological sensitisation

Blood tests for specific immunoglobulin G antibodies to the causative antigen are positive (e.g. avian precipitins for bird fancier's lung). However, antigen exposure without hypersensitivity pneumonitis can also test positive for precipitins.

Imaging

In contrast to idiopathic pulmonary fibrosis, hypersensitivity pneumonitis has a predilection for the upper and middle zones.

- The chest X-ray shows patchy diffuse infiltrates in acute hypersensitivity pneumonitis, and reticulonodular shadowing in chronic hypersensitivity.
- High-resolution CT shows ground glass consolidation, centrilobular nodules, mosaicism and fibrotic changes (**Figure 4.6**).

Bronchoscopy

The differential cell count in alveolar fluid

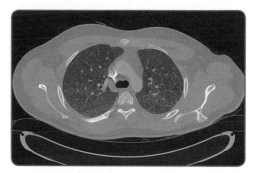

Figure 4.6 CT showing hypersensitivity pneumonitis.

collected by bronchoalveolar lavage usually shows > 40% lymphocytosis.

Lung biopsy

Transbronchial or surgical biopsies show small, poorly formed non-caseating granulomas, a mononuclear cell infiltrate and peribronchial fibrosis.

Management

The patient must avoid the causative antigen (if known). Treatment is with high-dose systemic corticosteroids (initially 0.5–1 mg/kg) but has inconsistent results and only a small number of patients benefit.

Prognosis

Acute hypersensitivity pneumonitis settles without consequences. However, repeated attacks lead to chronic damage. Chronic hypersensitivity pneumonitis progresses to end-stage pulmonary fibrosis (causing permanent scarring and symptoms) unless exposure to the antigen is prevented.

Patients with hypersensitivity pneumonitis are often reluctant to relinquish beloved pets, despite the high risk associated with continued exposure to the pet-derived antigen. Furthermore, antigens may persist in a home in which the pet has lived for a long time.

Sarcoidosis

Sarcoidosis is an inflammatory disorder of unknown cause. The disease is characterised by infiltration of affected tissues by non-caseating granulomas. It is most common in the lung but can affect multiple organs (Table 4.6).

Aetiology

The cause of sarcoidosis is unknown. Environmental agents, viruses and bacteria have all been suggested as triggers. Genetic background is relevant; sarcoidosis is associated with autoimmunogenic HLA-DRB1*0301 allele.

Pulmonary and extrapulmonary manifestations of sarcoidosis		
Organ or organ system	Symptoms	Frequency (%)
Lungs	Dry cough, breathlessness, bilateral hilar lymphadenopathy, pulmonary fibrosis and traction bronchiectasis	> 90
General	Systemic (usually mild) symptoms: fever, weight loss, night sweats and decreased appetite	80
Liver	Hepatomegaly and abnormal liver function test results	60
	Portal fibrosis and cirrhosis	Rare
	Portal hypertension	Rare
Spleen and blood	Splenomegaly	40
	Anaemia, neutropenia, lymphopenia and thrombocytopenia	Uncommon
Musculoskeletal system	Polyarthralgia (usually knees, ankles, wrists and elbows)	15–40
	Swelling and tenderness of fingers	
Kidneys	Nephrolithiasis, renal infiltration, obstructive uropathy, renal sarcoidosis (granulomas) and hypercalcaemia (renal calculi)	35
Eyes	Uveitis, episcleritis or scleritis, conjunctivitis, optic atrophy (rare) and extraocular muscle involvement	25
Skin	Erythema nodosum (tender erythematous nodules on anterior shin) in acute disease	25
	Lupus pernio (purple, firm, non-tender raised skin infiltates) in chronic disease	< 10
Heart	Electrocardiogram conduction defects or sudden fatal arrhythmias	5–25
	Restrictive cardiomyopathy	< 5
	Cardiac failure	Rare
Central nervous system	Cranial nerve palsies, optic neuritis and peripheral neuropathy	5–20
	Focal neurology due to central nervous system deposits	< 5
	Chronic aseptic meningitis	Rare
Salivary (including parotid) glands	Symmetrical enlargement and sicca syndrome, sometimes with facial palsy (Heerfordt's syndrome)	5
Endocrine system	Hypercalciuria and hypercalcaemia	5
	Hypopituitarism and diabetes insipidus (pituitary granulomas)	Rare
Ear, nose and throat	Sinus or nasal granulomas and destructive nasal lesions	Rare

Table 4.6 Pulmonary and extrapulmonary manifestations of sarcoidosis

Epidemiology

In the UK, the incidence of sarcoidosis is 5–10/100,000. The incidence is higher in Irish, West Indian and African-American populations. The most common age at presentation is between 20 and 40 years, and it is slightly commoner in women.

Pathogenesis

Sarcoidosis is caused by a cell-mediated immunological response that causes granulomas and fibrosis in affected organs.

Clinical features

A third of patients with sarcoidosis are asymptomatic.

- Acute sarcoidosis (Löfgren's syndrome) presents as bihilar lymphadenopathy frequently associated with erythema nodosum, low-grade fever and arthralgia
- Chronic sarcoidosis has an insidious onset. Its course is relapsing and remitting, and progressive in 30%.

Clinical presentation depends on the organ (or organs) affected. Lung disease causes a dry cough and dyspnoea.

Sarcoidosis is classified into four stages according to chest X-ray appearance (**Table 4.7**). Fine end inspiratory crackles may be heard, but often no lung signs are detectable. Common extrapulmonary presentations are shown in **Table 4.6.**

> **Sarcoidosis is occasionally almost asymptomatic,** with near-normal lung function despite extensive changes on chest X-ray.

Diagnostic approach

Diagnosis requires histological confirmation of non-caseating granulomas in affected tissue. Granulomas also occur in other conditions, such as tuberculosis, fungal infections and hypersensitivity pneumonitis. Therefore these have to be considered in the differential diagnosis.

Blood tests

Serum ACE concentrations are increased in up to 80% of patients and mirror disease activity. Hypercalcaemia occurs in 2–5%. Liver infiltration is common and is the reason for the mildly abnormal liver function test results (e.g. increased alkaline phosphatase).

Pulmonary function tests

Lung involvement causes a mixed obstructive–restrictive pattern of results. Transfer factor is reduced.

Imaging

Chest X-ray can show symmetrical smooth hilar lymphadenopathy (see **Figure 4.3**), pulmonary infiltrates (**Figure 4.7**), or both. Alternatively, fibrosis may be present predominantly in the upper and middle zones (**Table 4.7** and **Figure 4.8**).

The differential diagnosis of hilar lymphadenopathy is lymphoma and tuberculosis. High-resolution CT is essential for the diagnosis of sarcoidosis and to define the extent of the disease (**Figure 4.9**).

The involvement of other organs can be identified by ultrasound and CT of the abdomen, magnetic resonance imaging of the brain or heart, and echocardiography.

Stages of pulmonary sarcoidosis				
Stage	Chest X-ray findings	Symptoms	Frequency (%)	Remission rate (%)
0	Normal	None	10	
1	Bilateral hilar lymphadenopathy	None or mild cough	50	≤ 90
2	Parenchymal infiltrates and bilateral hilar lymphadenopathy	None, breathlessness or cough	25	≤ 70
3	Parenchymal infiltrates only	Progressive breathlessness	15	≤ 20
4	Advanced pulmonary fibrosis	Progressive breathlessness	5	≤ 5

Table 4.7 Stages of pulmonary sarcoidosis

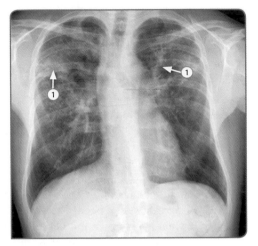

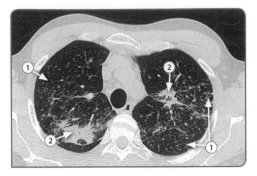

Figure 4.9 High-resolution computerised tomography showing chronic sarcoidosis. ① Micronodular infiltrate. ② Areas of more confluent infiltrations.

Figure 4.7 Chest X-ray showing pathological changes in chronic sarcoidosis: bilateral apical interstitial infiltrates ① with upper lobe volume loss. The volume loss of upper lobe has pulled up the upper hilar pole.

Other tests

Heart block and arrhythmias caused by cardiac sarcoidosis are identified by electrocardiography or 24-h Holter monitoring.

Tissue biopsy

The diagnosis of sarcoidosis is confirmed by the identification of non-caseating granulomas in biopsy samples. Commonly used approaches to biopsy include:

- endobronchial ultrasound or surgical biopsy of mediastinal lymph nodes
- bronchial and transbronchial biopsies (positive in 70% of lung cases)
- biopsies of skin lesions, parotids, extrathoracic lymph nodes or liver

Management

Treatment is unnecessary for most patients with sarcoidosis. However, patients with progressive lung disease; hypercalcaemia; or eye, cardiac, renal or neurological involvement require prolonged treatment with systemic corticosteroids, hydroxychloroquine and (rarely) methotrexate or infliximab, which all reduce inflammation and granulomatous infiltrations.

Prognosis

Acute sarcoidosis usually resolves within 2 years. Chronic progressive disease can cause severe disability and, in a minority, death. Cardiac sarcoidosis rarely causes fatal arrhythmias. Patients older than 40 years or of Afro–Caribbean ethnicity have a poorer prognosis.

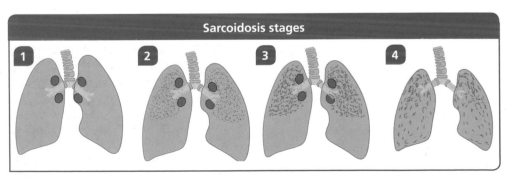

Figure 4.8 The four stages of sarcoidosis. Stage 1, bilateral hilar nodes with no lung parenchymal disease. Stage 2, hilar nodes with a parenchymal infiltrate. Stage 3, parenchymal infiltrates alone. Stage 4, extensive pulmonary fibrosis.

Pneumoconiosis

Pneumoconiosis is lung damage caused by inhalation of mineral dusts, usually through occupational exposure. The exposure must be prolonged or severe for the disease to develop, usually insidiously. The key to diagnosis is a history of occupational exposure.

Many types of pneumoconiosis exist. Only the commonest forms are discussed here. In the UK, patients whose lung function is impaired by pneumoconiosis are entitled to compensation (see page 184).

> In pneumoconiosis, the physician's role extends beyond diagnosis and treatment. They should also provide information about compensation schemes for industrial diseases.

Asbestos exposure also causes various other benign and malignant disorders.

- Pleural plaques: localised (focal) pleural thickening, often with calcification, that are visible on chest X-ray but are asymptomatic.
- Benign diffuse pleural thickening and exudative effusions: potential causes of mild dyspnoea, chest pain and restrictive lung function defects.
- Malignant mesothelioma: a primary neoplasm of the pleura caused only by asbestos exposure (see page 225).
- Bronchial carcinoma: asbestos exposure and smoking synergistically increase the risk of developing bronchial carcinoma, mainly adenocarcinoma.

Asbestosis

Asbestos fibres consist of metal silicates that induce tissue fibrosis and readily reach the lower respiratory tract when inhaled. Asbestos has heat-resistant properties and was used as a building and insulating material.

Occupational exposure occurred in dockworkers, pipe laggers, rail and ship workers, and those in the building trade (especially plumbers, roofers and carpenters). Unless precautions are taken, the risk of exposure continues during the renovation and demolition of buildings erected before the use of asbestos was banned as a building material.

Heavy exposure causes pulmonary fibrosis that is indistinguishable from idiopathic pulmonary fibrosis. Asbestosis is suggested by:

- presentation at a younger age than is usual for idiopathic pulmonary fibrosis
- the presence of pleural plaques
- the finding of asbestos bodies (asbestos fibres covered with ferritin) in fluid collected by bronchoalveolar lavage

No specific treatments are available for asbestosis.

Coal worker's pneumoconiosis

Coal worker's pneumoconiosis is caused by exposure to coal dust. The disease affects current and former coal miners. Some patients progress from simple to more complicated disease.

- Simple coal worker's pneumoconiosis: multiple diffuse small opacities on chest X-ray, with minimal effects on lung function.
- Complicated coal worker's pneumoconiosis (or progressive massive fibrosis): progressive dyspnoea and a cough with black sputum. This type of pneumoconiosis leads to respiratory failure. Chest X-ray shows expanding fibrotic masses in the upper lobes. Pulmonary function tests show irreversible mixed obstructive–restrictive defects.
- Caplan's syndrome: coal worker's pneumoconiosis associated with rheumatoid arthritis, with multiple cavitating peripheral nodules.

No treatment options are available except for removal from ongoing exposure to coal dust.

Silicosis

Silicosis is caused by inhalation of dusts containing silica (silicon dioxide). Exposure occurs in multiple occupations, including coal mining, sand blasting, quarrying and stonemasonry. Presentations include the following.

- Asymptomatic silicosis: upper lobe micronodular infiltrates on chest X-ray, associated with hilar lymphadenopathy with 'eggshell' calcification.
- Complicated silicosis: the micronodules coalesce to form a destructive lung disease similar to progressive massive fibrosis.
- Acute silicosis: rapidly progressive alveolar infiltrates occurring within a few months

of high-level exposure that usually cause fatal respiratory failure.

Silicosis increases the risk of pulmonary tuberculosis.

Other types of pneumoconiosis

Many types of pneumoconiosis cause micro-nodular infiltrations. Other, rarer types of pneumoconiosis include:

- Exposure to quartz can cause progressive massive fibrosis.
- Inhalation of beryllium causes berylliosis, which presents similarly to sarcoidosis.
- Acute exposure to cadmium and beryllium fumes causes a diffuse alveolitis.

Rare types of interstitial lung disease and lung infiltrations

A range of rare diseases produce distinct types of lung infiltrations and appearances on CT (**Table 4.4**). Specific causes are discussed below.

Eosinophilic and organising pneumonias

These two diseases are characterised by bilateral patches of consolidation caused by infiltration with eosinophils (in eosinophilic pneumonias) or intraluminal plugs of connective tissue (in organising pneumonia). Both diseases are usually idiopathic. However:

- eosinophilic pneumonia is also caused by drugs or infestation with parasites such as *Toxocara* or *Ascaris* (Löffler's syndrome)
- organising pneumonia is associated with connective tissue diseases, drugs (e.g. amiodarone), radiotherapy and infections

Patients have a short history of cough, dyspnoea and fever. An increased percentage of eosinophils (>25%) in fluid collected by bronchoalveolar lavage is diagnostic of pulmonary eosinophilia. Lung biopsy is required to confirm a diagnosis of organising pneumonia.

Both eosinophilic and organising pneumonias respond rapidly to systemic corticosteroids but can cause pulmonary fibrosis.

Lymphocytic interstitial pneumonia

Lymphocytic interstitial pneumonia is characterised by interstitial infiltration with lymphocytes. The disease is usually idiopathic, associated with HIV infection or autoimmune diseases. Fluid collected by bronchoalveolar lavage has a high lymphocyte count (lymphocytosis), but confirmation of the diagnosis requires a lung biopsy.

Treatment is with systemic corticosteroids.

Lymphangiomyomatosis and Langerhans cells histiocytosis

These diseases produce lung cysts (**Figure 4.10**). In lymphangiomyomatosis, this is caused by smooth muscle proliferation; in Langerhans cells histiocytosis, infiltration by Langerhans cells (a type of dendritic cell).

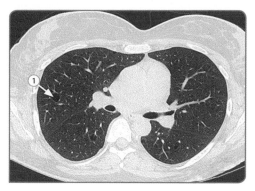

Figure 4.10 High-resolution computerised tomography of the chest, showing lung cyst ① caused by lymphangiomyomatosis.

Both diseases cause progressive respiratory failure but are differentiated as follows.

- Lymphangiomyomatosis affects only women and is associated with tuberous sclerosis. The disease causes spontaneous pneumothoraces and effusions (often chylous) as well as progressive respiratory failure. Treatment is by hormonal manipulation with intramuscular injections of medroxyprogesterone and/or calcineurin inhibitors (e.g. tacrolimus).
- Langerhans cells histiocytosis occurs almost exclusively in smokers. The treatment is smoking cessation.

Alveolar proteinosis

In alveolar proteinosis, alveoli become filled with lipoproteinaceous material. This pathological change causes cough and dyspnoea, and widespread alveolar infiltrates. Diagnosis is confirmed by bronchoalveolar lavage. Treatment requires whole-lung lavage or injections of granulocyte–macrophage colony–stimulating factor.

Amyloidosis

Amyloidosis can cause diffuse or nodular lung infiltrations. It can also cause endobronchial disease. A biopsy is required for diagnosis.

Lymphangitis carcinomatosis

Lymphangitis carcinomatosis is an infiltration of pulmonary lymphatics by malignant cells in patients with lung cancer or metastases. This process causes progressive dyspnoea and restrictive lung function, reticulonodular infiltrates are visible on chest X-ray. However, the disease has few respiratory signs.

No effective treatment is available.

Answers to starter questions

1. Diffuse abnormalities on chest X-ray have a wide differential diagnosis, ranging from infection to malignancy or any of the ILDs. A thorough history and clinical examination are necessary to identify associated diseases. For example, rheumatoid arthritis sometimes manifests as an ILD and a history of breast cancer might suggest previous radiotherapy as a cause of pulmonary fibrosis.

    The most useful initial investigations include:

    - blood tests such as autoantibodies, serum precipitins or serum ACE
    - high-resolution CT to fully define the lung shadowing and narrow the differential diagnosis
    - pulmonary function tests to assess disease severity
    Bronchoscopy and lung biopsy (depending on the clinical and high-resolution CT findings) may be needed to confirm the diagnosis.

Answers *continued*

2. Familiarity with the abbreviations used in discussions of interstitial lung disease aids understanding of this diverse group of diseases.

    The terms *interstitial lung disease (ILD)* and *diffuse parenchymal lung disease (DPLD)* are largely interchangeable. They describe diseases characterised by non-infective infiltration of the lung alveoli and interstitium.

    ■ Some ILDs are named as specific clinical syndromes: idiopathic pulmonary fibrosis (IPF) and hypersensitivity pneumonitis (HP).
    ■ ILDs are also described with their pathology: certain histological findings on lung biopsy can be present in several ILDs but are most closely associated with specific clinical syndromes. For example, usual interstitial pneumonia (UIP) occurs mainly with idiopathic pulmonary fibrosis (IPF) and non-specific interstitial pneumonia (NSIP) is often associated with connective tissue diseases.
    ■ Confusingly, some names have changed with time. Cryptogenic fibrosing alveolitis (CFA) is an old term that is largely interchangeable with IPF.

3. In pulmonary fibrosis, disease severity is judged using a combination of symptoms and objective markers. Functional impairment is assessed by asking how far patients can walk on the flat, how many stairs they can climb, and the effects of dyspnoea on their activities of daily living. Pulmonary function tests provide objective data, for example the degree of a restrictive defect and reductions in transfer factor (in severe disease, <40% of expected), distance walked and extent of desaturation in a 6-min walk test, and the presence or absence of cor pulmonale (e.g. pulmonary artery pressures on echocardiogram).

4. Tests done to identify the cause of a patient's ILD depend on the clinical context but include the following.

    ■ A screen for autoimmune diseases (including antinuclear antibodies, extractable nuclear antigens, anti–neutrophil cytoplasmic antibody, creatine kinase, rheumatoid factor, complement levels and immunoglobulin G), C-reactive protein, serum ACE (increased in some patients with sarcoidosis) and serum precipitins (to identify hypersensitivity pneumonitis).
    ■ Analysis of fluid collected by bronchoalveolar lavage helps differentiate hypersensitivity pneumonitis and sarcoidosis from idiopathic pulmonary fibrosis.
    ■ Lung biopsy is necessary to confirm a diagnosis. However, video-assisted thoracoscopic surgery is usually required, because a transbronchial biopsy is only rarely helpful unless the patient has sarcoidosis.

5. In the UK, patients exposed to asbestos are entitled to compensation include those with mesothelioma, primary carcinoma of the lung and diffuse pleural thickening affecting lung function. Patients with pleural plaques and unilateral pleural thickening do not qualify but other types of pneumoconiosis that affect lung function (especially complicated disease) do.

    Compensation is claimed directly from the employers. If the company has ceased trading, a one-off payment can be claimed from the state through the Pneumoconiosis, etc. (Worker's Compensation) Act 1979.

Chapter 5
Sleep and ventilatory disorders

Starter questions

Answers to the following questions are on page 193–194.

1. What should patients with obstructive sleep apnoea be advised about driving? Why?
2. What is high-quality sleep?
3. Why is obstructive sleep apnoea associated with an increased risk of heart disease and stroke?

Introduction

Sleep and ventilatory disorders are disorders that include ventilatory failure caused by obesity or neuromuscular disorders and sleep disordered breathing such as obstructive sleep apnoea.

In sleep disordered breathing there is an abnormality in either the quality or quantity of ventilation during sleep. Symptoms vary, from falling asleep inappropriately and feeling tired to snoring at night or experiencing episodes of nocturnal choking.

The commonest sleep disorder is obstructive sleep apnoea. In this condition, breathing is intermittently reduced or interrupted during sleep.

Case 5 Falling asleep at work

Presentation

Mr Carter, aged 45 years, has been referred by his general practitioner to the respiratory clinic, because he is finding it increasingly difficult to concentrate at the office. He even fell asleep in a meeting last week.

Initial interpretation

Tiredness and difficulty sleeping are common (**Table 5.1**). However, when people fall asleep at the wrong times, such as in the middle of a meeting at work, a more serious cause than just tiredness is likely.

History

Mr Carter has felt sleepy during the day for years, and he does not feel refreshed by a night's sleep. He snores so loudly that his wife sleeps in a separate bedroom, and his children hear him from their bed-

rooms. His wife says that sometimes during the night he seems to stop breathing briefly.

Since his weight has increased, Mr Carter has occasionally woken up choking and gasping for air. He says that his memory is not what it used to be. Given the opportunity, he naps during the day, frequently falling asleep while watching television in the evening.

Interpretation of history

Loud snoring, daytime somnolence, possible episodes of night-time apnoea and the inability to stay awake or concentrate at work all suggest significant obstructive sleep apnoea.

Further history

Mr Carter has no nasal problems and does not have hay fever. He has no history of

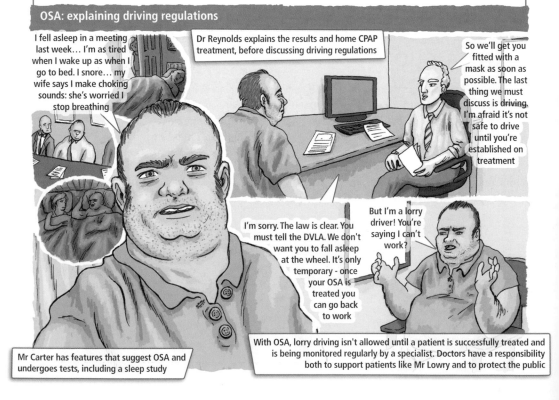

OSA: explaining driving regulations

I fell asleep in a meeting last week… I'm as tired when I wake up as when I go to bed. I snore… my wife says I make choking sounds: she's worried I stop breathing

Dr Reynolds explains the results and home CPAP treatment, before discussing driving regulations

So we'll get you fitted with a mask as soon as possible. The last thing we must discuss is driving. I'm afraid it's not safe to drive until you're established on treatment

I'm sorry. The law is clear. You must tell the DVLA. We don't want you to fall asleep at the wheel. It's only temporary - once your OSA is treated you can go back to work

But I'm a lorry driver! You're saying I can't work?

Mr Carter has features that suggest OSA and undergoes tests, including a sleep study

With OSA, lorry driving isn't allowed until a patient is successfully treated and is being monitored regularly by a specialist. Doctors have a responsibility both to support patients like Mr Lowry and to protect the public

Case 5 *continued*

Daytime sleepiness causes	
Category	Examples
Problems with nocturnal sleep	Fragmented sleep
	Sleep deprivation
	Irregular sleep pattern (e.g. because of shift work)
Drugs	Sedatives
	Beta-blockers
	Excess daytime caffeine
	Theophyllines
	Selective serotonin reuptake inhibitors
	Excess alcohol
Other medical conditions	Depression
	Narcolepsy
	Hypothyroidism
	Neurological conditions
Ventilatory disorders	Obstructive sleep apnoea
	Obesity hypoventilation syndrome
	Chest wall and neuromuscular disorders (see page 192 and Table 5.4)

Table 5.1 Causes of excess daytime sleepiness

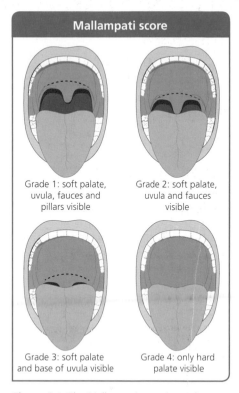

Mallampati score

Grade 1: soft palate, uvula, fauces and pillars visible

Grade 2: soft palate, uvula and fauces visible

Grade 3: soft palate and base of uvula visible

Grade 4: only hard palate visible

Figure 5.1 The Mallampati score is used to grade obstruction at the back of the throat: the higher the score, the smaller the passage.

depression or thyroid problems. However, his sleep routine is inconsistent; he rarely goes to bed at the same time each night. He does not take sleeping tablets but does smoke 20 cigarettes per day. He drinks four cups of coffee and two cups of tea daily, including one at bedtime. He drinks about 25 units of alcohol a week. He gets up twice each night to pass urine.

Examination

Mr Carter's body mass index is 32 kg/m², so he is obese. His collar size is 43 cm. Examination of his pharynx finds normal-sized tonsils and a Mallampati score of 3 is calculated (**Figure 5.1**).

He has a respiratory rate of 12 breaths/min. His blood pressure is 160/80 mmHg.

His oxygen saturation is 98% on room air. On auscultation, his chest is clear and he has normal heart sounds.

Interpretation of findings

Depression causes sleep problems but Mr Carter's mental health is good. Hypo- and hyperthyroidism also negatively affect sleep, so thyroid functions tests are warranted.

Poor sleep hygiene could contribute to Mr Carter's tiredness. The stimulating effects of nicotine and caffeine disrupt sleep, as does alcohol use.

Mr Carter's increased body mass index and large neck are classic characteristics

Case 5 *continued*

of patients with obstructive sleep apnoea. He has no other obvious reasons for his nocturnal upper airways obstruction. His Mallampati score of 3 supports a diagnosis of obstructive sleep apnoea, as does the hypertension, which is often associated with this condition.

Investigations

Investigations are done to identify any comorbidities that need attention and to determine the severity of the obstructive sleep apnoea. The results are as follows.

- Blood tests: thyroid function tests and full blood count are normal.
- Spirometry: normal results, with no evidence for coexisting chronic obstructive pulmonary disease (COPD)

- Chest X-ray: normal
- Epworth Sleepiness Scale score: 23
- Sleep study: pattern consistent with obstructive sleep apnoea (**Figure 5.2**)

Diagnosis

The Epworth Sleepiness Scale score of > 19 confirms severe sleepiness. The diagnosis is obstructive sleep apnoea.

The treatment is overnight continuous positive airway pressure (CPAP) which uses a small increase in both inspiratory and expiratory air pressure to splint the airways open. Mr Carter drives regularly, so is told that he must inform the appropriate authority of his diagnosis (in the United Kingdom, this is the Driver and Vehicle Licensing Agency, DVLA).

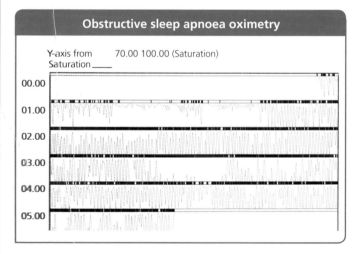

Figure 5.2 Result of overnight oximetry, showing the typical sawtooth pattern (70–100% oxygen saturation) of obstructive sleep apnoea.

Obstructive sleep apnoea

Obstructive sleep apnoea is the most common syndrome of sleep-disordered breathing. It is characterised by excessive daytime sleepiness and lack of concentration. These symptoms result from irregular overnight breathing caused by repeated partial or total collapse of the upper airway during sleep.

People with obstructive sleep apnoea are 2–7 times more likely to have a road traffic accident.

Patients often do not know that they have obstructive sleep apnoea, particularly if they sleep alone. Campaigns aim to increase awareness of the disease.

Epidemiology and aetiology

The prevalence of obstructive sleep apnoea is 1–2% in men and 0.5–1% in women aged 30–65 years. However, these figures may be underestimates, because obstructive sleep apnoea often remains undiagnosed.

The most common risk factors for obstructive sleep apnoea are listed in **Table 5.2**.

Pathogenesis

During sleep, the tone of the muscles in the upper pharynx reduces. This reduction in tone causes the upper airway to collapse (**Figure 5.3**). The resultant narrowing of the upper airway causes snoring (if it is partial) or apnoeic episodes (if it is total).

Increased inspiratory effort is needed to overcome the airway collapse. This effort causes a change from deep to light sleep (or awakening), so normal muscle tone returns and the patient starts breathing again. This cycle is repeated hundreds of times throughout the night, making sleep quality poor because it has been disturbed.

As sleep is disrupted, affected individuals feel unrefreshed in the morning. They are prone to daytime somnolence and decreased concentration and alertness.

Obstructive sleep apnoea risk factors	
Modifiable	Non-modifiable
Body mass index >30 kg/m²	Male sex
Collar size >43 cm for men and >41 cm for women	Age >40 years
	Perimenopause
Nasal congestion, polyps or deviated septum	Micrognathia or retrognathia
Diabetes	Acromegaly
Hypothyroidism	Family history of obstructive sleep apnoea
Sedative medications	Abnormal pharyngeal anatomy
Excess alcohol	

Table 5.2 Risk factors for obstructive sleep apnoea

Clinical features

Symptoms typical of obstructive sleep apnoea are:

- nocturnal choking attacks
- snoring
- daytime sleepiness
- feeling unrefreshed after waking
- nocturia
- personality change
- decreased concentration, short-term memory impairment, or both

Severe disease can lead to type 2 respiratory failure, especially if there is associated COPD (overlap syndrome). As well as severely

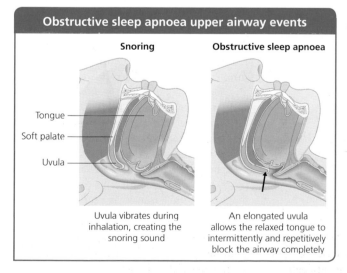

Obstructive sleep apnoea upper airway events	
Snoring	Obstructive sleep apnoea

Tongue
Soft palate
Uvula

Uvula vibrates during inhalation, creating the snoring sound

An elongated uvula allows the relaxed tongue to intermittently and repetitively block the airway completely

Figure 5.3 Upper airway events during obstructive sleep apnoea.

affecting quality of life, obstructive sleep apnoea is sometimes associated with life-threatening illnesses and complications, including:

- hypertension
- cardiac arrhythmia
- myocardial infarction
- stroke
- diabetes
- pulmonary hypertension

Diagnostic approach

Obstructive sleep apnoea is diagnosed using typical features in the history and on examination and by confirming apnoeic episodes with a sleep study. The most common differential diagnosis of obstructive sleep apnoea is snoring without evidence of apnoeic episodes ('simple snorers'). This is ruled out by doing a sleep study.

Clinical assessment may suggest obstructive sleep apnoea, but this diagnosis can only be confirmed by a sleep study.

During history taking, the Epworth Sleepiness Scale score is used to assess the severity of sleepiness (**Figure 5.4**).

Key features to assess during examination are weight and neck circumference, nasal patency and mandible size. Examine the upper airway; look for obvious obstruction and grade pharyngeal appearance using the Mallampati score (**Figure 5.1**). Examine the tongue for macroglossia, and assess dentition to look for obvious causes of obstruction.

Cardiovascular, respiratory and neurological examinations are carried out to identify coexisting diseases, some of which may be caused by obstructive sleep apnoea. Specific investigations include the following.

- Blood tests: thyroid function tests screen for hypothyroidism, as people who are hypothyroid can be at increased risk of OSA (and treatment of hypothyroidism could therefore help those with OSA) and the results of a full blood count would identify polycythaemia as high haemoglobin levels can occur in response to chronic low oxygen levels.

Epworth Sleepiness Scale

Do any of the following activities lead to sleep? Score your chance of dozing:

0 = none   2 = moderate
1 = slight   3 = high

☐ Watching TV

☐ Sitting and reading

☐ Sitting in a public place

☐ Sitting as a car passenger for an hour

☐ Sitting in traffic for a few minutes

☐ Lying down in the afternoon

☐ Chatting to someone

☐ Sitting after lunch (no alcohol)

Figure 5.4 Epworth Sleepiness Scale. The maximum score is 24. A score of > 10 suggests obstructive sleep apnoea. However, a lower score does not rule out the condition.

- Spirometry: to find evidence of obstructive or restrictive airways disease, which may co-exist and contribute to the severity of the OSA.
- Chest X-ray: to identify coexisting lung disease, such as asthma, COPD, fibrosis and pleural disease.

Sleep studies

Multiple methods are used to assess sleep, from simple overnight oximetry to polysomnography. Definitions used in the interpretation of sleep studies are given in **Table 5.3**.

Simple overnight (pulse) oximetry measures only oxygen saturation. However, the advantage is that it is possible in the patient's own bedroom using a recording saturation probe lent to the patient. This method can be diagnostic, and it is used as a screening tool to identify patients who require more complex sleep studies. The characteristic oximetry tracing in obstructive sleep apnoea is a sawtooth

Sleep study terms	
Term	Definition
Apnoea	Interval of > 10 s between breaths
Hypopnoea	Interval of > 10 s in which airflow is reduced to < 50% of baseline flow
Apnoea/hypopnoea index (AHI used to determine severity of obstructive sleep apnoea)	No. of apnoeic or hypopnoeic episodes per h
Mild	AHI of 5–14
Moderate	AHI of 15–30
Severe	AHI of > 30

Table 5.3 Definitions used in the interpretation of sleep studies

pattern (see **Figure 5.2**), although this pattern is also seen in COPD or congestive cardiac failure.

Polysomnography requires an overnight stay in a sleep laboratory. The polysomnographic equipment measures electrical activity in the brain (electroencephalography), heart (electrocardiography) and skeletal muscles (electromyography); it also does pulse oximetry. The test records oronasal airflow and thoracoabdominal movements, and audio or video recordings are made.

Management

Weight loss is the definitive treatment for OSA. Other treatment options include advising patients to avoid sedatives and reduce alcohol intake; these steps help decrease the severity of the condition. Patients should also stop smoking because it can worsen symptoms.

Remind patients not to drive if they are feeling sleepy. Tell them that they must inform the driver-licensing authority of the diagnosis.

> **A diagnosis of obstructive sleep apnoea is particularly important for patients who drive passenger vehicles or lorries.** They need not give up their job, but their obstructive sleep apnoea must be treated. Patients must be under specialist follow-up to retain their driving licence.

There is no drug treatment for obstructive sleep apnoea. Mechanical therapies are required to prevent upper airways obstruction during sleep.

- For mild obstructive sleep apnoea, a mandibular advancement device displaces the mandible anteriorly, thus increasing the diameter of the upper airway.
- Patients with moderate to severe obstructive sleep apnoea who have been unable to modify their lifestyle may need nocturnal CPAP. Severe obstructive sleep apnoea with type 2 respiratory failure may require home nocturnal non-invasive ventilation.

Surgery helps the few patients who have an underlying physical cause for their condition. A deviated septum can be corrected. Tonsillectomy removes enlarged tonsils, and adenoidectomy enlarged adenoids. Some obese patients require bariatric surgery to reduce their body mass index.

Prognosis

The prognosis is very good for those who tolerate treatment. However, left untreated, obstructive sleep apnoea can cause cardiovascular morbidity and mortality.

Obesity itself is associated with increased mortality, but obstructive sleep apnoea confers additional mortality risk in obese patients. Evidence suggests that treatment with CPAP may reduce this risk, particularly reducing cardiovascular mortality.

Obesity hypoventilation syndrome

Obesity hypoventilation syndrome is a complication of severe obesity. Its symptoms and signs are similar to those of obstructive sleep apnoea, and patients can have both conditions. However, the pathophysiology is distinct: at night, patients with obesity hypoventilation syndrome suffer from hypoventilation rather than intermittent upper airways obstruction.

Epidemiology and pathogenesis

The prevalence of obesity hypoventilation syndrome is unknown. However, an increase in awareness and the availability of diagnostic tests has led to an increase in the number of recorded cases.

About 15% of patients with suspected obstructive sleep apnoea have obesity hypoventilation syndrome.

The pathophysiology of obesity hypoventilation syndrome is not understood fully. Obesity impairs movement of the chest wall and is associated with overnight central hypoventilation. This results in significant under-ventilation and type 2 respiratory failure.

Clinical features

The pathophysiology of obesity hypoventilation syndrome differs from that of obstructive sleep apnoea, but the clinical presentation of the two conditions is similar. Patients experience hypersomnolence, personality changes, and problems with memory and concentration.

Patients with obesity hypoventilation syndrome have daytime hypercapnia. They can also present acutely with decompensated type 2 respiratory failure (see Chapter 11), which can cause early morning headaches, drowsiness and even coma.

Diagnostic approach

A diagnosis of obesity hypoventilation syndrome requires proof of nocturnal hypoventilation and daytime hypercapnia ($Pa\text{CO}_2$ >6kPa). Therefore a sleep study is essential and arterial blood gases must be checked.

Pulmonary function test results show a restrictive lung defect with preserved transfer factor. Chest X-ray, electrocardiographic and echocardiographic results may provide evidence of pulmonary hypertension and right-sided cardiac failure.

Management

Weight loss is the main treatment. Some patients require bariatric surgery to achieve sufficient weight loss.

Hypercapnia can be exacerbated by CPAP so overnight non-invasive ventilation may be needed. Acute episodes of type 2 respiratory failure necessitate non-invasive ventilation and treatment of cor pulmonale and any associated diseases (e.g. COPD and congestive cardiac failure).

Obesity hypoventilation syndrome has a good prognosis if treated, but severe cases are complicated by cor pulmonale.

Chest wall and neuromuscular disorders

Weakness of the respiratory muscles as a result of neuromuscular disease, and inefficient ventilation due to chest wall abnormalities, can cause chronic type 2 respiratory failure. Common causes are listed in **Table 5.4**. Hypoventilation in these conditions (and other causes of type 2 respiratory failure) is worse at night.

Once type 2 respiratory failure develops, overnight non-invasive ventilation is usually necessary in the long term. This intervention prevents acute deteriorations and for non-progressive conditions extends life expectancy considerably.

Other causes of sleep-disordered breathing

Other conditions that cause sleep-disordered breathing are:

- narcolepsy, a rare neurological disorder that affects regulation of the sleep–wake cycle
- periodic limb movement disorder, a condition in which the limbs have repetitive movements, which disrupt sleep

- central sleep apnoea, when the brain temporarily stops sending signals to the muscles that control breathing

However, these conditions are beyond the scope of this chapter.

Mechanical and neuromuscular causes of type 2 respiratory failure	
Category	Disorders
Neuromuscular	Myasthenia gravis
	Motor neurone disease
	Muscular dystrophies
	Guillain–Barré syndrome
	Diaphragmatic paralysis
Mechanical chest wall problems	Kyphoscoliosis
	Thoracoplasty (e.g. to treat tuberculosis)
	Obesity (which restricts chest wall movement resulting in hypoventilation)

Table 5.4 Neuromuscular and mechanical chest wall disorders that cause type 2 respiratory failure

Answers to starter questions

1. Obstructive sleep apnoea prevents deep sleep, so daytime concentration and alertness are impaired. Patients are two to seven times more likely than other drivers to have a road traffic accident. Therefore patients have a responsibility to inform both the driver-licensing authority and their insurance provider of their diagnosis. If they do not, their insurance may be invalid, and they could lose their licence. The DVLA website (United Kingdom) has comprehensive information on what needs to be done. It is not the physician's responsibility to inform the driver-licensing authority and the patient's insurance provider. Rather, physicians must inform patients of the need to do so.

Answers *continued*

2. High-quality sleep is subjective. Essentially, it leaves people feeling well rested and refreshed on waking in the morning, and they do not feel tired during the day. At night, it is normal to toss and turn occasionally, but genuinely poor sleep quality leads to decreased performance during the day. On average, people need about 8 h of sleep per night.

3. It is unclear why patients with obstructive sleep apnoea are at increased risk of heart disease and stroke. Some of the increased risk may be related to underlying obesity, which is common in people with this condition. It may also be related to the changes in cerebral blood flow and hypoxia that occur in obstructive sleep apnoea. The results of some studies have shown that treating the obstructive sleep apnoea reduces the increased risk.

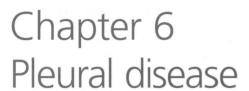

Chapter 6
Pleural disease

Starter questions

Answers to the following questions are on page 207

1. How does fluid or air enter the pleural space?
2. How can a pneumothorax be 'spontaneous'? What causes spontaneous pneumothorax?
3. How does analysis of pleural fluid help identify the cause of a pleural effusion?

Introduction

Pleural disease is common, affecting an estimated 3000 people per million each year worldwide. The most serious conditions are fluid in the pleural space, termed pleural effusion, and air in the pleural space, termed a pneumothorax. Pleural thickening is also common but is usually of little clinical consequence.

Case 6 Progressive breathlessness over 3 months

Presentation

Mr Smith, aged 69 years, has become increasingly breathless over 3 months. He has come to the accident and emergency department after becoming breathless while walking only 20 m.

Initial interpretation

In patients over 60 years of age the likely causes of dyspnoea are chronic obstructive pulmonary disease (COPD) and heart failure. Other possible explanations for a subacute presentation (occurring over days to months) of steadily progressive

Case 6 *continued*

dyspnoea are multiple pulmonary emboli, some forms of interstitial lung disease, progressive lobar collapse and an increasing pleural effusion of any cause.

History

Mr Smith has several medical conditions. His hypertension and diabetes are well controlled with medication. He also has ischaemic heart disease; 3 years ago, after an episode of severe angina, he had percutaneous coronary intervention (a non-surgical procedure to treat narrowed coronary arteries) and two stents were inserted. He has COPD but has never been admitted to hospital because of it. He takes a tiotropium inhaler daily

He has no cough, wheeze or fever and has not lost any weight recently. He has noticed increasing swelling of his ankles but is able to sleep in a horizontal position at night and has not woken feeling breathless. He saw his general practitioner 3 weeks ago and was prescribed furosemide 40 mg twice daily. The peripheral swelling has improved a little, but he remains breathless.

Interpretation of history

Pre-existing ischaemic heart disease and peripheral oedema suggest cardiac failure. There are no red flag symptoms of malignancy, such as weight loss, anorexia and pain. At this point, nothing in the history suggests multiple pulmonary emboli. Examination would help identify the cause of the breathlessness.

Further history

Mr Smith gave up smoking 10 years ago; before this he smoked 25 cigarettes per day for 32 years (40 pack-year history). He used to work as a theatre director and does not believe that he has ever been exposed to asbestos or other toxic substances. He has not travelled recently and has remained active, with no recent immobility.

Examination

Mr Smith is breathless on minimal exertion. However, at rest he has a respiratory rate of 16 breaths/min and normal oxygen saturation. His lymph nodes are not palpable and his trachea is central. He has pitting oedema up to his mid calves and his jugular venous pressure is raised. Over the right mid and lower zones there is decreased chest expansion, a dull percussion note and absent vocal resonance and breath sounds.

Interpretation of findings

A unilateral pleural effusion seems likely from the clinical examination. From the history the most likely causes are heart failure and malignancy. The absence of obvious weight loss or enlarged lymph nodes make malignancy less likely, but do not rule it out. The normal position of the trachea suggests that there is no collapse of the lobe underlying the effusion, which makes malignancy less likely. The presence of peripheral oedema is suggestive of heart failure, but could be due to lymph-oedema or dependant oedema.

Investigations

The chest X-ray shows a large right pleural effusion and an enlarged cardiac outline (**Figure 6.1**). The results of routine blood test are normal. A portable ultrasound scan of the chest confirms that the opacity is pleural fluid. Therefore a therapeutic and diagnostic pleural aspiration is done: 1.0 L of pale yellow fluid is removed, and samples are sent to the biochemistry, microbiology and cytology laboratories.

The results of biochemical analysis of the pleural fluid show a protein content of 20 g/L and a lactate dehydrogenase (LDH) concentration of 100 IU/L; serum protein content is 75 g/L and serum LDH

Case 6 *continued*

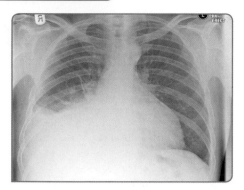

Figure 6.1 Chest X-ray showing a right-sided pleural effusion and enlarged cardiac shadow.

concentration is 250 IU/L. The results of microbiological tests of the fluid are negative. Cytological investigations find no malignant cells. An additional blood test shows an increased concentration of NT-proBNP (N-terminal pro brain natriuretic peptide).

Diagnosis

The low concentration of albumin and LDH show that the pleural fluid is a transudate. This finding makes heart failure the most likely diagnosis. Further evidence is provided by the increased concentration of NT-proBNP. An echocardiogram is requested and additional medications are prescribed to treat Mr Smith's condition.

Case 7 Sudden onset of breathlessness

Presentation

Anil is a 20-year-old student who presents with a sudden sharp pain on the left side of his chest and acute breathlessness.

Initial interpretation

Sudden onset of pain and breathlessness in a young person suggests primary spontaneous pneumothorax, pulmonary embolism or musculoskeletal chest wall pain.

Further history

Anil has no medical problems. He regularly smokes cannabis but does not use other recreational drugs.

Examination

Anil is able to talk in full sentences. His pulse rate is 105 beats/min and respiratory rate is 18 breaths/min. His blood pressure is 110/70 mmHg and oxygen saturation 98% on air. His trachea is deviated to the right. Chest expansion is reduced on the left, and the percussion note is hyper-resonant. No breath sounds are audible on the left side.

Interpretation of findings

The examination findings confirm a pneumothorax. The lack of breath sounds could be due to consolidation or lobar collapse, but the percussion note would then be dull and a sudden onset is unusual. In the absence of underlying lung disease or trauma, Anil's pneumothorax is classified as primary spontaneous pneumothorax (PSP). Importantly, there are no signs of a tension pneumothorax, which is a medical emergency (see Chapter 11).

Case 7 *continued*

Pneumothorax: inserting a chest drain

Dr Lovell explains the procedure and its risks

As the chest X-ray still shows a large pneumothorax, we need to put a chest drain in

Can I have a go?

"Have a go"?! How many have you done?

I'll insert the drain, don't worry, I've done more than 50. Joe needs to get more experience, so he'll assist if that's OK?

Ok

Anil has a primary spontaneous pneumothorax and needs a chest drain. It's important Anil has confidence in whoever performs the procedure

With the Seldinger technique a guidewire is inserted and the tract dilated before the drain is inserted and the wire removed

Yes, I'm OK

You're doing great. The wire's in: you'll just feel a bit of pushing as we enlarge the hole a bit for the drain. Are you OK?

Great. We're all done and it's bubbling well. It may make you cough to start with but your breathing should be easier soon

The drain is connected to an underwater seal. Chest X-ray is repeated to check drain position

Investigations

A chest X-ray confirms a left-sided pneumothorax (**Figure 6.2**) and reveals no underlying lung disease. The results of routine blood tests and electrocardiography are normal.

Diagnosis

The diagnosis is primary spontaneous pneumothorax. Smoking cannabis increases the risk of developing this condition. The pneumothorax is large enough to warrant intervention; pleural aspiration is done to reduce its size. If aspiration fails, a chest drain will be required (**Figures 6.3** and **6.4**).

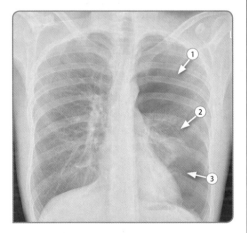

Figure 6.2 Chest X-ray showing a large left primary spontaneous pneumothorax. ① Absent lung markings. ② Lung collapsed against hilum. ③ Pleural line.

Case 7 *continued*

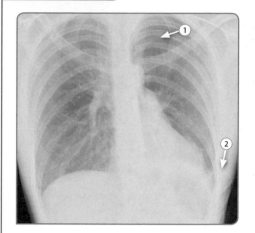

Figure 6.3 Chest X-ray showing a large left primary spontaneous pneumothorax after a chest drain has been inserted. ① Visible pleural line with lack of lung markings in the apex. ② Chest drain visible.

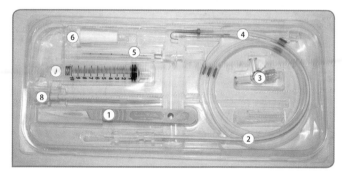

Figure 6.4 A Seldinger chest drain insertion kit. ① Scalpel. ② Chest drain ③ Three-way tap ④ Guidewire. ⑤ Large-bore hollow needle. ⑥ Connector (to drain tubing). ⑦ Syringe. ⑧ Dilator.

Pleural effusions

A pleural effusion is fluid in the pleural space. Pleural effusions are caused by a wide range of conditions (**Table 6.1**); the major clinical issues are identifying the cause and preventing symptomatic fluid accumulation in the pleural space.

Types

There are various types of pleural effusion.

- Transudate pleural effusions have a low protein content. They are usually caused by a systemic problem that increases fluid leak into the pleural space; the pleura itself is usually normal. Transudate pleural effusions are unilateral or bilateral.

- Exudate pleural effusions have a high protein content. They are usually caused by pleural disease driving fluid leak into the pleural space. Exudate pleural effusions are usually unilateral.

- Parapneumonic effusions are sterile exudate pleural effusions in patients with pneumonia.

- Complicated parapneumonic effusions are parapneumonic effusions that have become infected and are culture-positive, have a pH < 7.2, are loculated, or contain visibly turbid pleural fluid.

- Empyema is caused by a pleural infection. It is an accumulation of pus; the pleural fluid is visibly turbid or culture-positive. Empyema can be acquired

Causes of pleural effusions		
Classification	Common	Rarer
Transudates (often bilateral)		
Increased venous pressure	Cardiac failure Renal failure Iatrogenic fluid overload	Pericardial effusion Constrictive pericarditis
Hypoalbuminaemia (low concentration of albumin)	Liver cirrhosis Nephrotic syndrome	Protein-losing enteropathy
Transdiaphragmatic spread of peritoneal fluid	Liver cirrhosis	Peritoneal dialysis Ovarian hyperstimulation syndrome Meigs' syndrome (can be an exudate)
Exudate (usually unilateral)		
Infection	Parapneumonic* Complicated parapneumonic effusions Empyema Tuberculosis	Subphrenic or hepatic abscess Oesophageal rupture *Nocardia* infection *Actinomyces* infection
Malignancy (secondary)	Primary lung cancer Breast cancer Gastrointestinal tract cancers	Many other less common cancers
Malignancy (primary)	Mesothelioma	Lymphoma Sarcoma
Connective tissue disease	Rheumatoid arthritis Systemic lupus erythematosus	Vasculitis Familial Mediterranean fever
Haemothorax	Trauma Iatrogenic (e.g. caused by pleural procedures and central line insertion)	Bleeding disorders
Drug use or occupational exposure	Benign asbestos effusions	Drug use (e.g. practolol, methysergide and bromocriptine)
Other	Pulmonary embolus Pancreatitis (high pleural fluid amylase concentration)	Hypothyroidism Yellow nail syndrome Chylothorax

*It is essential to distinguish a parapneumonic effusion from an empyema (see Chapter 8).

Table 6.1 Causes of pleural effusions

in the community as a complicated parapneumonic effusion or can present without evidence of associated pneumonia. Alternatively, empyema can be acquired in hospital, where it is often caused by the introduction of an infectious agent during pleural procedures or lung surgery.

- Loculated pleural effusions are trapped by fibrous adhesions between the visceral and parietal pleura.
- Hydropneumothorax is the presence of both air and fluid in the pleural space.
- Haemothorax is the presence of blood in the pleural space. The condition is usually caused by trauma.

- Chylothorax is the accumulation of chyle (fat and lymphatic fluid) in the pleural space. This type of pleural effusion is usually caused by disruption of the lymphatic system as a result of lymphoma, cancer or trauma.

Epidemiology

Pleural effusions are very common. Most cases are transudate pleural effusions, parapneumonic effusions, pleural infections or malignancies.

Aetiology

The cause of the pleural effusion.
- In transudate pleural effusions, pleural fluid production is increased by either low oncotic pressure in the blood (as a result of low albumin concentration) or increased venous pressure.
- In exudate pleural effusions, there is a diseased pleura. Effusions form due to excessive production of protein and fluid by the pleura, leakage from capillaries, impaired lymphatic drainage, or any combination of these.

Clinical features

Patients with pleural effusions become breathless as the effusion enlarges. The daily rate of fluid accumulation dictates the speed at which the severity of dyspnoea increases.

The fluid itself causes no pain. However, inflammatory causes of effusions cause pleuritic chest pain, which also occurs if there is infiltration of a tumour into the pleura and chest wall.

Examination can identify signs of the pleural effusion itself (see Chapter 2), as well as signs of the underlying cause (**Table 6.1**). Large effusions are obvious clinically, but small ones are difficult to detect.

> **Small bilateral effusions are more difficult to detect clinically.** They produce less obvious asymmetry on examination.

Diagnostic approach

Bilateral effusions are highly likely to be transudates. If there is an obvious cause (e.g. hypoalbuminaemia) and no atypical features, no further investigation is required.

Pleural infection and malignancy are the most serious causes of unilateral effusions that must be excluded. Use a structured approach, as follows:

1. A chest X-ray is done to confirm the presence of an effusion (Figure 7.2).
2. Routine blood tests are required, as well as specific tests (e.g. rheumatoid factor and tumour markers), depending on clinical presentation.
3. At least 50 mL of pleural fluid is aspirated for measurements of protein content, LDH and glucose concentration, and pH. Samples are also needed for microbiological tests (including detection of acid-fast bacilli) and cytological investigations. Pleural aspiration are best performed under guidance by pleural ultrasound to avoid damage to surrounding organs (**Figure 6.5**). Ultrasound also detects fluid septations (common in pleural infection) and pleural thickening or nodularity (which suggest malignancy).
4. The results of pleural fluid analysis differentiate between transudates and exudates (**Table 6.2**) and are used to identify many cases of infection and pleural malignancy. Combined with clinical findings, a pleural aspirate is

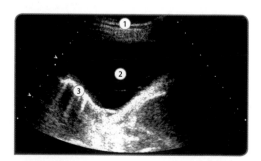

Figure 6.5 Ultrasound showing a pleural effusion. ① Ultrasound probe on chest wall. ② Pleural fluid. ③ Diaphragm.

Light's criteria

Pleural fluid protein content (g/L)	Transudate or exudate
<25	Transudate
>35	Exudate
25–35	Use Light's criteria (99% sensitivity, 98% specificity)
	The effusion is an exudate if it fulfils one or more of these criteria are fulfilled
	■ protein content pleural fluid:serum ratio >0.5
	■ lactate dehydrogenase (LDH) concentration pleural fluid:serum ratio >0.6
	■ pleural fluid LDH over two-thirds of the upper limit of normal for serum LDH

Table 6.2 Light's criteria for differentiating transudates and exudates

diagnostic in 75% of cases. A guide to interpreting the results of pleural fluid analysis is shown in **Table 6.3.** Obviously loculated fluid is often visible on chest X-ray (**Figure 6.6**).

5. If the pleural fluid is an exudate, computerised tomography (CT) of the thorax is needed to assess pleural thickness and nodularity. A CT scan also identifies masses that may be primary or secondary lung cancers. The scan is best done when most of the pleural fluid has been drained, leaving the underlying lung visible.

6. If the cause of an exudative effusion remains unclear, pleural biopsy is required. This is especially important if pleural nodularity or thickening is seen on CT, or if malignancy or tuberculosis is suspected. Pleura can be biopsied percutaneously under ultrasound or

Pleural fluid analysis

Cause	Appearance	Protein content (g/L)	LDH concentration pleural fluid:serum ratio	Glucose concentration (mmol/L)	pH	Cytological findings	Microbiological findings
Heart failure	Clear and straw-coloured	<25	Normal	Normal	>7.2	None	None
Parapneumonic	Turbid and yellow	>35	Normal	Normal	>7.2	Neutrophils	None
Empyema	Purulent	>35	Increased (>0.6)	<3.3	<7.2	Neutrophils	Gram stain–positive Culture-positive (30–50%)
Malignancy	Clear and straw-coloured, or blood-stained	>35	Increased (>0.6)	<3.3	<or >7.2	Malignant cells (60%)	None
Pulmonary embolism	Clear and straw-coloured, or blood-stained	>35	Normal	Normal	>7.2	Neutrophils	None
Rheumatoid arthritis	Clear and straw-coloured	>35	Increased (>0.6)	<3.3	<or >7.2	Lymphocytes	None
Tuberculosis	Clear or yellow	>35	Increased (>0.6)	<3.3	<or >7.2	Lymphocytes	Visible acid-fast bacilli (15%) Culture-positive (50%)

LDH, lactate dehydrogenase.

Table 6.3 Typical results of pleural fluid analysis for common causes of pleural effusions

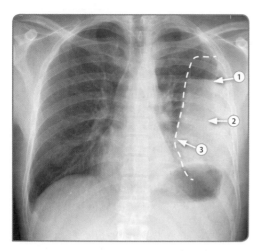

Figure 6.6 Chest X ray showing a loculated left hydropneumothorax. (1) The air–fluid level indicates a hydropneumothroax (air and liquid in the pleural space), in this case caused by introduction of air after partial drainage of a locule of infected pleural fluid. (2) Loculated pleural fluid. (3) Pleural line showing lack of the normal curve.

CT guidance, or by medical or surgical thoracoscopy. A pleurodesis can be done at the same time as thoracoscopy to prevent fluid reaccumulating.

Other potentially useful investigations are positron emission tomography CT scan (to identify distal tumours), CT pulmonary angiography (in cases of suspected pulmonary embolism), liver ultrasound or biopsy (if cirrhosis is suspected) and measurement of adenosine deaminase concentration in the pleural fluid (if tuberculosis is suspected).

Management

Pleural infection is discussed in Chapter 8. The aim of treatment of non-infective pleural effusions is to deal with the underlying cause. For example, diuretics and angiotensin-converting enzyme inhibitors are used to treat transudates caused by cardiac failure.

> **During the delay between discovery of a pleural effusion and identification of the cause,** keep the patient well informed but avoid worrying them unduly. Remember people vary in how much they want to know so be guided by your patient in how much information to give at each stage.

If treatment is not possible or is ineffective, which is often the case with malignant effusions, the options are as follows.

- Pleural aspiration or drainage is used to remove large quantities of fluid. Such procedures are often combined with diagnostic pleural aspirations and are repeated when fluid reaccumulates. Sites for aspiration or drainage are identified using pleural ultrasound to avoid damaging nearby structures.
- Pleurodesis or pleurectomy is used to obliterate the pleural space to prevent recurrence of the effusion. Medical or surgical pleurodesis introduces an irritant (e.g. talc) into the pleural space through the chest drain or a thoracoscopic procedure. Surgical pleurodesis is achieved by abrading the pleura or by removing it (pleurectomy).

Prognosis

Malignant effusions are, by definition, evidence of extensive disease. Only a small proportion of patients survive for 5 years.

Pneumothorax

At functional residual capacity, the intrapleural pressure is 5 cm H_2O more negative than atmospheric pressure. This pressure keeps the lung expanded. If air enters the pleural space (in a pneumothorax), the negative pressure is lost and the lung collapses.

Epidemiology

Primary spontaneous pneumothorax is two to three times more common in men. The incidence peaks at the age of 20 years.

Aetiology

Pneumothoraces are divided into the following types.

- Primary spontaneous pneumothorax without underlying lung disease is common in tall and thin young men, smokers and people who inhale recreational drugs. Subpleural blebs and bullae are present in most cases. This type of pneumothorax is also common in patients with Marfan's or Ehlers–Danlos syndrome.
- Spontaneous secondary pneumothoraces are related to an underlying lung disease (e.g. COPD and cystic fibrosis).
- In tension pneumothorax, air continues to leak into the pleural space after inspiration but is unable to escape during expiration. Intrapleural pressure builds up, causing mediastinal shift and impaired cardiac function. Tension pneumothorax is a medical emergency (see Chapter 11).
- In traumatic pneumothoraces, the lung is punctured by a penetrating injury to the chest (which can happen during medical interventions) or by ribs fractured by blunt trauma.

Clinical features

Pneumothoraces present with sudden onset of chest pain, breathlessness or both. Even a small secondary pneumothorax can cause severe life-threatening dyspnoea if the patient's respiratory reserve is limited by an underlying lung disease.

On examination, patients are breathless and signs of a pneumothorax are present (see Chapter 2). Hypotension and obvious tracheal deviation suggest a tension pneumothorax (see Chapter 11).

Diagnostic approach

The main differential diagnosis of the clinical presentation is pulmonary embolism. However, chest X-ray readily confirms a pneumothorax. Rarely, a CT scan is needed to identify a small pneumothorax or to distinguish between large bullae and a loculated pneumothorax.

Management

Small primary spontaneous pneumothoraces resolve spontaneously. They are monitored by repeated chest X-rays.

> **Guidelines suggest criteria such as estimated size of pneumothorax on imaging to decide whether to intervene.** However, clinical status is much more important. The risks and benefits of intervention must be weighed up in partnership with the patient.

Patients who are symptomatic, or who have larger primary spontaneous pneumothoraces, require intervention. First, pleural air is aspirated. If aspiration fails to improve the patient's condition, a chest drain is needed. The British Thoracic Society has produced a treatment algorithm for primary spontaneous pneumothorax (**Figure 6.7**). International guidelines are similar but differ in how they determine pneumothorax size (eg. measured at apex rather than hilum on chest X-ray).

Secondary pneumothoraces usually require chest drainage. In people with underlying lung disease, the effects of a pneumothorax on respiration are potentially severe (**Figure 6.8**).

Pleural aspiration fails if air continues to leak from the lung (in cases of bronchopleural fistula). Persisting air leaks cause continuous bubbling if a chest drain is in situ. Surgical intervention is warranted if they persist after 5–7 days. Surgery is also mandated in special circumstances, for example if the lung fails to re-expand, or in cases of bilateral pneumothoraces.

Preventive pleurectomy or pleurodesis is offered to patients with recurrent pneumothorax on the same side. These procedures are also offered to divers and pilots, because without surgical intervention they are unable to return to these activities and occupations.

Prognosis

The recurrence rate after one primary spontaneous pneumothorax is up to 50%. This figure increases after two. For secondary pneumothorax, the recurrence rate is higher. Most recurrences occur within 6 months to 2 years. Smoking increases the risk of recurrence.

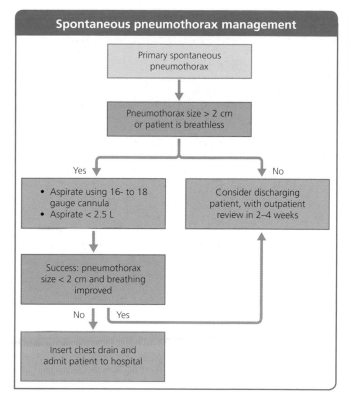

Spontaneous pneumothorax management

Primary spontaneous pneumothorax

↓

Pneumothorax size > 2 cm or patient is breathless

Yes ↓

- Aspirate using 16- to 18 gauge cannula
- Aspirate < 2.5 L

No →

Consider discharging patient, with outpatient review in 2–4 weeks

↓

Success: pneumothorax size < 2 cm and breathing improved

No ↓   Yes

Insert chest drain and admit patient to hospital

Figure 6.7 Management of a primary spontaneous pneumothorax. Adapted from British Thorax Society Pleural Disease Guideline Group. BTS pleural disease guideline. Thorax 2010; 65 (suppl 2): ii13-ii21.

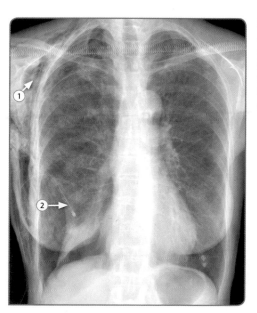

Figure 6.8 Chest X-ray showing a right-sided chest drain inserted for secondary spontaneous pneumothorax complicated by subcutaneous emphysema, in which air tracks up between soft tissue planes. ① Subcutaneous emphysema. ② Chest drain. The lungs are hyperinflated due to underlying COPD.

Benign pleural thickening

This condition is common and usually asymptomatic. Benign pleural thickening is often an incidental finding on examination (dullness to percussion and quiet breath sounds) or chest X-ray (**Figure 6.9**). Common causes are previous pleural infection, haemothorax, and asbestos exposure (**Table 6.4**).

Extensive pleural thickening causes restrictive lung defects and dyspnoea. Treatment is surgical pleurectomy, a procedure associated with significant morbidity and mortality. Pleurectomy is reserved for only the most severe cases.

The main differential diagnosis of benign pleural thickening is pleural malignancy, especially mesothelioma.

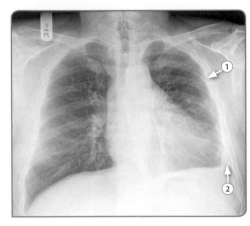

Figure 6.9 Chest X-ray showing left-sided pleural thickening. (1) Lung edge and ribs separated by a layer of additional tissue. (2) Characteristic filled-in squared-off costrophrenic angle.

Causes of pleural thickening	
Cause and common examples	Features
Infection	
Post-empyema	Usually basolateral; can calcify; non-progressive
Post-tuberculosis	Common: 'apical capping'; non-progressive
	Rare: extensive, with sheet-like calcifications; non-progressive
Active non-tuberculous mycobacteria infection or chronic aspergillosis	Slowly progressive apical disease with associated cavitation
Inflammation	
Asbestos exposure	Common: plaques – small patches of focal pleural thickening and calcifications, with holly leaf appearance on chest X-ray
	Less common: extensive confluent pleural thickening with or without benign exudate effusions
Post-pleurodesis	Diffuse, non-progressive
Post-haemothorax	Usually basolateral; can calcify; non-progressive
Caused by drug use (e.g. methysergide and bromocriptine)	Diffuse: may be associated with interstitial fibrosis
Malignancy	
Primary malignancy (e.g. mesothelioma) – related to asbestos exposure	Progressive pleural thickening; the mediastinal pleural reflection is affected
Secondary malignancy (e.g. lung adenocarcinoma)	Progressive pleural thickening associated with nodular changes and intrapulmonary masses

Table 6.4 Causes of pleural thickening and their clinical features

Answers to starter questions

1. The pleura produces pleural fluid, which is absorbed by the lymphatic system. The presence of a few millilitres of pleural fluid is normal. However, a pleural effusion forms if production is increased, absorption blocked, or both.

    Penetrating trauma allows air to enter the chest cavity. More commonly, air passes through an abnormal connection between the airways and the pleural space; when a subpleural bleb ruptures or a fractured rib damages the lung surface, air that was in the alveoli and bronchi enters the pleural space.

2. A spontaneous pneumothorax develops in the absence of trauma and lung disease, and therefore has no apparent cause. However, patients have an acute new defect in the lung that allows air into the pleural space. The defect is most commonly a ruptured localised bleb. The rest of the lung tissue is normal.

3. The pleural tap is one of the most informative tests for the cause of a pleural effusion. Pleural protein content and LDH concentration (see **Table 6.2**) differentiate a transudate from an exudate. These results therefore narrow the differential diagnosis. Cytological investigations identify about three-quarters of malignant effusions, and microbiological tests are used to diagnose pleural infection.

    Several rare causes of pleural effusion can be confirmed by specific tests on pleural fluid. For example, the concentration of amylase in pleural fluid is measured if pancreatitis is suspected.

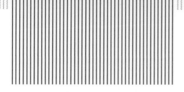

Chapter 7
Malignancy

Starter questions

Answers to the following questions are on page 231.

1. Why do only some people who smoke develop lung cancer?
2. Can lung cancer be cured?
3. Why is small-cell lung cancer harder to treat than non–small-cell lung cancer?
4. How does lung cancer spread?
5. If everyone stopped smoking cigarettes, would lung cancer still exist

Introduction

Malignant disease of the lungs is common and includes primary lung cancer, lung metastases and mesothelioma.

■ Primary lung cancer is one of the most common cancers and is a leading cause of cancer death worldwide. It is divided into two types, which require different approaches to treatment: small-cell lung cancer (SCLC) and non–small-cell lung cancer (NSCLC). NSCLC can be further divided into three pathological subtypes: adenocarcinoma, squamous cell carcinomas and large-cell carcinoma.

■ The lungs, pleura and mediastinal lymph nodes are common sites for metastases from a wide range of other primary malignancies. These include gastrointestinal tract cancers, breast cancer, renal cancer and melanoma.
■ Mesothelioma is a primary cancer of the pleura. This type of cancer is common in people exposed to asbestos during their previous occupation.

Several other rarer malignant and benign tumours also affect the respiratory tract.

Case 8 Breathlessness and weight loss

Presentation

Elsa Jeffard, aged 68 years, presents to her general practitioner (GP) with decreased appetite and a weight loss of 3 kg in the past month. She is known to have chronic obstructive pulmonary disease (COPD).

Initial interpretation

Decreased appetite is a common and non-specific symptom. Some patients choose to lose weight, but unintentional weight loss may be caused by a metabolic disorder; it is also associated with some chronic diseases and malignancy.

Unintentional weight loss of 3 kg in a month is a worrying symptom. It is probably too fast to attribute to the slow weight loss that occurs in some patients with COPD.

The combination of decreased appetite and unintentional weight loss suggests a significant new disease. It is essential to establish if the history includes any other features that suggest a malignancy.

History

When asked directly, Mrs Jeffard answers that she has had blood in her sputum. She has had no pain or new neurological symptoms.

Interpretation of history

People with COPD are at increased risk of developing lung cancer. Their risk is higher than that of smokers who do not have COPD. Haemoptysis in a patient who has smoked requires thorough investigation to ensure that lung cancer is not the cause.

It is essential to confirm that the blood is from the lungs and not from the gastro-intestinal tract (haematemesis). Use of anticoagulants (e.g. aspirin, clopidogrel and warfarin) should be checked, because these drugs increase the risk of bleeding.

Further history

On further questioning, it becomes apparent that Mrs Jeffard has been feeling unwell for the past few months. For the past 2 weeks, she has been bringing up fresh red blood most times she coughs, about a teaspoon at a time. She is certain that the blood comes only when she coughs. She has had no fevers or chest pain. She is a smoker with a 40 pack-year history.

Mrs Jeffard worked in a textile factory for 30 years before retiring 10 years ago. She reports no exposure to asbestos. She is using a salmeterol xinafoate–fluticasone propionate inhaler (two puffs twice daily), tiotropium (one puff once daily) and salbutamol (as required) for her COPD.

Examination

Mrs Jeffard has nicotine-stained fingers. She is also noted to have finger clubbing (Figure 2.5). She looks cachectic. Her respiratory rate is 14 breaths/min. She has an enlarged hard right-sided supraclavicular lymph node. On auscultation, a polyphonic end expiratory wheeze is heard throughout her chest. Cardiovascular, abdominal and neurological examinations are all normal.

Interpretation of findings

Examination provides some key signs associated with lung cancer.

- Nicotine-stained fingers show that the patient is a current smoker.
- Finger clubbing is often seen in patients with lung cancer (but it has numerous other causes; Table 2.14).
- Lymphadenopathy indicates spread of lung cancer and may provide an easily accessible biopsy site.

The polyphonic end expiratory wheeze is probably caused by COPD. However, a monophonic wheeze in a single area may

Case 8 *continued*

indicate bronchial obstruction, which could be caused by a tumour.

Combined with the history of weight loss, malaise and significant haemoptysis in a smoker, the examination findings make a diagnosis of lung cancer likely. Any patient who has haemoptysis and a smoking history requires a chest X-ray and urgent referral (within 2 weeks) to a chest physician. Other indications for referral include:

- cough
- chest or shoulder pain
- dyspnoea
- weight loss
- chest signs
- hoarseness
- finger clubbing
- symptoms suggesting metastasis from a lung cancer (e.g. in brain, bone, liver or skin)

- cervical or supraclavicular lymphadenopathy

Asbestos exposure is relevant, because it is associated with an increased incidence of lung cancer and with mesothelioma.

Investigations

Mrs Jeffard is referred by her GP for a chest X-ray, which shows a mass at the left hilum (**Figure 7.1**). An urgent respiratory appointment is arranged.

At the respiratory clinic, a staging computerised tomography (CT) scan and an ultrasound-guided biopsy of the enlarged supraclavicular lymph node are done. The CT scan confirms a lung mass at the left hilum, associated with enlarged mediastinal and right supraclavicular lymph nodes, and with liver lesions that are likely to be metastases.

Lung cancer: diagnosis and breaking bad news

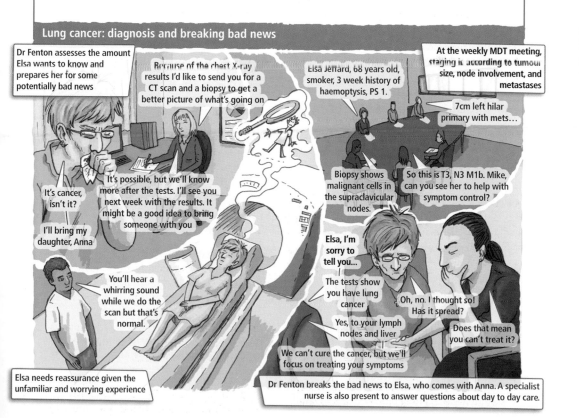

Dr Fenton assesses the amount Elsa wants to know and prepares her for some potentially bad news

Because of the chest X-ray results I'd like to send you for a CT scan and a biopsy to get a better picture of what's going on

Elsa Jeffard, 68 years old, smoker, 3 week history of haemoptysis, PS 1.

At the weekly MDT meeting, staging is according to tumour size, node involvement, and metastases

7cm left hilar primary with mets...

It's cancer, isn't it?

It's possible, but we'll know more after the tests. I'll see you next week with the results. It might be a good idea to bring someone with you

I'll bring my daughter, Anna

Biopsy shows malignant cells in the supraclavicular nodes.

So this is T3, N3 M1b. Mike, can you see her to help with symptom control?

You'll hear a whirring sound while we do the scan but that's normal.

Elsa, I'm sorry to tell you...

The tests show you have lung cancer

Oh, no. I thought so! Has it spread?

Yes, to your lymph nodes and liver

Does that mean you can't treat it?

We can't cure the cancer, but we'll focus on treating your symptoms

Elsa needs reassurance given the unfamiliar and worrying experience

Dr Fenton breaks the bad news to Elsa, who comes with Anna. A specialist nurse is also present to answer questions about day to day care.

Case 8 *continued*

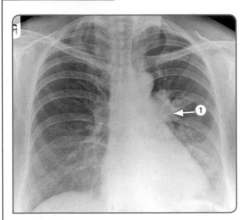

Figure 7.1 Chest X-ray showing ① a left hilar mass. The left hilum is denser than the right and the normal concavity of the hilar point has been lost, indicating the presence of abnormal tissue.

Diagnosis

Lymph node biopsy confirms the diagnosis of non–small-cell lung cancer. A management plan is agreed at the weekly meeting of the lung cancer multidisciplinary team.

In the clinic, the respiratory trainee who saw Mrs Jeffard before and a lung cancer specialist nurse discuss the diagnosis with Mrs Jeffard and her daughter. They both are shocked and upset by the news. However, the possibility of cancer has been at the back of her daughter's mind due to her mother's rapid weight loss and she is relieved to know what they are dealing with.

Breaking news of a lung cancer diagnosis can be very emotional for the patient and their family, as well as challenging for health care professionals. Good practice includes the following.

- Establishing a good rapport with the patient

- Choosing a quiet, private environment, ideally with family present

- First checking the understanding of the patient and family members

- Giving separate pieces of information gradually, allowing time for them to absorb each piece of information and to ask questions

- A 'warning shot' that there is bad news, before using the word 'cancer'

- Having a lung cancer nurse specialist present to offer additional support during and after the consultation

Case 9 Chest pain and breathlessness

Presentation

Mr Norman is a 68-year-old who has presented to his GP with worsening breathlessness on exertion. He has noticed that his exercise tolerance has gradually decreased over the past 3 months. He is now unable to climb a flight of stairs without stopping to catch his breath.

Mr Norman has also developed constant left-sided chest pain. The pain is dull, radiates all over the left side of his chest, and has been increasing in severity over the past few weeks.

Initial interpretation

Several cardiac and respiratory diagnoses cause breathlessness and chest pain. However, the progressive history over a short period is of great concern. Most causes of chest pain are intermittent.

Case 9 *continued*

Therefore constant pain is worrying, because it is a symptom of malignancy. It is essential to establish whether there are any associated features, such as weight loss.

Further history

Over the past 2–3 months, Mr Norman has had no appetite and has lost 6.5 kg in weight. He has been feeling generally lethargic but has had no night sweats, fevers, cough or haemoptysis. He retired recently after working as a plumber. He has worked with asbestos throughout his career but wore a mask only in recent years. He has a 20 pack-year smoking history.

Examination

Mr Norman is not cachectic. His respiratory rate is 14 breaths/min. He has reduced expansion, a dull percussion note, reduced breath sounds and vocal resonance on the left from the base to the middle of his back. The rest of the cardiovascular, abdominal and neurological examination findings are normal.

Interpretation of findings

The symptoms suggest a systemic disease. Malaise, anorexia and weight loss suggest an active inflammatory, infective or neoplastic process.

The lack of night sweats and fever suggests that the pathological process is not infective in origin. However, the absence of night sweats does not rule out infection. Neither does it exclude malignancy, which is sometimes associated with night sweats.

The social history is highly relevant. Exposure to asbestos confers a high risk of mesothelioma. A 20 pack-year smoking history, combined with asbestos exposure,

means that Mr Norman is also at high risk of lung cancer. His history, added to the signs of a left-sided pleural effusion, make mesothelioma or another cause of malignant effusions likely.

Investigations

Mr Norman is referred for a chest X-ray, which shows a large left pleural effusion (**Figure 7.2**). In the respiratory outpatient department, 500 mL of straw-coloured fluid is tapped under ultrasound-guidance. The sample is sent for microscopy and culture; for cytological analysis; and for measurement of protein, lactate dehydrogenase and glucose.

The pleural fluid protein and LDH levels were both raised, confirming this is an exudate effusion. The initial cytological analysis from the pleural tap does not show malignant cells.

A CT scan confirms pleural thickening, including over the mediastinum. A residual pleural effusion is visible.

Mr Norman is referred for video-assisted thorascopic surgery, and pleural biopsies are sent for histological examination.

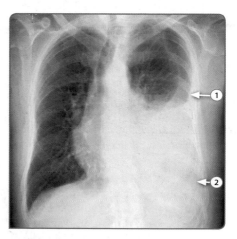

Figure 7.2 Chest X-ray showing a left-sided pleural effusion. ① Meniscus (sign of fluid). ② Loss of the costophrenic angle.

Case 9 *continued*

A pleurodesis (obliterating the pleural space by creating adhesions between the visceral and parietal pleura) is done at the same time.

Diagnosis

The histological results of the video-assisted thoracoscopic surgery biopsy confirm the presence of a mesothelioma. The case will be discussed and treatment planned at the meeting of the lung cancer multidisciplinary team.

Mesothelioma is an occupational lung disease. Therefore Mr Norman is entitled to compensation.

A unilateral effusion in a male middle-aged patient must always raise the suspicion of mesothelioma. An occupational history is essential. It must include former jobs, because the delay between asbestos exposure and presenting with mesothelioma is 20–30 years.

Primary lung cancer

Primary lung cancers are malignancies arising from the respiratory epithelium.

Epidemiology

Lung cancer is one of the most common cancers worldwide; it accounts for 13% of all new cancers. It is also the most common cause of cancer death, with one of the lowest survival rates of any type of cancer. Nearly 60% of people with lung cancer die within a year of diagnosis, and about 90% eventually die from the disease.

Cigarette smoking causes 9 out of 10 cases of lung cancer, and the rates of this disease increase in parallel to rates of smoking. The incidence of lung cancer is highest in Europe and North America, and lower in low- and middle-income countries (particularly in Africa).

Gender and age

Men have higher rates of lung cancer (**Figure 7.3**). In the UK, the estimated lifetime risk of lung cancer is 1 in 14 for men and 1 in 19 for women. The difference in incidence between the genders is falling in the USA and Europe, because more women are taking up smoking and there has been a decrease in men who smoke.

Incidence rises with age to peak at 80–84 years; 87% of lung cancer patients are older than 60 years at the time of diagnosis.

Types

Primary lung cancer is caused by one of four different histological types (**Table 7.1**):

- small-cell carcinomas (SCLC)
- adenocarcinomas
- squamous cell carcinomas
- large-cell carcinomas

Adenocarcinomas, squamous cell carcinomas and large-cell carcinomas are grouped as NSCLC and cause 80% of cases.

Small-cell lung cancer

One in five cases of primary lung cancer are SCLC. SCLC usually arises from the bronchi and is centrally located. It metastasises early. The most common sites of metastasis are the liver, adrenals, brain, bones and lymph nodes.

It is exceptionally uncommon for SCLC to present incidentally. Furthermore, because of the its aggressive nature, SCLC has usually spread from the primary site by the time the patient presents to a physician.

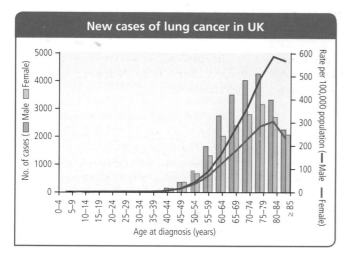

Figure 7.3 The average annual number of new cases of lung cancer and age-specific incidence rates in the UK (2006–2008).

Major cells types in primary lung cancer				
Type of lung cancer	Origin and histological findings	Location	Growth and metastasis	Percentage of lung cancers in the UK
Small-cell lung cancer	Peribronchial epithelium	Central airways	Rapid growth Early metastasis to mediastinal nodes, liver, bones and adrenals	20
Non–small-cell lung cancer				
Adenocarcinomas	Bronchial mucosal glands	Peripheral lung	Slower growth Metastasis common at presentation	40
Squamous cell carcinomas	Bronchial epithelium 'keratin pearls'	Central airways	Slower growth Later metastasis	30
Large-cell carcinomas	Histologically varied, undifferentiated cells	Peripheral lung	Slower growth Later metastasis	10

Table 7.1 General features of the four major cell types in primary lung cancer

Adenocarcinoma

Adenocarcinomas are slow-growing, usually peripheral tumours that arise from glandular epithelial cells. They cause about 40% of lung cancers.

Bronchoalveolar carcinoma is a rare subtype of adenocarcinoma arising from type 2 pneumocytes. Chest X-ray shows patches of slow-growing consolidation rather than focal, well-defined masses (**Figure 7.4**).

Most cases of adenocarcinoma are associated with smoking. However, adenocarcinoma is the most common form of lung cancer affecting non-smokers, especially females.

Adenocarcinoma has a varied response to treatment.

Squamous cell carcinoma

About 30% of cases of lung cancer are squamous cell carcinomas. These are usually located in the central part of the lung and proximal bronchus, where they cause haemoptysis.

Squamous cell carcinoma is the cancer most often associated with hypercalcaemia and cavitation. If the cells are well differentiated, squamous cell carcinoma tumours grow more slowly than other cancer types. Histologically,

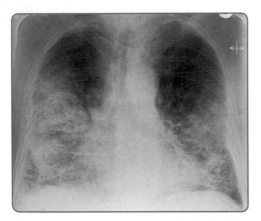

Figure 7.4 Chest X-ray showing widespread airspace shadowing caused by adenocarcinoma in situ.

squamous cell carcinoma cells usually show evidence of keratinisation ('keratin pearls').

Large-cell carcinoma

Large-cell carcinoma accounts for 10–15% of lung cancers. Histological investigation shows sheets of highly atypical cells with focal necrosis. The typical clinical manifestation of large-cell carcinoma is as a large peripheral mass on chest X-ray.

Aetiology

Cigarette smoking is the leading cause of lung cancer. The duration of the smoking history and the quantity of cigarettes smoked are both related to the likelihood of developing lung cancer, and they need to be defined when taking a history. The risk decreases after a patient stops smoking but does not return to that of a non-smoker.

Other risk factors for developing lung cancer include:

- passive smoking
- radon gas exposure
- asbestos exposure
- family history of lung cancer
- radiotherapy to the lungs
- exposure to cancer-causing chemicals (e.g. coal products, gasoline and diesel exhaust)

Prevention

Public health interventions are increasing in high-income countries in attempts to stop people starting to smoke, encourage smokers to quit, and to limit passive smoking. Interventions include the following:

- Banning smoking in public areas
- Banning tobacco advertising and product branding
- Antismoking messages on tobacco products
- Increasing tobacco tax
- Promoting smoking cessation advice, nicotine-replacement therapy and counselling in general practice

Evidence on the efficacy of bans on tobacco use is mixed. However, the promotion of smoking cessation in primary care is an effective and low-cost intervention to reduce the number of smokers.

There is only weak evidence that routine chest X-ray or CT screening for lung cancer in at-risk populations increases life expectancy.

Pathogenesis

Exposure to carcinogens and individual genetic susceptibility determine a person's risk of developing cancer. As with many other cancers, lung cancer is initiated by activation of oncogenes, with or without inactivation of tumour suppressor genes (e.g. p53). Mutations in the *K-ras* proto-oncogene are responsible for 10–30% of lung adenocarcinomas. Epidermal growth factor receptor (EGFR) mutations can arise in NSCLC. Cases of EGFR mutation–positive NSCLC are likely to respond to targeted anti-EGFR chemotherapy.

Clinical features

The common clinical features associated with lung cancer are:

- cough
- haemoptysis
- systemic symptoms (tiredness, weight loss and anorexia)
- symptoms and signs associated with metastases, often with no associated respiratory symptoms (discussed later in this chapter; **Table 7.2** and **Table 7.4**)

The following symptoms are less common.

- Shortness of breath, commonly caused by lobar collapse secondary to bronchial

obstruction; pleural effusions; or lymphangitis carcinomatosis or extensive intrapulmonary metastases
- Wheeze, caused by bronchial obstruction
- Progressive localised pain, resulting from chest wall or mediastinal invasion

Pancoast's tumours (**Figure 7.5**) are apical lung cancers that invade through the chest wall and brachial plexus. This process causes pain and weakness in the hand and arm, as well as an ipsilateral Horner's syndrome.

Non–small-cell lung cancer

The symptoms produced by the primary tumour depend on its location:

- Central tumours typically cause cough, breathlessness, wheeze, post-obstructive pneumonia and haemoptysis.
- Peripheral tumours also cause cough but are less likely to cause haemoptysis. Breathlessness may be caused by a pleural effusion. Severe pain may result from invasion of the parietal pleura and chest wall.

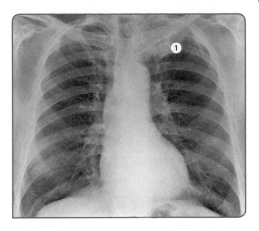

Figure 7.5 Chest X-ray showing a ① left Pancoast's tumour.

Small-cell lung cancer

This type of lung cancer has usually metastasised by the time of presentation. Patients typically report having had the following symptoms for a short duration (8–12 weeks).

- Shortness of breath
- Chronic cough

Invasion of local structures by lung cancer		
Symptom	Site of involvement	Presentation
Superior vena cava obstruction	Right paratracheal nodes or masses	Swelling of neck, face or arms Dizziness or headaches Fixed dilated neck veins Dilated collateral veins over chest wall
Recurrent laryngeal nerve palsy	Left hilar nodes or masses	Hoarse voice 'Bovine' cough
Phrenic nerve palsy	Mediastinal nodes or masses	Elevated hemidiaphragm Worsening dyspnoea
Horner's syndrome	Pancoast's (apical) tumour	Sympathetic chain involvement with partial ptosis, meiosis, hemifacial anhydrosis and enopthalmos
Brachial plexus invasion	Pancoast's (apical) tumour	Pain in hand or arm Weakness with wasting of small muscles of hand Paraesthesias and loss of sensation in hand and arm
Oesophageal compression	Mediastinal nodes or masses	Difficulty swallowing
Major airways obstruction	Intra- or extra-tracheal tumours	Stridor Dyspnoea
Chest wall involvement	Peripheral tumours	Chest wall pain and rib erosion Palpable masses eroding through the chest wall

Table 7.2 Symptoms and signs of invasion of local structures by lung cancer

- Bone pain
- Weight loss
- Fatigue
- Seizure (if brain metastases are present)

Paraneoplastic syndromes

Paraneoplastic syndromes arise when the tumour produces hormones or other substances that indirectly cause pathological changes. Fever is the most common paraneoplastic syndrome. However, more complex effects result from endocrine, neurological or immune mechanisms. Common paraneoplastic syndromes associated with lung cancer are listed in **Table 7.3**.

Metastases

Common sites of metastasis from lung cancers include brain, bone, adrenal glands, liver and kidneys. The clinical presentation depends on the site of spread (**Table 7.4**).

Paraneoplastic syndromes			
Lung cancer type	Paraneoplastic syndrome	Mechanism	Clinical features
All	Cachexia	Hypermetabolism	Rapid weight loss Fatigue Anorexia
	Trousseau's syndrome (malignancy-associated hypercoagulability)	Increased production of procoagulants	Venous thrombosis
	Full blood count abnormalities		Anaemia of chronic disease Thrombocytosis
	Dermatological		Acanthosis nigricans Dermatomyositis Gynaecomastia
Non–small-cell lung cancer	Hypertrophic pulmonary osteoarthropathy	Periostosis caused by unknown mechanisms	Painful swollen and tender wrists and ankles Tibial and radial periosteal reaction on X-ray Finger clubbing
Squamous cell carcinoma	Hypercalcaemia	Parathyroid hormone–like hormone production	Increased blood calcium levels Fatigue, bone pain, confusion, polyuria and constipation ECG abnormalities Hyper-reflexia
Small-cell carcinoma	SIADH	Antidiuretic hormone secretion	Confusion, coma and seizures Hyponatraemia Low serum and high urine osmolality
	Cushing's syndrome	Ectopic adrenocorticotropic hormone production	Central obesity and cushingoid features, and striae Oedema and hypertension Muscle weakness and myopathy Hypokalaemia and hyperglycaemia
	Eaton–Lambert syndrome	Anti–calcium channel antibodies	Limb weakness Autonomic dysfunction
	Neurological	Autoantibodies	Neuropathies Cerebellar dysfunction Cognitive dysfunction

SIADH, syndrome of inappropriate antidiuretic hormone hypersecretion.

Table 7.3 Paraneoplastic syndromes associated with lung cancer

Common sites of lung cancer metastasis			
Site	Clinical features	Investigation	Management
Mediastinal lymph nodes	Mediastinal masses on X-rays If large, bronchial, nerve or oesophageal compression	CT and PET Endobronchial ultrasound biopsies Mediastinoscopy or mediastinotomy	Usually no specific treatment required Radiotherapy for large nodal masses causing pressure effects
Cervical and axillary lymph nodes	Palpable mass in neck or axilla	Percutaneous biopsies	Usually no specific treatment required Radiotherapy for large nodal masses threatening skin erosion
Brain	Morning headache Nausea and vomiting Focal neurology Papilloedema	CT and MRI (ring-enhancing lesions with surrounding oedema)	High-dose corticosteroids for oedema Radiotherapy
Vertebral and paraspinal	Back pain Cord compression (incontinence, leg weakness and paraesthesia)	CT and MRI Radionuclide bone scanning PET	Radiotherapy High-dose corticosteroids for cord compression
Bone	Bone pain Pathological fracture	Bone profile (increased alkaline phosphatase) Radionuclide bone scanning CT and MRI PET	Analgesia Radiotherapy Surgery for fractures
Adrenal gland	Usually asymptomatic	CT, PET and MRI	No specific treatment necessary
Contralateral lung	Usually asymptomatic	Chest X-ray, CT and PET	No specific treatment
Pleura	Progressive breathlessness Signs of a pleural effusion	Chest X-ray, CT and PET Pleural tap for cytology Pleural biopsy	Therapeutic aspiration Medical or surgical pleurodesis Indwelling pleural catheter
Liver	Right upper quadrant pain Nausea and vomiting Palpable irregular liver	Liver function tests CT and ultrasound scans	No specific treatment

CT, computerised tomography; MRI, magnetic resonance imaging; PET, positron emission tomography.

Table 7.4 Common sites of lung cancer metastasis

Because of the wide range of possible sites for metastases and paraneoplastic conditions, lung cancer presents in myriad different ways to many types of physicians. A high index of suspicion is necessary. Chest X-ray is a standard investigation for any smoker older than 50 years with unexplained symptoms possibly caused by lung cancer.

Diagnostic approach

The general approach to diagnosis in a patient with suspected lung cancer is as follows.

1. Chest X-ray to look for a cancer
2. Further imaging to stage the extent of local disease and detect metastases
3. Confirm the diagnosis by obtaining a biopsy of the suspected tumour for histopathology
4. Blood tests to help identify metastases and paraneoplastic syndromes, as well as to assess the patient's background health
5. Pulmonary function tests to assess lung reserve if curative therapy is potentially possible

The timing, sequence and methods of investigation vary between patients, depending on the clinical presentation, radiological findings, and patient's health. A definitive diagnosis is made only on the results of histological or cytological investigations. Therefore a biopsy should be done or samples sent for cytological analysis in almost all cases.

The differential diagnosis of a solitary lung mass is shown in Table 2.30. The main diagnoses to consider are lung metastases, chronic infections (tuberculosis, bacterial or fungal), benign lung tumours and other benign lesions (e.g. healed granulomas and enfolded lung).

Investigations

Investigations are carried out in an order that gives the most information about diagnosis

and stage the extent of the cancer with the least risk to the patient. A commonly used algorithm is shown in **Figure 7.6**.

Chest X-ray

A posteroanterior or anteroposterior chest X-ray is always indicated and is the first investigation when lung cancer is suspected. Tumours often cause a shadow (see **Figure 7.1**).

The appearance of primary lung cancer varies from discrete nodules to large areas of hazy opaque shading. Enlarged lymph nodes indicate the presence of a tumour even if a

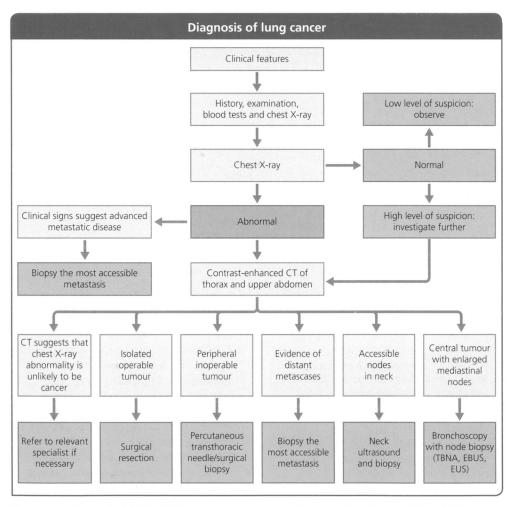

Figure 7.6 Diagnostic algorithm for lung cancer. CT, computed tomography; EBUS, endobronchial ultrasound; EUS, endoscopic ultrasound; TBNA, transbronchial needle aspiration.

shadow is not visible. Other associated signs, such as a collapsed lung, pleural effusion or pleural thickening, may also be identified (**Figure 7.2**). Old chest X-rays are useful for comparison to assess if a shadow is new or has changed.

Detectable lesion size

A lesion has to be >1 cm in diameter before it can be recognised on X-ray. A quarter of patients with lung cancer initially have a normal chest X-ray. In others, the abnormality on an earlier chest X-ray is only identified when a later chest X-ray shows an obvious tumour. When a diagnosis is finally made, patients or their relatives can be angry that recent earlier chest X-rays were reported as normal.

Sputum cytology and bronchoalveolar lavage

Cytological analysis of sputum can identify lung cancer without the need for invasive tests. However, this investigation often gives false negatives. Therefore it is generally used only if patients cannot undergo more invasive tests.

Biopsy

Tissue is sampled using the following methods.

- Bronchoscopy with endobronchial biopsies for proximal lesions or endobronchial ultrasound to biopsy peribronchial lesions and mediastinal nodes
- Percutaneous (needle) biopsy with X-ray, CT or ultrasound guidance for peripheral tumours, or for supraclavicular, axillary and anterior mediastinal lymph nodes
- Thoracentesis (needle aspiration) for pleural effusions
- Surgical biopsy for some tumours (with video-assisted thoracoscopic surgery) and lymph nodes (with mediastinoscopy or mediastinotomy) not accessible by CT-guided or bronchoscopic biopsies.

Bronchoscopy

If the tumour is visible on bronchoscopy, endobronchial biopsies and washings or brushings provide tissue for histological or cytological diagnosis, respectively. Endobronchial ultrasound is used to biopsy mediastinal lymph nodes and peribronchial lesions. Peripheral cancers cannot be biopsied by bronchoscopy, but cytological analysis of bronchial washings sometimes finds tumour cells.

Blood tests

The results of blood tests help show how ill a patient is overall, and therefore whether or not they are fit enough for treatment. Blood tests can suggest dissemination, for example increased alkaline phosphatase with liver or bone metastases. They can also identify metabolic or hormonal paraneoplastic syndromes, for example hyponatraemia from excess antidiuretic hormone secretion by a SCLC, or hypercalcaemia. The common blood tests indicated in suspected lung cancer are shown in **Table 7.5**.

Blood tests in lung cancer	
Blood test	Reason(s)
Full blood count	To check for anaemia, platelet and white blood cell count
	To identify marrow involvement (leucoerythroblastic picture)
Renal function	To assess kidney function (before chemotherapy)
	To measure sodium and potassium levels (SIADH and ectopic ACTH production)
Liver function	To find evidence for liver metastases (increased alkaline phosphatase, bilirubin and alanine transaminase)
Bone profile	To find evidence of bone involvement (increased alkaline phosphatase and hypercalcaemia)
Calcium	Because calcium is increased in bone involvement and paraneoplastic syndromes
Clotting	To assess safety for biopsy and assess bleeding risk

ACTH, adrenocorticotropic hormone; SIADH, syndrome of inappropriate antidiuretic hormone hypersecretion.

Table 7.5 Blood tests in suspected lung cancer

Pulmonary function tests

Respiratory comorbidities such as COPD are common in patients with lung cancer and may prevent curative surgery or radiotherapy. Therefore, spirometry is done in all patients being considered for treatment with curative intent. If the degree of the patient's breathlessness is disproportionate to the spirometry results, other lung pathology is present (e.g. lung fibrosis) or lobectomy or pneumonectomy is being considered, transfer factor should also be measured. Tracheal obstruction caused by tumours is diagnosed on flow–volume loops.

Computerised tomography and magnetic resonance imaging

A CT scan of the lungs, the liver and adrenal glands is essential in all patients with suspected lung cancer. The scan defines the position and size of the primary lesion. These findings show whether lung cancer is a likely diagnosis, which biopsy approach is most suitable, and whether the primary lesion is treatable with curative therapy.

Computerised tomography is also used to identify metastases in the hilar, mediastinal, cervical and axillary lymph nodes; the ipsilateral and contralateral lung; the pleura; the liver; the adrenals; the thoracic spine; and the ribs. If neurological symptoms or signs are present, CT, MRI, or both CT and MRI of the brain are necessary to detect cerebral metastases.

Positron emission tomography and bone scans

Total body positron emission tomography (PET)–CT scans reliably identify primary lung cancer and metastases >1 cm in diameter, which are visible as hotspots. PET scans are used before curative surgery or radiotherapy to ensure that there are no occult metastases. Radioisotope bone scans are used to identify potential bone metastases in patients with bone pain or increased blood calcium or alkaline phosphatase.

Staging

Staging determines the extent of the cancer and its location. Accurate staging of lung cancer is essential for deciding the most appropriate treatment option. For example, in a patient with primary lung cancer who is being considered for surgical resection, it is essential to ensure there is no mediastinal lymph node involvement; this is done by surgical or endobronchial ultrasound-guided biopsies. It is also necessary to ensure that no other unsuspected metastases are present; PET is used for this.

The staging of NSCLC is described in **Table 7.6**, and the staging of SCLC in **Table 7.7**. SCLC is now staged in the same way as NSCLC. However, clinical oncologists still think of it in terms of radiotherapy fields and consider disease to be either limited or extensive.

Management

Treatment for lung cancer depends on the following factors.

- Whether the patient has NSCLC or SCLC. Local treatment with curative intent (surgery or radiotherapy) may be appropriate for NSCLC. SCLC has normally disseminated at presentation but responds to chemotherapy.
- How far the cancer has spread (its stage).
- The patient's ability to tolerate surgery, radiotherapy or chemotherapy. This is assessed with pulmonary function tests, blood and radionucleotide tests of renal function, and assessment of the patient's performance status (e.g. using the World Health Organisation performance scale) (**Table 7.8**).

Management of each patient diagnosed with lung cancer is planned in a multidisciplinary meeting. The patient should have access to a lung cancer nurse specialist who provides expert support and aids communication between health care professionals and the patient.

Surgery

For non–small-cell lung cancer, surgical resection is the only treatment likely to cure the patient. Resection is by:

TNM classification for non small-cell lung cancer			
Score	Tumour size (T)	Nodal involvement (N)	Metastases (M)
X	Cannot be assessed	Cannot be assessed	Cannot be assessed
0	No evidence of tumour	No evidence of node metastases	No evidence of extrathoracic metastases
1a	Maximum dimension ≤ 2 cm	Ipsilateral peribronchiolar or hilar nodes	Additional nodules in contralateral lung or ipsilateral pleural effusion
1b	Maximum dimension 2–3 cm		Evidence of extrathoracic metastases (e.g. to liver, brain, bone or adrenals)
2a	Maximum dimension 3–5 cm	Ispilateral mediastinal or subcarinal nodes	
2b	Maximum dimension 5–7 cm		
3	Maximum dimension > 7 cm or additional nodule in same lobe	Contralateral or extrathoracic nodes	
4	Invading mediastinum, great vessels, trachea, oesophagus or vertebral body		

Table 7.6 Tumour size, nodal involvement and metastases (TNM) staging classification system for non–small-cell lung cancer

Classification of small-cell lung cancer	
Disease stage	Features
Limited	All detectable tumour can be treated within a 'tolerable' radiotherapy field
	Disease usually confined to one hemithorax and involves only ipsilateral hilar, supraclavicular or mediastinal lymph nodes
Extensive	Disease at sites beyond the definition of limited disease
	Includes:
	■ Metastatic lesions in contralateral lung
	■ Distant metastatic involvement (e.g. brain, bone, liver or adrenals)

Table 7.7 Staging classification for small-cell lung cancer

WHO performance scale	
Grade	Criterion
0	Fully active and able to carry out all normal activities
1	Ambulatory and able to carry out non-strenuous activities
2	< 50% in bed during waking hours, and capable of self-care
3	> 50% in bed during waking hours, and capable of only limited self-care
4	Bedbound and completely dependent

Table 7.8 World Health Organisation (WHO) performance scale

- lobectomy (removal of the lobe containing the cancer)
- pneumonectomy (removal of the entire lung); this is necessary if the cancer crosses the oblique fissure

However, surgery is used only for localised disease that is not invading mediastinal structures (stage 1 and selected cases of stage 2). Also, the patient has to have adequate lung function and performance status to suggest that they could tolerate the necessary loss of lung tissue. Occasionally, segmentectomy or wedge resection is used to limit lung loss.

Most small-cell lung cancers have disseminated at presentation. Therefore they are not appropriate for surgical resection.

Radiotherapy

In non–small-cell lung cancer, radical high-dose radiotherapy is used as a potentially curative treatment for localised disease that is not amenable to surgery (e.g. because of the patient's poor lung function or invasion of the chest wall).

Lower dose palliative radiotherapy is commonly used to control the following symptoms.

- Pain caused by chest wall or mediastinal invasion, or by bone metastases
- Haemoptysis
- Tumours causing bronchial obstruction
- Brain, skin, spinal or other extrapulmonary metastases

Radiotherapy is also given for the rare case in which a tissue diagnosis has not been obtained but the radiological findings strongly suggest localised lung cancer. Examples would be a new peripheral lung mass in a patient with severe COPD precluding biopsy (because of the risk of a fatal pneumothorax) or surgery (because of an unacceptably high surgical mortality).

Brachytherapy is localised radiotherapy delivered inside the airway to prevent the tumour causing dyspnoea as a result of bronchial obstruction. Brachytherapy is used if the maximum dose of external beam radiotherapy has already been given.

In small-cell lung cancer, palliative radiotherapy is used for similar indications as those for NSCLC.

Chemotherapy

Non–small-cell lung cancer is partially sensitive to chemotherapy agents. Chemotherapy improves survival and quality of life in patients with NSCLC when given to patients with stage 3 and 4 disease and is considered for patients with inoperable cancer due to spread to the mediastinal lymph nodes.

The potential survival benefit must be balanced against the risk of additional toxicities. Commonly used drugs include docetaxel, gemcitabine, paclitaxel and vinorelbine.

Testing for the presence of EGFR mutations in lung adenocarcinoma identifies patients who may have impressive responses to treatment with EGFR inhibitors (e.g. erlotinib).

Small-cell lung cancer responds rapidly to chemotherapy, with dramatic shrinkage of tumour masses. However, although long-term cure is achieved in a minority of patients, most relapse within a few months. Patients with limited SCLC are offered chemotherapy with or without adjuvant radiotherapy. Chemotherapy is used only in extensive disease if patients are sufficiently fit. Cisplatin is commonly used for SCLC. Radiotherapy is useful for palliation of local symptoms if relapse occurs after first-line treatment.

> **Small-cell lung cancers may respond quickly to chemotherapy, but a rapid response increases the risk of tumour lysis syndrome.** This syndrome is more common in patients with extensive disease. It is characterised by electrolyte disturbance and renal failure. Treatment includes allopurinol and intravenous fluids.

Interventional radiology

Radiofrequency ablation is a new technique in the treatment of localised bronchogenic carcinoma that is unsuitable for surgical resection. A treatment probe is inserted into the tumour, and heat generated from high-frequency alternating current is used to destroy cancer cells.

Management of metastases

Dexamethasone reduces the oedema surrounding brain metastases, and often produces impressive, albeit temporary, improvements in a patient's neurological status. If a patient's performance status is good, brain metastases are treated with whole-brain radiotherapy. In limited stage SCLC, prophylactic cranial irradiation reduces and delays the onset of symptoms associated with brain metastases. It also improves survival.

Radiotherapy is also used to help control pain in patients with bone metastasis, and in those with vertebral metastases causing, or with the potential to cause, spinal cord compression. Adrenal metastases, although common, are usually asymptomatic and do not require treatment.

Palliative care

Unfortunately, most patients with lung cancer die of the disease. Therefore control of symptoms through expert palliative care is an important part of its management. Early integration of palliative care can significantly improve both quality of life and mood. Domiciliary services allow the patient to remain in their own home.

Adequate pain control, using opiate analgesics if necessary, is essential. Weight loss, loss of appetite, depression and difficulty swallowing are managed by multidisciplinary groups, including palliative care professionals.

Smoking cessation

Patients are advised to stop smoking as soon as a diagnosis of lung cancer is suspected. They should be informed that smoking increases the risk of pulmonary complications after lung cancer surgery. Nicotine replacement therapy and other therapies are offered to smokers, however, surgery should not be postponed.

Prognosis

In non–small-cell lung cancer, prognostic factors include the size and type of tumour, symptoms and the extent of tumour spread. The worse the performance status, the worse the prognosis and the fewer the available treatment options. Five-year survival by stage is shown in **Table 7.9.**

Small-cell lung cancer is widespread by the time that most patients present, making it incurable. Mean survival time at the point of diagnosis is only 6 weeks. As with NSCLC, weight loss and poor performance status are associated with a worse prognosis.

Prognosis of lung cancer			
Stage	TNM type	1-year survival (%)	5-year survival (%)
1	T1–2 N0	70	35.3
2	T1–2 N1	59	20.9
	T3 N0		
3	T1–2 N2–3	34	6.3
	T3 N1–3		
	T4 N0–3		
4	Any M1 disease	16	Unknown (poor)

Table 7.9 Prognosis of lung cancer

Mesothelioma

Mesotheliomas are malignancies that arise from mesothelial cells, which are located in the pleura, peritoneum, pericardium and testes. Pleural mesothelioma is the most common. The main histological subtypes are:

- sarcomatous
- epithelial
- mixed sarcomatous–epithelial

Tumour growth

Tumours start as malignant plaques, most often towards the bottom of the chest. The cells subsequently coalesce to form a sheet. This sheet can grow to involve the diaphragm and lung surfaces.

As the disease progresses, it invades the chest wall and mediastinum. Further extension can involve the brachial plexus, ribs, oesophagus and even the superior vena cava. Metastases beyond the thorax are not uncommon, but they are usually asymptomatic.

Epidemiology

The epidemiology varies extensively with geography, depending on the use of asbestos (**Table 7.10**).

Aetiology

Carcinogens

The primary carcinogen responsible for mesothelioma is asbestos. Occupations that involve working with asbestos include mining; any jobs in the building trade; and

Epidemiology of mesothelioma	
Factor	Note(s)
Gender	More common in males than in females
Age	Most common in 50- to 70-year-olds
Occupation	Building trade (carpenters, electricians, builders, etc.)
	Insulation (boilermakers, ship and rail workers, etc.)
	Processing (asbestos mining, dockworkers, etc.)
Incidence	Marked global variability
	Worldwide, 0.9 cases per 100,000 persons per year
Prognosis	Inexorably progressive
	Median survival of 8–14 months

Table 7.10 Epidemiology of mesothelioma

employment on the docks, the railways, or in the automobile industries. In some areas, environmental exposure is a problem, for example from local asbestos mines. These increase the incidence of mesothelioma by 2- to 10-fold compared with areas with no environmental increase in asbestos exposure.

Genetics

Chromosome 22 monosomy (one rather than two copies of the whole chromosome) is the most common genetic abnormality associated with mesothelioma; it is found in up to 40% of cases. The disorder leads to malignancy by causing loss of tumour suppressor gene function.

Clinical features

Presentation is usually with a pleural effusion, progressive breathlessness and chest pain. Other non-specific symptoms include tiredness, night sweats, loss of appetite and weight loss. The chest pain associated with mesothelioma is often severe and difficult to treat. The history of asbestos exposure is often many years before and may not be obvious to the patient.

The risk of mesothelioma is proportional to the extent of asbestos exposure but even a very low-level exposure can cause disease. For example, children of dockers can develop mesothelioma through exposure to asbestos fibres on their father's clothes, or someone may inhale fibres during a single episode when asbestos is fitted to or stripped from a building.

Diagnostic approach

A suggested diagnostic pathway is shown in **Figures 7.6** and **7.7**.

Investigations

Chest X-ray and computerised tomography

Common findings include decreased chest cavity size, thickening of the pleura and a pleural effusion. This effusion may be large. A CT scan confirms the chest X-ray findings and shows circumferential irregular or nodular pleural thickening, pleural effusion and a shrunken underlying lung (**Figure 7.8**).

Pleural fluid

The presence of high protein but normal lactate dehydrogenase is typical, along with few white and red blood cells. It is uncommon for cytological examination to detect malignant cells.

Pleural biopsies

Diagnosis requires adequate histological samples of involved pleura by radiologically guided or thoracoscopic biopsy. Not infrequently, the initial pleural biopsy does not confirm mesothelioma. Therefore repeated biopsies may be necessary.

Staging

Mesothelioma is categorised into four stages (**Table 7.11**).

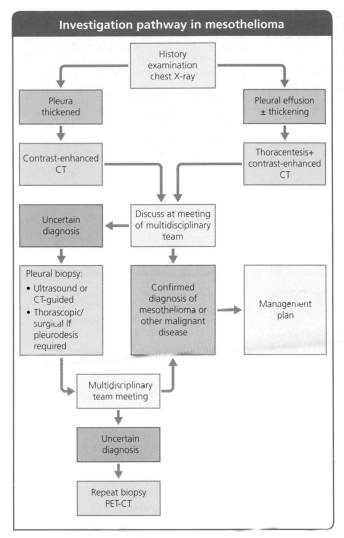

Investigation pathway in mesothelioma

History examination chest X-ray

Pleura thickened

Pleural effusion ± thickening

Contrast-enhanced CT

Thoracentesis+ contrast-enhanced CT

Uncertain diagnosis

Discuss at meeting of multidisciplinary team

Pleural biopsy:
- Ultrasound or CT-guided
- Thorascopic/ surgical if pleurodesis required

Confirmed diagnosis of mesothelioma or other malignant disease

Management plan

Multidisciplinary team meeting

Uncertain diagnosis

Repeat biopsy PET-CT

Figure 7.7 Pathway for investigation of possible mesothelioma. CT, computed tomography; PET, positron emission tomography.

Mesothelioma staging	
Stage	Features
1	No lymphadenopathy
	Remains within parietal pleura
2	As for stage 1, except:
	■ resection margins are positive
	■ local lymphadenopathy may be present
3	Disease has extended to:
	■ chest wall, mediastinum or heart
	■ through the diaphragm or peritoneum
	May involve extrapleural lymph nodes
4	Widespread metastatic disease

Table 7.11 Staging of mesothelioma

Management

Treatment of mesothelioma is determined by stage at presentation and the patient's performance status. Options include surgery, chemotherapy and radiotherapy.

Surgery

Surgery is an option, for example pleurectomy plus perhaps resection of the lung, pericardium and diaphragm. However, surgical resection is difficult because of the large surface area involved, and mortality is high. Surgery is indicated only for some patients with early-stage disease and good performance status.

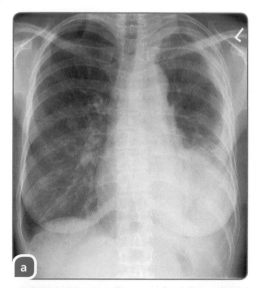

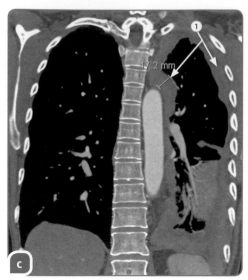

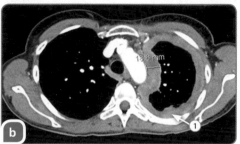

Figure 7.8 (a) Chest X-ray showing left mesothelioma. (b) Computerised tomography (CT saggital section) of mesothelioma showing reduced volume of the left hemithorax, and ① circumferential pleural thickening. (c) CT coronal section of mesothelioma showing ① circumferential pleural thickening.

Radiotherapy

Radiotherapy is used to palliate chest pain and to reduce the size of tumour masses growing through the chest wall. However, it does not improve survival.

Chemotherapy

Mesothelioma responses to chemotherapy are generally poor. Clinical trials are ongoing.

Prognosis

Mesothelioma is usually fatal. Median survival is 11 months. Factors indicating poor prognosis include:

- weight loss
- increased white cell count, lactate dehydrogenase and platelets
- low haemoglobin
- non-epithelial histology
- chest pain
- age > 75 years
- male sex
- poor performance status

Lung metastasis

The lung has an extensive lymph and blood supply, so it is a common site for metastasis of intra- and extrathoracic tumours. Tumours that commonly metastasise to the lung include lung, colon, breast, bladder and renal cancers, as well as melanoma (**Table 7.12**).

Nearly half of all patients with cancer develop lung metastases. Lung metastases are a

Tumours that metastasise to the lung	
Primary tumour	Frequency at presentation of primary tumour (%)
Choriocarcinoma	60
Bronchus*	30
Kidney	20
Osteosarcoma	15
Testis or germ cell	12
Thyroid	7
Bladder	7
Melanoma	7
Prostate	5
Head and neck*	5
Ovary	5
Colorectal*	<5
Cervix	<5
Breast*	4
Uterus, pancreas, oesophagus, stomach or hepatoma	<1

*Common causes of lung metastases.

Table 7.12 Tumours that metastasise to the lung

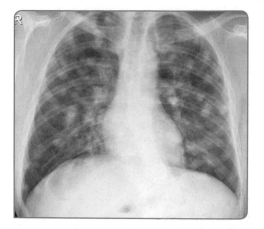

Figure 7.9 Chest X-ray showing multiple lung metastases.

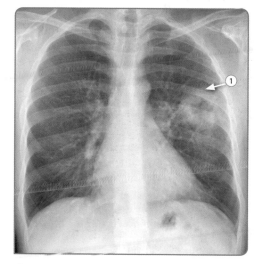

Figure 7.10 Chest X-ray showing a cavitating mass. ① Thick walled cavity in the left mid-zone.

prognostic factor confirming advanced malignant disease.

Clinical features

There are four main patterns of involvement.

- Intrapulmonary metastases. The X-ray appearances are of single or multiple round nodules of varying size (**Figure 7.9**). Some primary tumours cause cavitating lung metastases (**Figure 7.10**). In many cases, lung metastases are identified by staging radiology or incidental chest X-rays, and there are no respiratory symptoms initially. Symptoms include cough, haemoptysis, chest pain and breathlessness.
- Pleural effusions. These are caused by pleural metastases (see Chapter 6).
- Mediastinal lymphadenopathy. This is usually asymptomatic and identified by the finding of enlarged mediastinal lymph nodes on chest X-ray, CT or PET. Massively enlarged nodes can occur with lymphomas.
- Lymphangitis carcinomatosis. Cancer cells infiltrate along the pulmonary lymphatics. This causes marked progressive breathlessness, decreased transfer factor, and patches of reticular nodular shadowing on chest X-ray (**Figure 7.11**). Lymphangitis carcinomatosis has a characteristic appearance on CT.

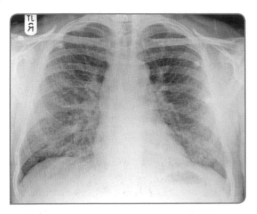

Figure 7.11 Chest X-ray showing lymphangitis with widespread basal reticular opacities.

Management

A biopsy may be necessary to confirm the histological diagnosis. Treatment depends on the primary tumour. Occasionally, surgery is possible if the primary tumour has been removed and has not spread, and if the lung metastasis is easily accessible. Other possible treatments include chemotherapy, hormonal therapy (for breast and prostate cancer), radiotherapy and radiofrequency ablation.

> Accurate detection of the presence of lung metastases is essential, because they qualify as stage 4 disease (cancer that is usually incurable). If patients have already had chemotherapy, an important differential diagnosis is infection as a consequence of chemotherapy-related immunosuppression.

Carcinoid and other lung tumours

Carcinoid tumours are rare lung tumours that originate from neurosecretory cells in the bronchial mucosa. They cause <3% of all lung cancers and are usually found growing in a major bronchus. Carcinoids usually grow slowly and invade locally and recur after excision. However, they rarely metastasise. Carcinoids produce hormones (e.g. adrenocorticotropic hormone, serotonin and bradykinin), which cause paraneoplastic syndromes. The incidence of carcinoid tumours is unrelated to smoking.

Adenoid cystic carcinomas are benign salivary gland tumours that affect the bronchial tree. Hamartomas are benign peripheral tumours consisting of different types of well-differentiated tissue.

Clinical features

Carcinoid or adenoid cystic carcinomas cause cough, lobar collapse and recurrent infections distal to the bronchial obstruction. In most cases, a mass or lobar collapse is visible on chest X-ray. CT is necessary to define the appearances and local extent accurately, as well as for staging (**Figure 7.12**).

Serotonin release can cause carcinoid syndrome, with diarrhoea and skin flushing. Hamartomas are almost always incidental findings on chest X-ray.

> Slowly progressive airways obstruction caused by a benign tumour is often mistakenly diagnosed as asthma. If the tumour is not obvious on chest X-ray, it is identified by CT or bronchoscopy.

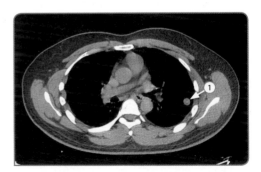

Figure 7.12 CT showing a pulmonary hamartoma ①.

Management

Surgical removal, if possible, is the best treatment option for carcinoids and cystic adenoid carcinomas. If the tumour is inoperable, or if metastasis has occurred, chemotherapy may be indicated.

Somatostatin analogues (e.g. octreotide) are useful in decreasing symptoms associated with carcinoid syndrome. Hamartomas can be observed; surgical resection is curable but rarely necessary.

Answers to starter questions

1. Smoking is by far the main cause of lung cancer. However, an individual's susceptibility to the carcinogens in smoke varies. Carcinogens increase the number of DNA mutations in a cell, increasing the chance of a cell proliferating or growing abnormally as systems of self-regulation and repair are damaged. This risk is also influenced by individual genetic components (e.g. in DNA repair systems) that make some people more susceptible to, or protect them from, the mutagenic effects of cigarette smoke than others.

2. Cure is possible if lung cancer is identified early, when the tumour is small, has not metastasized, and all of it can be surgically removed. However, clinically undetectable metastases may have occurred by the time of surgery, so recurrence is possible.

3. With all types of cancer, some respond better to one type of treatment over another. SCLC usually responds well to chemotherapy. However, by the time it is found it has usually spread, and the tumour bulk is large, making it difficult to treat.

4. Metastasis occurs when single cancer cells pass into the bloodstream or lymph. From there, they can be transported all over the body and can settle anywhere and start to proliferate forming satellite tumours distal to the primary tumour. Very small metastases (micrometastases) cannot be seen by present imaging methods. This is the main reason why patients with operable lung cancer often relapse despite successful surgery.

5. If everyone in the world stopped smoking, the incidence of lung cancer would be significantly reduced. However, even when all the people who smoked have eventually died, lung cancer would still persist, because 10% of cases are unrelated to cigarette smoking. A tobacco ban is unlikely because of the large sums of money governments and tobacco companies make from the sale of cigarettes worldwide.

Chapter 8
Lung infections

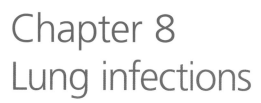
Starter questions

Answers to the following questions are on page 271–272.

1. What do the abbreviations CAP, HAP, VAP, CPE and NTM stand for?
2. What does a positive sputum culture result mean for the most common respiratory pathogens?
3. Is the term atypical pneumonia useful?
4. When should antituberculous therapy be started for a patient with suspected tuberculosis?
5. How is severity assessed in cases of community-acquired pneumonia?
6. Why does influenza cause considerable mortality?

Introduction

Infections of the respiratory tract are largely defined by the anatomical site affected (**Table 8.1**). The most common are acute upper respiratory tract infections (URTIs) and bronchitis (**Figure 8.1**). These infections are usually mild and self-limiting. However, the lungs are continually exposed to microorganisms in inspired air as well as material aspirated from the upper respiratory tract. Therefore more severe lung infections, such as pneumonia, are also a common worldwide cause of morbidity and mortality.

Respiratory infection syndromes		
Site of infection	Name	Definition and notes
Upper respiratory tract		
Nasal passages	Rhinitis	The 'common cold'
Pharynx, larynx and/or tonsils	Pharyngitis, laryngitis and tonsillitis	A sore throat; these illnesses often overlap with rhinitis
Lower respiratory tract		
Bronchi and trachea	Bronchitis and tracheitis	Commonest lower respiratory tract infection in adults
		Major cause of exacerbations of chronic obstructive pulmonary disease and bronchiectasis
Bronchioles	Bronchiolitis	Common childhood illness caused by respiratory syncytial virus infection
		In adults, generally associated with bronchitis or pneumonia
Alveoli and interstitium	Community-acquired pneumonia	Pneumonia acquired outside hospital
	Hospital-acquired pneumonia	Pneumonia acquired during or within 7 days of hospital admission
	Ventilator-acquired pneumonia	Pneumonia acquired by mechanically ventilated patients
	Pneumonia in the immunocompromised patient	Pneumonia in patients with *severe* immune defects
	Lung abscess	Cavitating lung infection, usually with a fluid level
	Subacute lung infections	Slowly progressive focal pneumonia or cavitating lung infections
	Pulmonary tuberculosis	Subacute lung infections caused by *Mycobacterium tuberculosis*
Pleural space	Parapneumonic effusions	Sterile exudative pleural effusion associated with pneumonia
	Complicated parapneumonic effusions	Infected or loculated parapneumonic effusion
	Empyema	Culture-positive pleural effusion or one with visibly turbid fluid
	Pleural tuberculosis	Pleural effusion caused by tuberculosis

Table 8.1 Clinically important respiratory infection syndromes

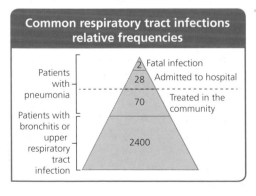

Common respiratory tract infections relative frequencies

Figure 8.1 The relative frequencies of common respiratory tract infections.

Case 10 Three days of cough and fever

Presentation

Mrs Martin, aged 45 years, visits the emergency department with a 3-day history of high fevers and cough.

Initial interpretation

A new fever suggests an infection, and the cough localises the infection to the respiratory tract. The clinical assessment needs to determine which part of the respiratory tract has been affected and define the severity of the infection.

History

Mrs Martin was previously well. The cough produces two teaspoons of green phlogm daily. Over the past 24 h, she has become short of breath and developed a pain on her right side. The pain is worse when she breathes in.

Interpretation of history

Shortness of breath suggests that the infection is affecting the alveoli. Therefore pneumonia is possible, in this case community-acquired pneumonia (CAP); Mrs Martin was out of hospital when the infection developed.

The pain on inspiration could be pleuritic chest pain caused by inflammation of the pleura overlying the pneumonia. Alternatively, it could be musculoskeletal pain from a pulled muscle or even a rib fracture caused by coughing.

Further history

Mrs Martin smokes 15 cigarettes a day and drinks 30 units of alcohol per week. There is no significant past history. She has not recently travelled abroad.

Examination

Mrs Martin's temperature is 39.5°C, her pulse rate 110 beats/min and her blood pressure 95/50 mmHg. She is centrally cyanosed with a respiratory rate of 30 breaths/min. She has a patch of painful vesicles over her lip.

The trachea is central, but there is reduced expansion on inspiration of the right chest. There is dullness to percussion over the right lung base. On auscultation, focal coarse crepitations are heard at the right base, with an area of bronchial breathing and a pleural rub. The rest of the examination is normal.

Interpretation of findings

Smoking and excess alcohol intake are major risk factors for CAP (**Table 8.9**). A travel history is important, because travel exposes patients to rarer or resistant pathogens.

The high temperature and heart rate suggest an active infection. The increased respiratory rate and cyanosis strongly suggest that this infection is pneumonia. This diagnosis is confirmed by the signs of consolidation and pleural inflammation (the rub) over the right lower lobe.

The lip vesicles are a recurrence of herpes simplex, which is commonly associated with pneumonia.

Investigations

Chest X-ray confirms consolidation of the right lower lobe (**Figure 8.2**). Oxygen saturation is 84% on air. Blood gases show a Pao_2 of 8.3 kPa and a $Paco_2$ of 3.9 kPa on 40% oxygen.

Some of her blood tests results are abnormal: white cell count 2.1×10^6/mL; platelets 115×10^6/mL; haemoglobin, 15.3 g/L; urea 9.8 mmol/L; albumin 24 g/L; alkaline phosphatase 160 IU/L; and alanine transaminase 93 IU/L. Urea and electrolytes and coagulation test results are normal. C-reactive protein concentration is markedly raised at 395 mg/L.

Case 10 *continued*

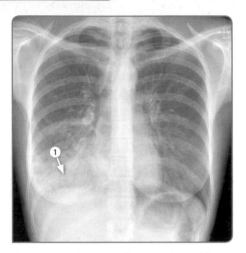

Figure 8.2 Chest X-ray from a patient with community-acquired pneumonia affecting the right lower lobe. ① Consolidation of the right lower lobe.

Diagnosis

The symptoms and signs indicate a CAP. This diagnosis is confirmed by the new consolidation seen on chest X-ray.

Blood test abnormalities are common in patients with CAP. Increased C-reactive protein and low albumin reflect the acute-phase inflammatory response. The low white cell and platelet counts, and the increased urea and test results showing deranged liver function are the result of sepsis.

A CURB-65 score of 3 is calculated from the values for urea (>7.6 mmol/L), respiratory rate (>30 breaths/min) and diastolic blood pressure (<60 mmHg) (**Table 8.2**). This score indicates severe disease with a 17% mortality (**Table 8.3**). Significant hypoxia and high C-reactive protein are additional markers for severe CAP.

Mrs Martin needs:

- high-flow oxygen (to increase oxygen saturation to 94–98%)
- immediate administration of empirical intravenous antibiotics (co-amoxiclav and clarithromycin for a patient with CURB-65 score of 3)

- intravenous fluid to treat the hypotension
- painkillers to relieve the chest pain

Furthermore, careful monitoring is needed, perhaps on the intensive care unit.

Blood and sputum cultures, urine antigen tests for *Legionella* and *Streptococcus pneumoniae* (to identify possible causative pathogens), and an HIV test (an important underlying risk factor) are necessary (**Tables 8.11** and **8.12**).

CURB-65 score	
Symptom	Criterion*
Confusion	
Urea	> 7 mmol/L
Respiratory rate	> 30 breaths/min
Diastolic blood pressure	< 60 mmHg
Age	> 65 years

*One point for each. Additional markers of severity are bilateral consolidation, marked hypoxia, extensive comorbidities and C-reactive protein >250 mg/L.

Table 8.2 Calculation of the CURB-65 score

Management according to the CURB-65 score		
Score	Mortality (%)	Action
0 or 1	1	Patient could be treated at home
2	13	Admit patient to hospital
3	17	Admit patient to hospital. Severe disease: consider intensive care
4	42	Admit patient to hospital. Severe disease: consider intensive care
5	57	Admit patient to hospital. Severe disease: consider intensive care

Table 8.3 Management of CAP according to the CURB-65 score

Case 11 Three months of cough and fever

Presentation

Mr Khan, who is 40 years old, has been referred to the respiratory department with a 3-month history of a new cough with occasional fevers.

Initial interpretation

Cough persisting for 3 months would be unusual for most acute lung infections. Post-infective bronchial hyper-reactivity or asthma could explain this symptom. However, these would not cause fever, which suggests a differential diagnosis of subacute lung infection (e.g. tuberculosis), an inflammatory lung disease or cancer.

History

Mr Khan has had night sweats, feels tired, lacks appetite and energy, and has lost 8 kg in weight. On several occasions, he has coughed up small amounts of fresh red blood.

Interpretation of history

The history describes marked systemic symptoms. If Mr Khan belongs to a high-risk group, these symptoms would strongly suggest tuberculosis.

Further history

Mr Khan does not smoke or drink. He has no recognised HIV risk factors and no

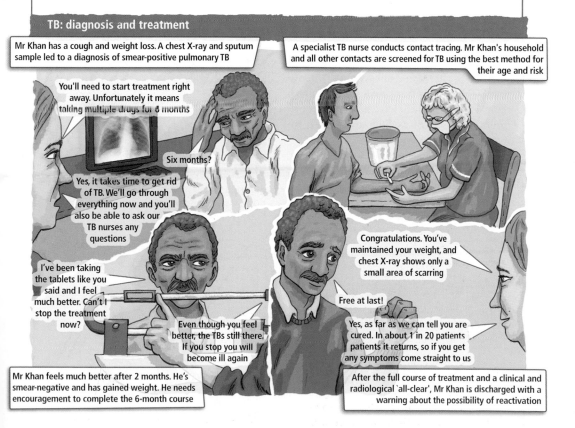

TB: diagnosis and treatment

Mr Khan has a cough and weight loss. A chest X-ray and sputum sample led to a diagnosis of smear-positive pulmonary TB

A specialist TB nurse conducts contact tracing. Mr Khan's household and all other contacts are screened for TB using the best method for their age and risk

You'll need to start treatment right away. Unfortunately it means taking multiple drugs for 6 months

Six months?

Yes, it takes time to get rid of TB. We'll go through everything now and you'll also be able to ask our TB nurses any questions

I've been taking the tablets like you said and I feel much better. Can't I stop the treatment now?

Even though you feel better, the TBs still there. If you stop you will become ill again

Congratulations. You've maintained your weight, and chest X-ray shows only a small area of scarring

Free at last!

Yes, as far as we can tell you are cured. In about 1 in 20 patients patients it returns, so if you get any symptoms come straight to us

Mr Khan feels much better after 2 months. He's smear-negative and has gained weight. He needs encouragement to complete the 6-month course

After the full course of treatment and a clinical and radiological 'all-clear', Mr Khan is discharged with a warning about the possibility of reactivation

Case 11 *continued*

significant previous medical history. He was born in Pakistan and moved to the UK 3 years ago. He has no personal history of tuberculosis, but his aunt had the disease when he was 7 years old.

Examination

Mr Khan looks pale, thin and unwell. His temperature is 37.5°C. No other abnormal signs are present, and the chest examination is unremarkable.

Interpretation of findings

Birth in a country with a high incidence of tuberculosis is the most significant risk factor for tuberculosis (**Table 8.20**). The risk of reactivation of latent tuberculosis is increased by emigration for up to 5 years.

Most patients with tuberculosis do not recall exposure to anyone with a known case of the disease. However, Mr Khan's family history confirms exposure to tuberculosis. He is likely to have had latent (dormant) tuberculosis, which reactivated to cause the present symptoms.

Tuberculosis is likely because of the demographic factors combined with the history of systemic and respiratory symptoms over months. Patients with pulmonary tuberculosis often have no specific signs, unless they have extensive or destructive disease.

Investigations

Chest X-ray shows a patchy consolidation with small areas of cavitation in the right upper lobe (**Figure 8.3**). Mr Khan has an increased erythrocyte sedimentation rate (100 mm/h) and C-reactive protein (57 mg/L), and a mild normochromic normocytic anaemia (haemoglobin, 10.2 g/L). His HIV test is negative. Microscopy identifies acid-fast bacilli in two out of three morning sputum samples (**Figure 8.4**).

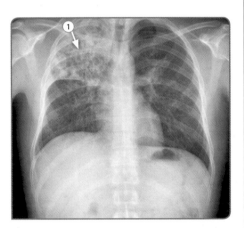

Figure 8.3 Chest X-ray from a patient with pulmonary tuberculosis. ① Patchy consolidation with cavitation in the right upper lobe.

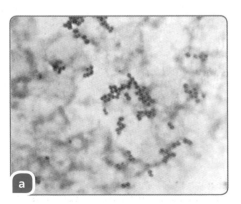
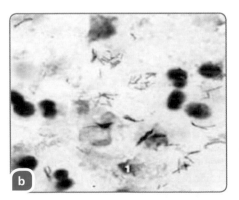

Figure 8.4 Sputum microscopy to identify causative organisms. (a) *Staphylococcus aureus* in clusters (Gram stain x1000). (b) Ziehl-Nielsen stain for Acid Fast Bacilli showing *M. tuberculosis*.

Case 11 *continued*

Diagnosis

The chest X-ray appearances strongly suggest active pulmonary tuberculosis. Other chronic infections are possible but are much rarer causes of this presentation than TB. These findings, along with the history and risk factors, mean that conventional quadruple antituberculous therapy should start before microbiological confirmation of the disease.

In Mr Khan's case, the presence of acid-fast bacilli in the sputum confirms a mycobacterial infection. In this context, the bacterium is almost certainly *Mycobacterium tuberculosis*, the cause of tuberculosis, rather than a non-tuberculous mycobacteria (NTM).

The mycobacterial species is confirmed only by culture, which takes 4–6 weeks. Patients with visible acid-fast bacilli in their sputum are highly infectious. Therefore Mr Khan needs to avoid contact with young children and people who are immunosuppressed. His family and close contacts need to be screened to see whether they also have tuberculosis.

Antituberculosis treatment cures 95% of uncomplicated disease. However, treatment lasts ≥6 months, so adherence is often a problem.

Microbiology of the respiratory tract

Many different microorganisms cause respiratory tract infections. However, a limited number of pathogens dominate: influenza A, *S. pneumoniae* and *M. tuberculosis* cause the vast majority of deaths from lung infection worldwide.

The features of common respiratory microbial pathogens are summarised in **Table 8.4**, and their treatment in **Table 8.5**. Common routes of infection are shown in **Figure 8.5**.

Viruses

Influenza

Influenza A, B and C, and parainfluenza, are highly contagious RNA respiratory viruses that cause flu, an acute URTI or bronchitis with marked systemic symptoms.

Influenza A is the most common of these viruses. It is responsible for annual winter epidemics in the northern hemisphere. Influenza often exacerbates underlying chronic lung or cardiac disease, causing significant mortality in the elderly.

Occasionally, influenza can be complicated by primary viral or secondary bacterial pneumonias. These complications are more common during worldwide epidemics (termed pandemics, the most recent was in 2009) of a new viral variant, and cause large numbers of deaths. Avian flu is caused by influenza A strains prevalent in domestic fowl that sporadically spread to humans. Although rare, avian flu infection has a high mortality because it causes primary viral pneumonia.

Other respiratory viruses

Other common respiratory viruses include respiratory syncytial virus, measles, rhinovirus, coxsackie virus, metapneumovirus, coronavirus and adenovirus. These cause URTIs, bronchitis, bronchiolitis (respiratory syncytial virus) and occasionally pneumonia. A highly contagious and virulent coronavirus caused the severe acute respiratory syndrome (SARS) epidemic in 2003.

Cytomegalovirus and other herpesviruses

Herpesviruses are DNA viruses that rarely cause severe diffuse bilateral interstitial pneumonias. The herpesvirus family

Respiratory pathogens			
Pathogen	Microbiology	Usual source of infection	Main clinical presentations
Viral			
Influenza and parainfluenza	RNA viruses	Inhalation of infected droplets	Upper and lower respiratory tract infections*
Other respiratory viruses (e.g. respiratory syncytial virus, rhinovirus and adenovirus)	Variable	Inhalation of infected droplets	Upper and lower respiratory tract infections*
Cytomegalovirus	DNA herpesvirus	Close contacts who have the infection Reactivation of latent infection	Pneumonia in immunocompromised patients
Bacterial			
Corynebacterium diphtheriae	Gram-positive and pleomorphic	Close contacts	Diphtheria (pharyngitis and tonsillitis)
Bordetella pertussis	Gram-positive coccobacilli	Inhalation of infected droplets	Whooping cough (a severe bronchitis)
Streptococcus pyogenes	Gram-positive cocci	Close contacts	Pharyngitis
S. pneumoniae	Gram-positive cocci	Microaspiration	Lower respiratory tract infections* Empyema
Haemophilus influenzae	Gram-negative coccobacilli	Microaspiration	Lower respiratory tract infections* Acute epiglottitis
Moraxella catarrhalis	Gram-negative coccobacilli	Microaspiration	Lower respiratory tract infections*
Staphylococcus aureus	Gram-positive cocci	Microaspiration	Lower respiratory tract infections* HAP and VAP Empyema Lung abscess
Gram-negative bacilli (e.g. Klebsiella pneumoniae, Escherichia coli, and Proteus species)	Enteric Gram-negative bacilli	Microaspiration	Lower respiratory tract infections* HAP and VAP Subacute lung infections Lung abscess
Anaerobes (e.g. Bacteroides and Peptostreptococcus)	Variable	Microaspiration	Aspiration pneumonia Empyema Lung abscess
Pseudomonas aeruginosa	Gram-negative bacilli	Environmental sources	Lower respiratory tract infections* HAP and VAP
Legionella pneumophila†	Gram-negative bacilli Intracellular pathogen	Inhalation of infected water source	Flu-like illness (Pontiac fever) Lower respiratory tract infections*
Chlamydophila pneumoniae†	Small intracellular pathogen	Inhalation of infected droplets	Lower respiratory tract infections*
Mycoplasma pneumoniae†	No cell wall Smallest free-living organism	Inhalation of infected droplets	Lower respiratory tract infections*

Respiratory pathogens *Continued*			
Pathogen	Microbiology	Usual source of infection	Main clinical presentations
Mycobacterium tuberculosis	Slow-growing Intracellular pathogen	Inhalation of infected droplets Reactivation of latent infection	Tuberculosis
Non-tuberculous mycobacteria	Slow-growing Intracellular pathogens	Environmental sources	Subacute lung infections (similar to tuberculosis) Bronchiectasis
Fungal			
Aspergillus species	Filamentous fungi	Inhalation of spores	Mycetomas Allergic bronchopulmonary aspergillosis Subacute lung infections Pneumonia in immunocompromised patients
Pneumocystis jirovecii (*Pneumocystis* pneumonia)	Single-cell fungus No cell wall	Overgrowth of lung commensal	Pneumonia in immunocompromised patients
Endemic fungi (e.g. Histoplasma)	Restricted geography Intracellular pathogens	Inhalation of spores Reactivation of latent infection	Flu-like illness Subacute lung infections (similar to tuberculosis)

HAP, hospital-acquired pneumonia; VAP, ventilator-acquired pneumonia.

*Bronchitis (including infective exacerbations of chronic obstructive pulmonary disease) and community-acquired pneumonia.

†Atypical organisms that cause community-acquired pneumonia.

Table 8.4 Features of the commonest clinically relevant respiratory pathogens

includes cytomegalovirus (CMV) and varicella-zoster virus.

- Reactivation of latent CMV infection causes pneumonia in severely immunosuppressed patients.
- Primary varicella-zoster virus infection (chicken pox) in adults often causes pneumonia.

Bacteria

Streptococcus pneumoniae

S. pneumoniae is a pharyngeal commensal bacterium (colonises an anatomical site without causing disease) in 10% of adults and >50% of children. It is also the predominant bacterial cause of CAP. Bacteria reach the lungs by silent aspiration of the nasopharyngeal contents (microaspiration).

Resistance of *S. pneumoniae* to common antibiotics is a problem in some countries (e.g. Spain and Mexico). Childhood vaccination against 13 of the bacterium's 93 known serotypes is routine in increasing numbers of Western and developing countries.

Haemophilus influenzae and Moraxella catarrhalis

The common nasopharyngeal commensal organisms *H. influenzae* and *M. catarrhalis* are major causes of acute or chronic bronchial infection in patients with chronic obstructive pulmonary disease or bronchiectasis; they are less common causes of CAP. *H. influenzae* rarely cause a life-threatening acute epiglottitis.

Staphylococcus aureus

S. aureus is a skin and upper respiratory tract commensal that causes CAP (often aggres-

Drug treatments of respiratory pathogens		
Pathogen	Standard treatment options	Resistance pattern
Viral		
Influenza and parainfluenza	Neuraminidase inhibitors, amantadine and ribavarin	Resistance rare
Other respiratory viruses	Limited options	Resistance rare
Cytomegalovirus	Ganciclovir and foscarnet	Resistance rare
Bacterial		
S. pneumoniae	ß lactams, macrolides and tetracyclines	Resistance to penicillins and macrolides common in some countries (e.g. Spain)
H. influenzae	ß lactams, tetracyclines and fluoroquinolones	Often resistant to amoxicillin and macrolides
M. catarrhalis	ß lactams, tetracyclines, macrolides and fluoroquinolones	Often resistant to amoxicillin
S. aureus	Flucloxacillin, fusidic acid, co-amoxiclav and macrolides	Often resistant to amoxicillin
MRSA	Teicoplanin and vancomycin	
Gram-negative bacilli	Co-amoxiclav, fluoroquinolones, second- and third-generation cephalosporins, extended spectrum penicillins, aminoglycosides and carbapenems	Often resistant to amoxicillin and macrolides
Anaerobes	Penicillins, clindamycin and metronizadole	
P. aeruginosa	Ciprofloxacin, 3rd generation cephalosporins, extended spectrum penicillins, aminogylcosides, carbopenems	Resistant to almost all oral antibiotics except ciprofloxacin Frequent resistance to other antibiotics
L. pneumophila*	Macrolides and fluoroquinolones	Resistant to ß lactams
C. pneumoniae*	Macrolides, tetracyclines and fluoroquinolones	Resistant to ß lactams
M. pneumoniae*	Macrolides, tetracyclines and fluoroquinolones	Resistant to ß lactams
M. tuberculosis	Anti-mycobacterial antibiotics, fluoroquinolones, aminoglycosides	Resistance common in some countries (e.g. Baltic states)
Non-tuberculous mycobacteria	Anti-mycobacterial antibiotics, fluoroquinolones, macrolides and aminoglycosides	Resistance is common and treatment often difficult
Fungal		
Aspergillus species	Amphotericin, voriconazole, posaconazole, itraconazole and echinocandins	Resistant to fluconazole
P. jirovecii (Pneumocystis pneumonia, PCP)	Co-trimoxazole, pentamadine, and clindamycin plus primaquine	Resistance to first-line treatment is rare

MRSA, methicillin-resistant S. aureus.

*atypical pneumonia organisms.

Table 8.5 Antimicrobial treatments of common respiratory pathogens

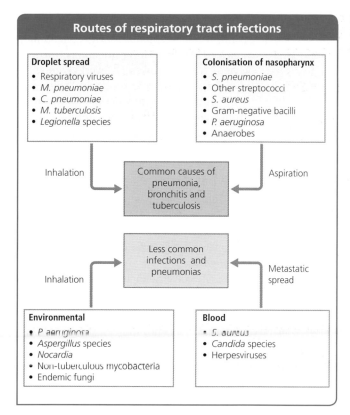

Figure 8.5 Common routes of infection for respiratory tract infections.

sive, with cavitating multifocal consolidation), hospital-acquired pneumonia (HAP) and hospital-acquired empyemas. The bacterium also spreads to the lung via the blood from infected indwelling venous catheter or right-sided endocarditis.

Methicillin-resistant *S. aureus* (MRSA) is resistant to all first-line antibiotics. It is a common cause of hospital-acquired infections.

Legionella pneumophila

Legionella are environmental bacteria found in sources of water such as air conditioning units or cooling towers. If contaminated water is inhaled, *Legionella* invades alveolar macrophages to cause a flu-like illness (Pontiac fever) or CAP.

Chlamydophila pneumoniae and Mycoplasma pneumoniae

C. pneumoniae and *M. pneumoniae* infect the respiratory mucosa to cause bronchitis, bronchiolitis and CAP. *C. psittaci* causes psittacosis, a rare CAP caught from birds.

Chlamydophila and *Mycoplasma*, along with *Legionella*, are sometimes called 'atypical organisms'. This name reflects their unusual microbiological characteristics and their requirement for special culture conditions.

Gram-negative bacilli

Gram-negative bacteria, including *Klebsiella pneumoniae* and *Escherichia coli*, are unusual causes of CAP. However, these bacteria are common oropharyngeal commensals in hospital patients, so they frequently cause HAP, ventilator-acquired pneumonia (VAP), and pneumonia in the immunocompromised patient. *K. pneumoniae* is an uncommon cause of aggressive upper lobe CAP, especially in patients with a history of alcohol abuse.

Anaerobes

Anaerobic bacteria (e.g. *Peptostreptococcus* and *Bacteroides* species) are commonly associated with aspiration pneumonia, empyema and lung abscess, often as a mixed infection with other bacteria. Anaerobic bacterial infections are characterised by production of a foul-smelling pus.

Pseudomonas aeruginosa

P. aeruginosa is an environmental bacterium that is a common cause of HAP, VAP, pneumonia in immunocompromised patients, and bronchial infections in bronchiectasis. It is resistant to most oral antibiotics and rapidly becomes resistant to intravenous antibiotics.

Other Gram-negative environmental organisms that cause VAP and infections in bronchiectasis patients are species of *Burkholderia*, *Stenotrophomonas* and *Acinetobacter*.

Mycobacterium tuberculosis

M. tuberculosis causes tuberculosis. The bacterium is slow-growing and has a unusual lipid cell wall structure. It replicates in macrophages and is resistant to most conventional antibiotics.

M. tuberculosis infects humans only. The related *Mycobacterium bovis* infects cattle and badgers as well as humans. Another related organism, bacille Calmette–Guerin (BCG), is a laboratory-altered strain of *M. bovis* used as a live attenuated vaccine against tuberculosis.

> **Identification of the following pathogens in a respiratory sample always confirms the presence of active infection: *M. tuberculosis*, *L. pneumophila*, *M. pneumoniae*, *C. pneumoniae* and the respiratory viruses.** In contrast, isolation of *S. aureus*, *P. aeruginosa*, *S. pneumoniae*, *H. influenzae* or *Aspergillus* species from sputum means either active infection or asymptomatic colonisation, depending on the clinical context.

Non-tuberculous mycobacteria

Non-tuberculous mycobacteria are species found in the environment (e.g. in water and soil) that occasionally cause lung infections resembling tuberculosis. Species that often cause human disease include *Mycobacterium kansasii, xenopi, avium* and *intracelluare*.

Rarer bacterial pathogens

Nocardia and *Actinomycosis* are uncommon causes of subacute lung infections. *Coxiella burnetii* (which causes Q fever), *Francisella tularensis*, *Bacillus anthracis* and *Yesinia pestis* are rare causes of pneumonia acquired through contact with infected animals.

Fungi

Aspergillus species

Aspergillus is a ubiquitous environmental fungus. Inhalation of its airbourne spores uncommonly causes a lung infection. The species that most commonly causes disease is *A. fumigatus*.

Possible consequences of *Aspergillus* exposure or infection are:

- the formation of mycetomas in pre-existing lung cavities
- allergic bronchopulmonary aspergillosis (ABPA)
- aggressive focal pneumonias or sinusitis (usually in immunosuppressed patients)

Pneumocystis jirovecii

P. jirovecii is an unusual fungus as it lacks a cell wall and grows as single cells. It is an asymptomatic coloniser of the lung. In immunocompromised patients, it causes a specific type of pneumonia called *Pneumocystis* pneumonia (PCP).

Endemic fungal pathogens

Histoplasma, Coccidioides and *Blastomycetes* cause flu-like illnesses in specific geographical areas, for example the Ohio River valley in the USA for *Histoplasma*. Rarely they cause more aggressive infections that mimic tuberculosis, especially in the immunocompromised patient.

Microbiological diagnosis

Identification of the pathogen responsible for the infection confirms the clinical diagnosis and helps guide the choice of antibiotics.

A range of methods are used to make a microbiological diagnosis. Each has its advantages and disadvantages (**Table 8.6**).

The choice of method for microbiological diagnosis depends on the pathogen and clinical scenario. Therefore the decision is guided by the results of clinical assessment. Generally, more extensive testing is reserved for patients with severe disease, as well as immunocompromised patients. In the latter, the range of potential causative pathogens is broader.

Microbiological diagnosis for specific types of respiratory pathogen is summarised in **Table 8.7**.

Microbiological diagnostic tests: advantages and disadvantages		
Method	Advantages	Disadvantages
Microscopy (e.g. Gram stain and test for acid-fast bacilli; **Figure 8.4**)	Rapid (< 24 h) Positive despite antibiotics	Requires expertise Does not identify the species No drug sensitivities
Culture on media	Definitive identification of organism Allows testing of antibiotic sensitivities	Slow (24 h for most bacteria but up to 6 weeks for tuberculosis or NTM) Negative after antibiotics Unsuitable for viruses, *Mycoplasma* and *Chlamydophila* Positive result can reflect colonisation rather than infection
Cell culture	For pathogens that are difficult to grow on conventional media (e.g. viruses, *Mycoplasma*, *Chlamydophila*)	Slow (days) Expensive Technically difficult
Antigen tests	Rapid (< 24 h) Specific Positive despite antibiotics	Requires specific laboratory expertise No drug sensitivities
Serology	Positive for pathogens that are difficult to grow Positive despite antibiotics	Very slow; most tests require paired samples 3 weeks apart
Nucleic acid amplification tests	Rapid (< 24 h) Positive despite antibiotics	Require specific laboratory expertise Positive result can reflect colonisation or latent rather than active infection
Cytology	Rapid (< 24 h) Positive despite antibiotics	Requires specific laboratory expertise Cytological appearances diagnostic for selected pathogens only (e.g. *Pneumocystis*, fungi, *Nocardia*, *Actinomycetes* and cytomegalovirus)
Histopathology	Diagnostic for some infections (e.g. tuberculosis) Samples can also be cultured	Can be slow (days) No drug sensitivities Histological appearances diagnostic only for selected pathogens (e.g. tuberculosis, NTM, fungi, *Nocardia* and *Actinomycetes*)
NTM, non-tuberculous mycobacteria.		

Table 8.6 Advantages and disadvantages of different methods for making a microbiological diagnosis

Common microbiological tests for respiratory pathogens

Pathogen	Sample source(s)	Microbiological test(s)
Influenza, parainfluenza or respiratory virus*	Nasopharyngeal aspirates	Immunofluorescence or DNA amplification tests
	Blood	Serology
Cytomegalovirus	Blood	Serology (identifies latent infection)
	Blood	Antigen and nucleic acid amplification (viral load)
	Bronchial washings or bronchoalveolar lavage	Cytology (immunofluorescence)
S. pyogenes (pharyngitis)	Throat swab	Microscopy (Gram stain) and culture
	Blood	Serology (antistreptolysin O titre)
M. pneumoniae or C. pneumoniae*	Blood	Serology
S. pneumoniae	Sputum, bronchial washings, blood or pleural fluid	Microscopy (Gram stain) and culture
	Urine	Urinary antigen test (70% sensitivity)
S. aureus, H. influenzae and P. aeruginosa	Sputum, bronchial washings, blood or pleural fluid	Microscopy (Gram stain) and culture
L. pneumophila*	Blood	Serology
	Urine	Urinary antigen test (70% sensitivity)
M. tuberculosis	Sputum, bronchial washings or bronchoalveolar lavage, or pleural fluid	Microscopy (acid-fast bacilli) and prolonged culture
	Sputum, bronchial washings or bronchoalveolar lavage, pleural fluid	Nucleic acid amplification tests
	Blood	Interferon-γ release assay (identifies latent infection)
	Skin test	Mantoux or Heaf test (identifies latent infection)[†]
	Lymph node, lung or pleural biopsy	Histology (shows caseating granulomas and sometimes positive staining for acid-fast bacilli)
Aspergillus	Sputum, bronchial washings or bronchoalveolar lavage	Microscopy (fungal stains) and culture
	Blood, bronchial washings or bronchoalveolar lavage	Galactomannan antigen
	Blood	Serology (for fungal sensitisation, not invasive disease)
	Lung biopsy	Histology (to look for visible fungal hyphae)
P. jirovecii	Induced sputum, bronchial washings or bronchoalveolar lavage	Cytology and nucleic acid amplification test

*Culture is difficult and requires specific techniques, so it is restricted to selected patients.

†Also positive in patients with previous bacille Calmette–Guerin vaccination.

Table 8.7 Common microbiological tests for respiratory pathogens

Upper respiratory tract infection, tracheitis and bronchitis

Acute URTIs and infections of the bronchial tree (**Table 8.1**) are usually mild and self-limiting. Exceptions are acute epiglottitis and diphtheria, which cause life-threatening upper airways obstruction.

Types

Upper respiratory tract infections include rhinitis (the 'common cold'), pharyngitis, tonsillitis, epiglottitis and laryngitis (sore throat).

Infections of the bronchial tree include bronchitis and tracheitis. These two illnesses are very similar, so the term bronchitis is used for both.

Epidemiology

Upper respiratory tract infections and bronchitis are common. Many people have one or more episodes in a year, and infants frequently have multiple URTIs in the same period. Whooping cough, acute epiglottitis and diphtheria are all rare.

Aetiology

The dominant pathogen varies with the site of disease (**Table 8.8**). Influenza and respiratory viruses are the most common causes overall.

- *H. influenzae* causes acute epiglottitis
- *Corynebacterium diphtheria* causes diphtheria
- *Bordetella pertussis* causes whooping cough.

Prevention

Influenza A, diphtheria and whooping cough can be prevented by vaccination.

Pathogenesis

Infection of the respiratory tract causes an inflammatory response resulting in increased nasal secretions, cough and sputum. In diptheria, a toxin creates a pharyngeal pseudomembrane, and acute epiglottitis causes swelling of the epiglottis; both obstruct the upper airways.

A major clinical challenge for physicians based in the community is distinguishing the mild infections (URTI and bronchitis) from the potentially serious CAP. For every patient presenting with pneumonia, at least 20 present with an URTI or bronchitis (**Figure 8.1**). Marked fever, pleuritic chest pain, increased respiratory rate, focal lung signs and low oxygen saturations all point towards a diagnosis of CAP and the need for antibiotic therapy.

Upper respiratory tract, bronchi and bronchiole infections			
Rhinitis	Pharyngitis, tonsillitis, laryngitis	Bronchitis/tracheitis	Bronchiolitis
Rhinovirus	Influenza, parainfluenza	Influenza, parainfluenza	RSV (children)
RSV	*S. pyogenes*	*H. influenzae*	Influenza, parainfluenza
Adenovirus	*H. influenzae* (epiglottitis)	*M. catarrhalis*	*M. pneumoniae*
Coxsackie viruses	Diphtheria	*S. pneumoniae*	*C. pneumoniae*
Influenza viruses		*S. aureus*	
		M. pneumoniae	
		C. pneumoniae	
		Whooping cough	

Table 8.8 Microbial causes of infections of the upper respiratory tract, bronchi and bronchioles (in approximate order of frequency)

Clinical features

Different URTIs and bronchial tree infections present with different clinical features.

- Rhinitis causes nasal discharge and sneezing.
- Pharyngitis, epiglottitis and laryngitis cause a sore throat. The throat sometimes contains visible pharyngeal erythema and pus; the tonsils may be enlarged and cervical lymphadenopathy apparent.
- Bronchitis causes a cough; purulent phlegm indicates a bacterial infection. There are usually no chest signs, unless the infection has exacerbated an underlying airways disease. Patients have variable degrees of fever, anorexia and malaise.
- Whooping causes a cough that lasts about 12 weeks and is associated with a distinct inspiratory whooping noise.
- Diphtheria or acute epiglottitis may cause dyspnoea, drooling and stridor indicating acute upper airways obstruction

Diagnostic approach and management

The diagnosis is usually clinically obvious. Upper airway samples, such as nasopharyngeal aspirates, throat swabs and sputum, are used to confirm viral or bacterial causes of infection (**Table 8.7**). However, these tests are often unnecessary, because the infections are usually self-limiting.

Antibiotics are necessary for:

- diphtheria
- acute epiglottitis

- bronchitis in patients with underlying chronic lung disease or immunosuppression
- some patients with more severe bacterial bronchitis

Chest X-ray is sometimes required to distinguish between bronchitis and a pneumonia; the latter should always be treated with antibiotics. Diphtheria is treated with intravenous antitoxin.

Prognosis

Most URTIs and bronchitis infections are self-limiting within 10 days. *S. pyogenes* pharyngitis is rarely complicated by rheumatic fever or glomerulonephritis. During diphtheria epidemics, up to half of patients die.

Most cases of influenza cause a self-limiting and short-lived bronchitis. However, influenza can cause substantial morbidity and mortality through the following mechanisms.

- Decompensation of pre-existing chronic lung and heart diseases
- Temporary impairment of host immunity against bacterial infection leading to CAP as a complication of influenza
- Devastating primary viral pneumonia with a very high mortality; this is very rare, except with some types of influenza (e.g. avian influenza, 'bird flu')

Bronchiolitis

Respiratory syncytial virus (RSV) infection of the bronchioles (bronchiolitis) is the most common lower respiratory tract infection of infants. In adults, bronchiolitis is caused by *M. pneumoniae*, *C. pneumoniae* and respiratory viruses. However, bronchiolitis in adulthood is usually associated with bronchitis, CAP or both, and is covered in pages 247 and 249.

Clinical features

Bronchiolitis in infants presents as cough, wheeze and dyspnoea. Widespread wheezes and crepitations are heard on auscultation of the chest.

Diagnostic approach

Diagnosis is based on the clinical assessment.

Chest X-ray is often normal but sometimes shows bronchial wall thickening and atelectasis. Respiratory syncytial virus is frequently detected in nasopharyngeal aspirates samples.

Management

Treatment of RSV bronchiolitis is supportive, with oxygen, nebulised β-agonists and antibiotics for secondary bacterial infections.

Prognosis

RSV bronchiolitis is mostly self-limiting. However, 5% of infants with the infection need to be admitted to hospital. RSV infection predisposes children to developing asthma.

Community-acquired pneumonia

Acute infection of the alveoli is called pneumonia, the hallmark of which is clinical and chest X-ray evidence of consolidation. Community-acquired pneumonia (CAP) is pneumonia acquired while not in hospital. It is the most common severe respiratory infection.

Types

CAP is classified as follows.

- Lobar pneumonia: infection of contiguous anatomical units such that whole segments or lobes are affected. Most cases of CAP present as lobar pneumonia.
- Bronchopneumonia: widespread small patches of consolidation in both lungs (**Figure 8.6**). This type of pneumonia is common in patients with *S. aureus* CAP as

well as in those dying from other diseases (e.g. cancer). Primary viral pneumonia has a similar appearance.
- Interstitial pneumonia: this type of pneumonia presents with bilateral subtle interstitial infiltrates on chest X-ray. In the past, such non-lobar infiltrates would have been considered characteristic of what was called 'atypical pneumonia'. However, use of this outdated term should be avoided, because the causative bacteria, *M. pneumoniae* and *C. pneumoniae*, often produce lobar pneumonia as well. Similar appearances occur in immunocompromised patients with CMV or *Pneumocystis* pneumonia.

- Aspiration pneumonia: pneumonia caused by aspiration of stomach contents as a result of vomiting. This usually occurs while the patient's level of consciousness is lowered by alcohol, drugs or sedation (Figure 2.35). The stomach contents cause a chemical pneumonitis that somtimes progresses to CAP or HAP, often caused by a mix of organisms including anaerobic bacteria.

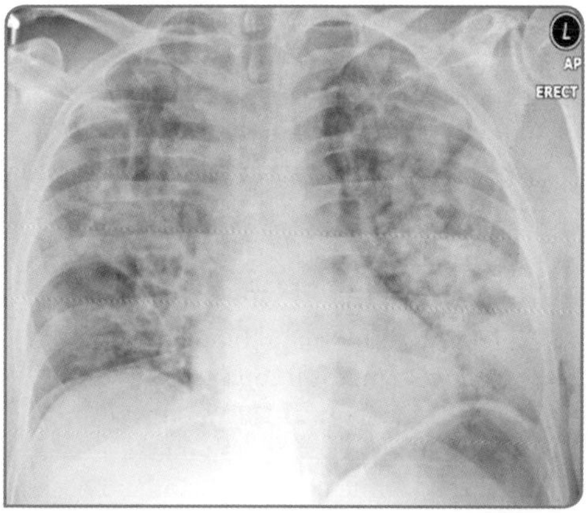

Epidemiology

The incidence of CAP is 2–5/1000 per year. The risk is much higher in children under 5 years of age and the elderly (65 years or older, increasing exponentially with increasing age). Risk factors for CAP are shown in **Table 8.9**.

Figure 8.6 Chest X-ray showing bronchopneumonia.

Risk factors for community-acquired pneumonia

Category	Risk factor
Age	Annual incidence (1000)
	■ < 65 years: 0.8
	■ 65–74 years: 3.5
	■ 75–84 years: 8.8
	■ > 85 years: 22
Smoking	Attributable risk 32%
Alcohol abuse	Even without associated cirrhosis
Comorbidity	Central nervous system disease
	Chronic lung disease
	Renal impairment
	Cirrhosis
Immune defects	HIV infection (even with a normal CD4 count)
	Inhaled corticosteroids in patients with chronic obstructive pulmonary disease
	Complement deficiencies
	Antibody deficiencies (e.g. multiple myeloma)
Occupation	Exposure to welding fumes
Medical history	Previous episode of community-acquired pneumonia

Table 8.9 Risk factors for community-acquired pneumonia

Aetiology

Many microbial pathogens cause CAP. However, most cases are caused by *S. pneumoniae*, influenza A and the 'atypical' bacteria *M. pneumoniae* and *C. pneumoniae* (**Table 8.10**).

Prevention

Community-acquired pneumonia is prevented by vaccination against *S. pneumoniae* in children, and against influenza A in both adults and children.

Pathogenesis

Pathogens stimulate a pulmonary inflammatory response which causes the alveoli to fill with extracellular fluid, as well as red and white cells. In a minority of patients bacteria spread from the lungs into the blood to cause septicaemia (sometimes with septic shock) or to the pleura causing empyema. The consolidation allows right-to-left shunting of deoxygenated blood from the pulmonary artery to the pulmonary vein, resulting in hypoxia (**Figure 8.7**).

Clinical features

Patients with CAP present with systemic symptoms (fever, malaise and anorexia), usually combined with chest symptoms (cough, purulent phlegm and dyspnoea). These symptoms have a short history, usually <3 weeks and often 2–3 days. Some patients have 'rusty' phlegm (purulent phlegm mixed with blood). They may also report pleuritic chest pain. Occasionally, there are no symptoms localising infection to the lungs.

On examination, the patient can have pyrexia, tachycardia, increased respiratory rate with signs of respiratory distress, central cyanosis and confusion. Herpes labialis is occasionally found around the mouth. Examination of the lung finds the following signs over areas of consolidation:

■ reduced expansion
■ dullness to percussion (especially if an associated pleural effusion is present)
■ coarse crepitations
■ bronchial breathing (occasionally)
■ a pleural rub (occasionally)

Diagnostic approach

The diagnosis of CAP requires evidence of infection combined with clinical or radiological evidence of new consolidation. CAP is often the obvious diagnosis. The tests required (**Table 8.11**) include the following.

■ Chest X-ray to identify consolidation and exclude lung complications
■ Oxygen saturation and blood gases to assess oxygen requirements
■ Blood tests to confirm a systemic inflammatory response: an increased or decreased white cell count, and increased C-reactive protein (>50 mg/L in most cases)

Microbial causes of pneumonia syndromes

CAP (mixed infection 25%)	HAP	VAP	Pneumonia in immunosuppressed patients	Subacute lung infections /lung abscess
Influenza A (15%)	Gram negative bacilli e.g.:	P. aeruginosa	Causes of HAP (≥30%), e.g.:	(Pulmonary TB) †
Other respiratory viruses (5%)	*E. coli* *Proteus* species	Gram negative bacilli, e.g.:	P. aeruginosa (10%) S. aureus / MRSA	P. aeruginosa
S. pneumoniae (30–50%)	*Klebsiella* species	*E. coli* *Proteus* species	(10–15%) Gram negative	Gram negative bacilli
M. pneumoniae (5–10%)		*Klebsiella* species	bacilli (10–15%)	Anaerobes
C. pneumoniae (10–15%)	S. aureus / MRSA		Streptococci (5%)	S. aureus
H. influenzae (<7%)	S. pneumoniae	Acinetobacter	Respiratory viruses and influenza (10%)	Nocardia
M. catarrhalis (<2%)	P. aeruginosa	Citrobacter	CMV (5%)	Actinomycetes
S. aureus (<2%)		S. aureus / MRSA	P. jirovecii (PCP, 5%)	Aspergillus
Gram negative bacilli (<2%)			Aspergillus, other fungi (25%)	Travel pathogens, e.g. parasites, endemic fungi
Legionella (3–5%)			Nocardia (<2%)	
Mixed pathogens* (25%)			No pathogen identified (20–50%)	
No pathogen identified (20%)				

* mixed pathogens: a combination of two or more pathogens, usually a virus, *M. pneumoniae*, or *C. pneumophila* in combination with *S. pneumoniae*, *S. aureus*, or *H. influenzae*

† usually considered a separate infectious disease but an important differential diagnosis for these conditions

Table 8.10 Microbial causes of pneumonia syndromes (in approximate order of frequency)

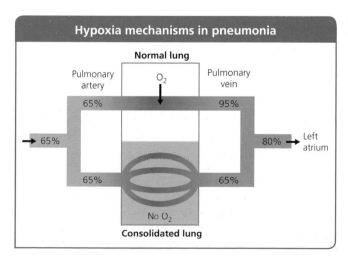

Figure 8.7 Mechanism of hypoxia during pneumonia.

Investigations for community-acquired pneumonia		
Test	Common abnormality (or abnormalities)	Usefulness
All admitted patients		
Chest X-ray	Consolidation with or without effusion	Confirms diagnosis or helps exclude alternative diagnoses
		Identifies extent of disease
		Identifies complications (e.g. complicated parapneumonic effusions and lung abscess)
C-reactive protein	Usually > 50 mg/L and often very high	Identifies a systemic inflammatory response to infection
		C-reactive protein > 250 mg/L associated with a 10% increase in mortality
		Helps monitor response to treatment
White cell count	< 2 10^9/L or > 10 10^9/L	Indicates a systemic inflammatory response
Platelet count	< 150 10^9/L or >450 10^9/L	Indicates active infection and potentially disseminated intravascular coagulation (a complication of severe sepsis)
Urea and electrolytes	Increased urea and creatinine	Indicates kidney injury requiring treatment
		Increased urea is a CURB-65 risk factor (**Tables 8.2 and 8.3**)
	Low sodium	Common in severe CAP but usually self-limiting and asymptomatic
Liver function tests	Increased alanine transaminase and alkaline phosphatase	Common in severe CAP but usually self-limiting and asymptomatic
	Low albumin	Indicates a systemic inflammatory response
Blood cultures	Positive in 20% of admitted patients	Can identify causative bacterial pathogens
		Positive blood cultures indicate severe disease with ≥ 20% mortality
Sputum culture*		Can identify causative bacterial pathogens (excluding atypical organisms)
Sputum microscopy*	Gram stain	Can identify causative bacterial pathogens (excluding atypical organisms)
		Not offered routinely by many hospitals
Nasopharyngeal aspirates*	Identifies viral infections	Identifies patients requiring neuraminidase treatment
		Positive patients are infective and require isolation
HIV test		Risk factor for CAP
		Required if P. jirovecii infection suspected because this infection is only common in immunocompromised patients,
Additional tests for severe disease		
Clotting	Increased prothrombin time	Suggests disseminated intravascular coagulation
Urine antigen tests	Positive in 70% of cases of S. pneumoniae or Legionella CAP	Rapid identification S. pneumoniae and L. pneumonia
Selected patients		
Blood serology	For diagnosis of viral or atypical pathogens	Needs convalescent sample, so retrospective only

Investigations for community-acquired pneumonia *Continued*		
Test	Common abnormality (or abnormalities)	Usefulness
Pleural ultrasound	For diagnosis of parapneumonic effusions	Establishes size of effusions and presence of loculations in CPEs
Pleural fluid tap	pH, lactate dehydrogenase and glucose	Confirms presence of infected pleural fluid (a CPE)
	Cytology, culture or Gram stain for bacterial pathogens	Identifies causative bacterial pathogens
Computerised tomography scan (rarely needed)	Consolidation with or without effusion	To exclude alternative diagnoses (e.g. CTPA for pulmonary emboli or lung cancer)
		Identifies complications (empyema or lung abscess)

CAP, community-acquired pneumonia; CPE, complicated parapneumonic effusion; CTPA, computerised tomography pulmonary angiography.

*May not be routinely available for CAP patients in some hospitals.

Table 8.11 Microbiological and other investigations for patients admitted to hospital with community-acquired pneumonia (CAP)

- General blood tests to assess severity and identify complications (e.g. urea and electrolytes, liver function tests, glucose, full blood count and clotting screen)
- Microbiological tests to identify the microbial cause: sputum and blood cultures, urinary antigen tests for *Legionella* or *S. pneumoniae*, and nasopharyngeal aspirates for respiratory viruses

Many other conditions have similar presentations to that of CAP (**Table 8.12**). Specific tests may be necessary to help exclude these other diagnoses, including: electrocardiogram and echocardiogram (for cardiac failure and pulmonary emboli), computerised tomography pulmonary angiogram (for pulmonary emboli and other lung conditions) and bronchoscopy (for lobar collapse and lung cancer).

> The signs and new chest X-ray changes of consolidation may be obscured in patients with chronic lung disease. Suspect pneumonia if the patient has a new fever, increased inflammatory markers and an unexplained decrease in oxygen saturation.

Management

Most cases of CAP are mild and can be treated out of hospital. Patients with more severe disease require admission to hospital. Of these, a fifth may need to be admitted to intensive care, mainly to treat severe hypoxia or septic shock.

Treatment of CAP involves the following:

- Empirical antibiotics (**Table 8.13**), with the first dose given as soon as possible
- Oxygen to maintain saturations >95%; this often requires high-flow oxygen through a Venturi mask or even continuous positive airway pressure or intubation and mechanical ventilation
- Intravenous fluids, especially if the patient is hypotensive or has poor urine output; septic shock often needs treatment with inotropes
- Non-steroidal anti-inflammatory drug or paracetamol analgesia for pleuritic chest pain and to lower the pyrexia

The severity of CAP is assessed using the CURB-65 score (**Tables 8.2** and **8.3**). CURB-65 identifies patients who can be treated as outpatients, and those with severe disease who need to be considered for admission to intensive care. The CURB-65 assessment also dictates the choice of empirical antibiotics (**Table 8.13**).

Progress is monitored by:

- checking temperature, heart and respiratory rates, and oxygen saturation

Differential diagnosis of community-acquired pneumonia		
Category	Examples	Notes and clinical recognition
Other lung infections	Subacute lung infection	For example, lung abscess, mycobacteria, *Nocardia* and *Aspergillus*
	P. jirovecii pneumonia (*Pneumocystis* pneumonia)	Often missed if the patient is not known to be HIV-positive
	Metastatic lung infection	For example, *S. aureus* endocarditis in an intravenous drug user
Non-infectious disease	Pulmonary embolus	Causes wedge-shaped patches of peripheral consolidation and hypoxia
	Lung cancer	Bronchial obstruction causes distal consolidation
	Pulmonary oedema	Bilateral shadowing, history of heart disease and low-level inflammation*
	Acute respiratory distress syndrome	For example, caused by septicaemia or aspiration; bilateral shadowing, severe hypoxia
	Alveolar cell carcinoma or lymphoma	Persistent slowly growing dense consolidation and low-level inflammation*
	Non-infective inflammatory lung disease: ■ pulmonary eosinophilia ■ organising pneumonia ■ hypersensitivity pneumonitis ■ vasculitis ■ allergic bronchopulmonary aspergillosis	All-cause lung shadowing with a significant inflammatory response; specific blood tests, bronchoscopy and perhaps lung biopsy are needed for diagnosis

*Inflammation is recognised by the presence of pyrexia, increased C-reactive protein and erythrocyte sedimentation rate, and increased or decreased white cell or platelet counts.

Table 8.12 Differential diagnosis of community-acquired pneumonia

Empirical antibiotic therapies			
CAP	HAP	VAP	Subacute lung infection/ lung abscess
Outpatient (CURB-65 score < 1) ■ Amoxicillin ■ or macrolide Inpatient (CURB65 <3) ■ Amoxicillin and macrolide Severe CAP (CURB65 >3) ■ Coamoxiclav ■ or cefuroxime and macrolide +/– flucloxacillin*	< 7 days after admission ■ Coamoxiclav ■ or cefuroxime > 7 days after admission (resistant organisms likely) ■ Ciprofloxacin ■ or 3rd generation cephalosporin or extended spectrum penicillin ■ +/– teicoplanin**	■ Ciprofloxacin ■ or 3rd generation cephalosporin ■ or extended spectrum penicillin +/– teicoplanin**	■ Co-amoxiclav ■ or amoxicillin and metronizadole ■ or clindamycin

*If non-methicillin resistant *S. aureus* infection suspected.

†Methicillin-resistant *S. aureus* infection suspected.

Table 8.13 Empirical antibiotic therapies for community-acquired pneumonia (CAP), hospital-acquired pneumonia (HAP), ventilator-acquired pneumonia (VAP) and subacute lung infection

- chest examination
- repeating previously abnormal blood tests

Most patients with CAP improve within 72 h of being given antibiotics; they become apyrexial and less hypoxic. If the patient fails to improve clinically, or if their high C-reactive protein concentration persists, they need clinical reassessment and a repeat chest X-ray. Complications of CAP and important reasons why patients fail to improve are listed in **Table 8.14**.

Prognosis

The mortality for patients admitted to hospital with CAP is 5–10% although recent audits in the UK suggest it may be over 20%. This figure increases to ≥25% for patients with septicaemia or requiring intensive care treatment. The consolidation usually resolves within 6 weeks. Persisting consolidation needs further investigation by bronchoscopy and computerised tomography (CT) to exclude a proximal bronchial obstruction (e.g. caused by a lung cancer).

Complications of community-acquired pneumonia		
Category	Examples	Notes and clinical recognition
Inadequate treatment	Antibiotic dose too low or wrong route of administration	For example, patient with malabsorption (rare)
	Atypical organism and no macrolide treatment	
	Antibiotic-resistant *S. pneumoniae*	Suspect if patient has recently travelled to countries with high levels of resistance
	Resistant organism (e.g. MRSA, *P. aeruginosa*)	<1% cases of community-acquired pneumonia but resistant to most ß lactams and macrolides
	Bronchial obstruction	For example, resulting from lung cancer
Non-infective complications	Atrial fibrillation	Irregularly irregular tachycardia
	Abnormal liver function tests	Usually not clinically important
	Confusion	Marker of severe disease
	Neurological signs	Rare, caused by autoimmune complication of infection
	Renal impairment	Marker of severe disease
	Acute respiratory distress syndrome	Bilateral widespread consolidation and increasing oxygen requirements (see Chapter 11)
	Septic shock	Hypotension, cool peripheries, poor urine output and lactic acidosis
	Pulmonary embolism	Sudden increase in oxygen requirements, shock, signs of a deep vein thrombosis
Infective complications	Herpes labialis	Usually not clinically important
	Septicaemia (5–10% of cases)	Positive blood cultures, associated with septic shock and ≥20% mortality
	Complicated parapneumonic effusions or empyema (7% of cases)	Loculated pleural fluid, or visibly turbid pleural fluid or pH <7.2
	Lung abscess or pulmonary gangrene	Rare: persisting fever and high C-reactive protein, with cavitation on chest X-ray
	Pericarditis	Rare: chest pain, abnormal electrocardiogram and pericardial effusion
	Septic arthritis	Rare: hot, tender swollen joint

Complications of community-acquired pneumonia *Continued*		
Category	Examples	Notes and clinical recognition
	Intravenous catheter site infection	Consider MRSA
	Clostridia difficile diarrhoea	Associated with broad-spectrum antibiotics use
Misdiagnosis	See Table 8.12	
MRSA, methicillin-resistant *S. aureus*.		

Table 8.14 Causes of failure to improve and complications of community-acquired pneumonia

Hospital-and ventilator-acquired pneumonia

Pneumonia is a relatively frequent complication of being admitted to hospital for any reason.

Types

Pneumonia acquired in hospital is divided into two main groups:

- Hospital-acquired pneumonia: pneumonia acquired in hospital or within a week of discharge from hospital. Excludes patients who are severely immunocompromised.
- Ventilator-acquired pneumonia: pneumonia developing in a patient who is intubated and mechanically ventilated

Epidemiology

Hospital-acquired pneumonia is the most common fatal nosocomial infection. The risk of developing VAP is 1% for each day a patient is mechanically ventilated.

Aetiology

Both HAP and VAP are caused by a different range of bacteria to those causing CAP. In HAP and VAP, *S. aureus* and Gram negative pathogens predominate (**Table 8.10**).

Prevention

Rapid postoperative mobilisation, physiotherapy and oropharyngeal decontamination with chlorhexidine help prevent HAP and VAP, as does reducing the unnecessary use of nasogastric tubes, intubation and proton pump inhibitors.

Pathogenesis

Previous antibiotic use results in Gram-negative bacilli and *S. aureus* colonisation of the oropharynx, often with antibiotic-resistant strains. Microaspiration of these bacteria can lead to infection of the lungs. The risk of microaspiration is increased by poor cough reflexes as a result of sedation or surgical scars, recumbent position and intubation.

Clinical features

The presentation of HAP is similar to that of CAP. VAP presents with new pyrexia, increasing oxygen requirements, new crepitations on chest auscultation, and purulent secretions in the endotracheal tube.

In cases of suspected HAP or VAP, several other possible diagnoses need to be excluded including

- lobar collapse caused by sputum plugging of a bronchus
- atelectasis resulting from inadequate inspiration
- pulmonary embolism or pulmonary oedema
- fluid overload with pulmonary oedema

Diagnostic approach

The diagnostic approach to HAP is similar to that for CAP, except that the CURB-65 assessment is inappropriate. The diagnosis of VAP is often difficult, because the signs are non-specific, and positive bacterial cultures from endotracheal samples often reflect colonisation rather than infection.

Management

Both HAP and VAP are managed similarly to CAP. However, different empirical antibiotic regimens are used (**Table 8.13**).

Prognosis

In HAP and VAP, mortality is 30%. However, many deaths are caused by the underlying illnesses rather than the pneumonia.

Pneumonia in the immunocompromised patient

Diseases affecting the blood, transplantation and treatment of cancers or inflammatory conditions severely impair the immune system (**Table 8.15**), often resulting in pneumonia.

Epidemiology

Pneumonia affects 25% of patients with neutropenia and ≥40% of bone marrow transplant recipients.

Aetiology

The weakened immune system allows a much larger range of pathogens to cause pneumonia. Therefore, as well as the usual causes of HAP, immunocompromised patients develop pneumonia due to fungal and viral pathogens (**Tables 8.10** and **8.15**).

Pneumonia in the immunocompromised patient		
Category	Examples	Likely respiratory pathogens
Neutropenia	Chemotherapy	Gram-negative and Gram-positive bacteria
	Aplastic anaemia	*Aspergillus* species
	Early phase after HSCT	(if neutropenic for > 10 days)
	Marrow infiltrations (e.g. acute leukemias and lymphoma)	
Defects in cell-mediated immunity	After HSCT	*Pneumocystis* pneumonia
	Lymphomas	Cytomegalovirus
	High-dose systemic corticosteroids	Respiratory viruses
	Immunosuppression for organ transplants	Tuberculosis and non-tuberculous mycobacteria
		Nocardia
Antibody deficiency	Multiple myeloma	Encapsulated bacteria (e.g. *S. pneumoniae* and *H. influenzae*)
	After HSCT	
	B-cell depletion therapy with rituximab	Respiratory viruses
	Chronic lymphocytic leukaemia	
	Chronic variable immunoglobulin deficiency	
HSCT, haematopoietic stem cell transplant.		

Table 8.15 Pneumonia in the immunocompromised patient

Prevention

Patients with no evidence of previous CMV infection are not given blood or organs from CMV-positive donors. Selected high-risk patients receive antibacterial, antifungal and/or antiviral agents as prophylaxis.

Pathogenesis

Immune defects allow unusual pathogens to replicate within the lungs and cause pneumonia. Frequent previous antibiotic use also selects for infection with resistant bacteria.

Clinical features

Bacterial pneumonia in the immunocompromised patient presents similar to HAP (see **Table 8.16**). Fungal and viral pneumonias differ in their clinical features.

Aspergillus pneumonia

Aspergillus pneumonia causes patches of consolidation or macronodules (**Figure 8.8**). These changes develop over days and are associated with pyrexia, cough and occasionally haemoptysis. There are often no signs. *Aspergillus* infections also cause invasive sinusitis and tracheobronchitis, and occasionally spread to the brain, joints or skin.

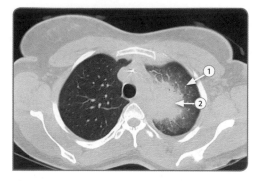

Figure 8.8 Computerised tomography scan showing invasive aspergillosis: a rounded patch of dense consolidation with a surrounding halo of lower attenuation. ① Halo of less dense consolidation. ② Dense consolidation.

Pneumocystis pneumonia

Pneumocystis pneumonia (**Figure 8.9**) classically causes a dry cough, progressive dyspnoea over 3–4 weeks and oxygen desaturation on exercise. There are usually few lung signs and only mild pyrexia.

Respiratory viruses

Common respiratory viral causes of URTI result in much more severe disease in immuncompromised patients, often resulting in pneumonia. Respiratory viral pneumonias in immunocompromised patients

Clinical presentation of pneumonia in immunocompromised patients	
Pathogen	Common presentation
Bacterial causes	Rapid onset of lobar consolidation with increased inflammatory markers and hypoxia
Aspergillus	Fever, cough, haemoptysis with progressive macronodular consolidation
	CT indicators: halo or crescent signs (**Figure 8.8**)
Pneumocystis pneumonia	Progressive dyspnea over weeks, dry cough and hypoxia with perihilar infiltrates on chest X-ray
	CT indicators: ground glass infiltrates with peripheral and basal sparing (**Figure 8.9**)
Cytomegalovirus pneumonitis	Progressive dyspnea, cough and hypoxia with widespread infiltrates on chest X-ray
	CT indicators: bilateral ground glass infiltrates and patchy consolidation
Respiratory viruses	URTI symptoms followed by cough and dyspnoea with widespread infiltrates on chest X-ray
	CT indicators: diffuse tree-in-bud changes (**Figure 8.10**)
CT, computerised tomography; URTI, upper respiratory tract infection.	

Table 8.16 Clinical presentation of pneumonia in immunocompromised patients

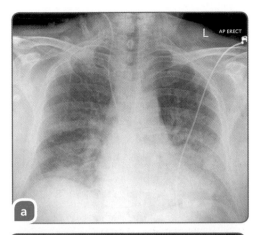

a

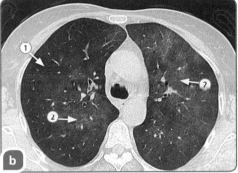

b

Figure 8.9 Radiological findings for *Pneumocystis* pneumonia. (a) Chest X-ray showing bilateral hilar insterstitial shadowing. (b) Computerised tomography scan showing bilateral ground glass infiltrates with sparing of the subpleural region. ① Subpleural sparing. ② Bilateral ground in glass intilitrates.

(**Figure 8.10**) all present similarly, with URTI symptoms followed by cough and dyspnoea that frequently persists for weeks. Widespread squeaks, crepitations and wheeze are heard on chest ausculatation.

Cytomegalovirus

Immunosuppression allows latent CMV infection to reactivate and invade the lung. Pneumonia caused by CMV presents with fever, cough, dyspnoea and hypoxia. Bilateral widespread crepitations are audible. The patient usually has evidence of CMV reactivation in their blood tests.

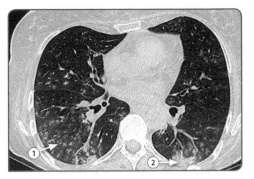

Figure 8.10 Computerised tomography scan showing changes caused by respiratory virus infection, in this case metapneumovirus infection in a recipient of a haemotopoietic stem cell transplant. ① Tree-in-bud changes suggesting small airways inflammation. ② Small patches of more confluent consolidation.

Diagnostic approach

The chest X-ray changes are often non-specific. However, CT shows features associated with specific pathogens (**Table 8.16** and **Figures 8.8–8.10**). Blood and sputum cultures are necessary. Additional microbiological tests are frequently needed, depending on the suspected pathogen(s) (**Table 8.7**); they include bronchoscopy or lung biopsy.

In many cases, the infective pathogen is not identified. Non-infective respiratory problems also commonly affect the immunocompromised patient. These include pulmonary oedema, acute respiratory distress syndrome, pulmonary haemorrhage, and drug and radiation toxicity. They need to be considered in the differential diagnosis.

Management

General management includes oxygen, intravenous fluids, antipyretics and, if possible, reducing the degree of the patient's immunosuppression. Empirical treatment choices are complex because of the range of potential pathogens, and also because non-infective respiratory problems are also common in these patients. Antimicrobial treatments for individual pathogens are listed in **Table 8.5**.

Patients usually need combinations of treatments against the most likely pathogens.

Prognosis

Mortality in *Aspergillus* and CMV pneumonia is ≥ 30%; it is 10% in *Pneumocystis* pneumonia. Respiratory viruses have a lower mortality but often persist for weeks in immunosuppressed patients.

> **There are too many pathogens causing pneumonia in immunocompromised patients for empirical therapy to cover all possibilities.** Clinical assessment can reduce the number of potential pathogens for targeted empirical therapy by answering the following questions.
>
> - What type of immune defect is present? (**Table 8.14**)
> - Is the radiological presentation diffuse (e.g. for CMV, *Pneumocystis* pneumonia or respiratory viruses) or focal (bacterial pathogens or *Aspergillus*)?

HIV infection

The HIV virus does not directly cause lung disease. However, untreated infection with HIV eventually causes profound immunosuppression and dysregulates immunological responses. Consequently, HIV-infected patients frequently develop secondary infective and non-infective lung diseases (**Table 8.17**).

Types

Patients with HIV infection and preserved CD4 counts are at risk of tuberculosis and *S. pneumoniae* CAP. Once the CD4 count decreases to < 200 cells/µL, they are at risk of opportunistic infections (commonly *Pneumocystis* pneumonia), pulmonary lymphoma or Kaposi's sarcoma. AIDS is defined as HIV infection complicated by the consequences of severely impaired immunity, such as *Pneumocystis* pneumonia or Kaposi's sarcoma. Long-term HIV infection increases the incidence of several chronic lung diseases (**Table 8.17**).

Epidemiology

HIV infection is spread by the exchange of bodily fluids. Homosexual and bisexual men, as well as intravenous drug users, are at increased risk of being exposed to the virus.

HIV is also widespread in sub-Saharan Africa where 1 in 20 are affected. In 2009, 31 million people were HIV-positive.

Aetiology

The HIV virus invades and kills CD4 cells, reducing T-cell–mediated immunity. As the CD4 count decreases, the risk of developing opportunistic infection or viral-related tumours (Kaposi's sarcoma and lymphomas) increases.

Prevention

The spread of HIV infection is substantially reduced by condom use, needle exchange programmes for intravenous drug users, screening of donated blood, and antiretroviral drug therapy for pregnant HIV-positive women (to prevent vertical transmission to the fetus).

Clinical features

Acute HIV infection causes a flu-like seroconversion illness followed by a long period without symptoms. The lung complications of HIV infection have a similar presentation to the same disease in non–HIV-positive patients.

Lung complications of HIV infection	
Infectious complications	Non-infectious complications
CD4 count > 200/mL	Chronic obstructive pulmonary disease
Tuberculosis	Bronchiectasis
S. pneumoniae	Pulmonary hypertension
S. aureus	Lung cancer
P. aeruginosa	Kaposi's sarcoma (herpes virus-related vascular tumours)
H. influenzae	Non-Hodgkins lymphoma
Plus when CD4 count < 200/mL	Interstitial lung diseases:
	■ non-specific alveolitis
Pneumocystis pneumonia (PCP)	■ lymphocytic interstitial pneumonitis
Cytomegalovirus pneumonitis	■ organising pneumonia
NTM (Mycobacterium avium or M. intracellulare)	
Endemic fungal pathogens	
Aspergillus species	
NTM, non-tuberculous mycobacteria.	

Table 8.17 Lung complications of HIV infection

Pneumocystis pneumonia presenting in someone who is not known to be HIV-positive can be misdiagnosed as CAP. However, it does not respond to empirical CAP antibiotics. Oral *Candida* or hairy leukoplakia, and bilateral interstitial infiltrates with marked exertional hypoxia and few lung signs, are clues to the real diagnosis.

cal testing. Treatment is with antiretroviral drugs; these are highly effective at suppressing viral replication but do not eliminate infection.

The response to antiretroviral treatment is assessed using the total CD4 count and polymerase chain reaction to measure HIV viral load. The management of lung complications in HIV-positive patients is similar to that for lung complications in patients without HIV.

Diagnostic approach and management

Infection with HIV is diagnosed by serologi-

Parapneumonic effusions and empyema

Bacterial infection of the pleural space is relatively common and causes significant mortality and morbidity. It most commonly occurs as a complication of CAP, but can also occur spontaneously. Infection of the pleural space causes a pleural effusion and often results in connections forming between the visceral and parietal pleurae called adhesions, which make draining fluid difficult.

Types

Pleural infections are classified as the following partially overlapping categories:

■ Parapneumonic effusions: sterile exudative pleural effusions in patients with pneumonia.
■ Complicated parapneumonic effusion (CPE): a parapneumonic effusion with

evidence of infection (usually bacterial) of the fluid.

- Empyema: an effusion with visibly turbid or culture positive pleural fluid, that is either acquired in the community as a CPE or spontaneously or acquired in hospital as a complication of HAP, or pleural procedures or lung surgery.

Epidemiology

Complicated parapneumonic effusion complicates 7% of cases of CAP. Empyema is a rare complication of most pleural procedures or surgery but becomes more common when pleural drains are maintained for long periods (e.g. over 7 days).

Aetiology

The common bacterial causes are different for community- and hospital-acquired pleural infections and are listed in **Table 8.18**.

Microbial causes of pleural infection	
Cause	Proportion of cases (%)
Community-acquired empyema	
S. pneumoniae	25
S. milleri	25
Anaerobes	20
S. aureus	11
Gram-negative bacilli	9
Other streptococci	5
Actinomycetes	rare
Hospital-acquired empyema	
S. aureus (usually MRSA)	35
P. aeruginosa	10
Gram-negative bacilli	10
S. pneumoniae, streptococci	< 10%
Anaerobes	8
MRSA, methicillin-resistant S. aureus.	

Table 8.18 Microbial causes of pleural infection (excluding tuberculosis)

Pathogenesis

Pleural effusions complicating pneumonia evolve through the following steps:

1. Parapneumonic effusion: pneumonic consolidation causes pleural inflammation and a sterile exudative pleural effusion.
2. Complicated parapneumonic effusions and empyema: bacteria translocate to the pleural space, where they cause inflammation and recruitment of white cells. Fibrinous adhesions form between the visceral and parietal pleura. These adhesions create divisions in the pleural space called loculations, which prevent drainage of pleural fluid (Figure 6.6).
3. Frank empyema: the high white cell content in the infected pleural fluid makes it visibly turbid.

Clinical features

Patients present with fever, anorexia, malaise, pleuritic chest pain and breathlessness. On examination, they often have a pyrexia and signs of a pleural effusion.

> **Suspect a diagnosis of pleural infection in any patient with evidence of infection and a pleural effusion, especially if the fluid is loculated.** Classic blood test abnormalities suggesting prolonged pleural infection are a normochromic normocytic anaemia, increased platelet count, reduced albumin and increased C-reactive protein.

Diagnostic approach

Uninfected parapneumonic effusions need to be distinguished from CPEs by a pleural tap. Infected pleural fluid is visibly turbid, has a pH < 7.2 or is culture- or microscopy-positive for a bacterial pathogen. However, radiological evidence of loculated pleural fluid (best identified using pleural ultrasound or CT) strongly suggests pleural infection (Figure 6.6). Blood tests show evidence of infection with an increased CRP.

Pleural tuberculosis is an important differential diagnosis for empyema or CPE. It presents similarly but is treated with different antibiotics and no pleural drainage. Consider this possibility in patients with an exudate pleural effusion risk factors for tuberculosis.

Management

Parapneumonic effusions usually resolve spontaneously. However, CPEs and empyema require treatment. The principles of their management are as follows.

- Prolonged antibiotic therapy for 3–6 weeks. The choice of antibiotics depends on the culture results and whether the infection was acquired in the community or in hospital (**Table 8.19**).
- Insertion of a chest drain to remove pleural fluid. Drainage improves control of the infection and minimises the extent of pleural thickening once the patient has recovered. However, loculated fluid often drains poorly, and 30% of patients need surgical pleural drainage. Intrapleural medical therapy does not improve drainage for most patients.

Antibiotic treatment of pleural infection	
Community-acquired empyema	Hospital-acquired empyema
Co-amoxiclav *or* clindamycin	Initial intravenous therapy ■ Carbapenem or third-generation cephalosporin or extended spectrum penicillin ■ with or without teicoplanin (if MRSA possible) Oral continuation therapy ■ Ciprofloxacin and either clindamycin or metronizadole ■ with or without rifampicin and trimethoprim (if MRSA possible)

Table 8.19 Empirical antibiotic treatment of pleural infection (over 3–6 weeks).

Prognosis

Empyema has 30% mortality. Incomplete pleural drainage often results in persistent pleural thickening and a permanent restrictive lung function defect. CPE or empyema complicating CAP increases the average length of a hospital admission by over a week.

Subacute lung infections and lung abscess

Some respiratory pathogens cause a less acute infection than pneumonia, and progress over weeks and months rather than days. These infections frequently cause focal lung destruction, creating lung cavities.

Types

These infections are divided into two main categories with overlapping microbial causes:

- Subacute lung infections: pneumonias that present with a longer history (over weeks and months) and usually have more focal chest X-ray abnormalities than are seen in cases of CAP.
- Lung abscess: a subacute infection that has a partially fluid-filled lung cavity. They

occur as a complication of pneumonia, aspiration or subacute lung infection.

Aetiology

Tuberculosis is the most common cause of subacute lung infection and is discussed in the next section. Other causes are rare and include bacterial, fungal and parasitic respiratory pathogens (**Table 8.10**).

Clinical features

The clinical features are:

- Patients with subacute lung infection present with fever, night sweats, malaise, weight loss, and cough, often with purulent phlegm or haemoptysis. Chest X-ray and CT show patches of consolidation and nodules that frequently cavitate or have associated pleural effusions.

■ Patients with lung abscesses produce large quantities of foul-smelling purulent phlegm. Chest X-rays and CT scans show a thick-walled cavity (or cavities) with air–fluid levels (**Figure 8.11**).

Identification of the microbial cause requires multiple sputum cultures for mycobacteria, fungi and anaerobic organisms. Bronchoscopy or percutaneous biopsy is frequently necessary to identify the causative organism and exclude non-infective causes. These include tuberculosis, lung cancer, ABPA, vasculitis and cavitating pulmonary emboli.

Management

Prolonged antibiotic therapy for 3–6 weeks is required. Empirical antibiotic therapies are shown in **Table 8.13**, but achieving a microbiological diagnosis is important as many causes require specific treatment (e.g. fungi, *Nocardia*).

Lung abscesses sometimes need CT-guided drainage or surgical resection.

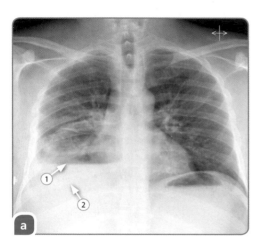
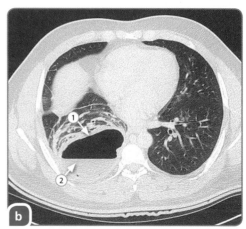

Figure 8.11 (a) Chest X-ray showing a lung abscess. ① Air–fluid level extending behind the heart. ② Loss of the right hemidiaphragm. (b) CT showing lung abscess. ① Thickened abscess wall. ② Air fluid level.

Tuberculosis

Tuberculosis is the most common fatal bacterial infection worldwide. However, in high-income countries this disease is only common in specific high-risk groups.

Types

There are various types of tuberculosis.

■ Primary infection: initial pulmonary infection with *M. tuberculosis*; this type is often asymptomatic but can cause progressive, potentially fatal infection
■ Latent tuberculosis: dormant *M. tuberculosis* infection that can reactivate decades after initial infection
■ Post-primary or reactivation tuberculosis: progression of latent tuberculosis to active disease
■ Pulmonary tuberculosis: active tuberculosis affecting the lungs
■ Extrapulmonary tuberculosis: active tuberculosis affecting other organs
■ Miliary tuberculosis: active tuberculosis disseminated by the blood throughout the body (**Figure 8.12**)
■ Bovine tuberculosis: tuberculosis caused by *M. bovis* and acquired from ingesting infected cows' milk

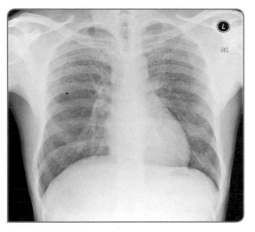

Figure 8.12 Chest X-ray showing miliary tuberculosis with hundreds of small dot-like opacities throughout both lungs.

- Multi–drug-resistant tuberculosis: Infection with *M. tuberculosis* that is resistant to rifampicin and isoniazid

Epidemiology

Worldwide, 9 million new cases of tuberculosis are diagnosed annually, and 30% of the world's population have latent tuberculosis. Latent tuberculosis has a 5% risk of progression to active disease within 2 years of infection, and a 5% lifetime risk thereafter.

The risk of infection differs between parts of the world; the incidence of tuberculosis is highest in Asia and sub-Saharan Africa. In Europe and North America, most cases of tuberculosis are in immigrants born in countries with a high incidence of the disease, or in specific high-risk groups (including drug users, prison inmates and people who are HIV-positive; **Table 8.20**). Emigration increases the risk of reactivation of latent tuberculosis.

Aetiology

Tuberculosis infections are caused by *M. tuberculosis* or *M. bovis*.

Prevention

Vaccination with BCG is partially effective at preventing tuberculosis. Sputum smear-positive patients are highly infective and

Risk factors for tuberculosis	
Risk factors	Details
Birth in high-incidence country	Annual incidence rates ■ Asia, sub-Saharan Africa and Eastern Europe > 100 per 100,000 ■ South America: 25–100 per 10,000 ■ Europe and North America: < 25 per 100,000 ■ Selected Western cities (e.g. London): 50 per 100,000
Smoking	
Alcohol and recreational drug use	
Diabetes	
Immune defects	HIV infection (with normal CD4 count) Systemic corticosteroids Defects of T-cell mediated immunity
Recent immigration	
Malnutrition	
Overcrowding or homelessness	
Living in prison	

Table 8.20 Risk factors for tuberculosis

should avoid contact with children. Close contacts of patients with active tuberculosis are screened for latent or active tuberculosis. Cases of latent tuberculosis are treated with isoniazid for 6 months, or isoniazid and rifampicin for 3 months, to reduce the risk of progression to active infection.

Pathogenesis

M. tuberculosis is spread by respiratory droplets from patients with pulmonary tuberculosis. The bacteria invade alveolar macrophages, where they evade normal phagosomal killing mechanisms and spread to other sites through the lymphatic system.

A cell-mediated immune response tries to control the infection by creating a granuloma, consisting of T cells and macrophages, around infected cells. In a minority, primary infection progresses to cause disease, but in most cases the host immune response succeeds in controlling the infection, which then becomes latent. Impaired immunity allows latent tuberculosis to reactivate, replicate and cause active disease (**Figure 8.13**). Reactivation may occur many years after the initial infection.

M. tuberculosis **is an example of an intracellular pathogen that evades extracellular immune defences by replicating within host cells.** It survives in macrophage phagosomes by inhibiting the normal phagolysomal killing mechanisms. The host can overcome this inhibition if the macrophage responses are boosted by helper Th1 CD4 T cells. However, a strong immune response can also cause tissue damage and fibrosis, which are common in reactivated pulmonary tuberculosis.

Clinical features

Tuberculosis presents as a subacute infection with a history over weeks or months of systemic disturbance as well as symptoms from the affected organ (or organs). Systemic symptoms of tuberculosis are night sweats, fevers, malaise, anorexia and weight loss.

Pulmonary tuberculosis causes a cough and often haemoptysis, which occasionally is severe and life-threatening (see Chapter 11). Dyspnoea is a feature of extensive disease. Examination of the lungs is often normal but sometimes identify patches of crepitations and bronchial breathing. Common sites and presentations of extrapulmonary tuberculosis are summarized in **Table 8.21**.

Diagnostic approach

Consider tuberculosis in all patients from a high-incidence country or in a specific high-risk group who present with focal lung disease or systemic symptoms. Diagnosis requires a positive culture of *M. tuberculosis* or *M. bovis*. However, only 70–80% of cases are culture-positive, so the remaining cases are treated as presumed tuberculosis.

The differential diagnosis of pulmonary tuberculosis includes other causes of subacute lung infection (**Table 8.10**), lung cavitation (e.g. cancer or vasculitis), X-ray changes in the upper lobes (e.g. sarcoidosis and ABPA), or granuloma formation (sarcoidosis and fungal infections).

The following tests are used to confirm pulmonary tuberculosis.

- Chest X-ray: patchy nodular shadowing mainly in the upper lobes and associated with dry cavitation (**Figure 8.3**). The mediastinal nodes are often enlarged (**Figure 8.15**).
- Sputum acid-fast bacilli (three morning samples): positive in half of patients.
- Sputum culture: positive in 70–80% of cases and allows drug sensitivity testing. However, culture takes up to 6 weeks, and patients frequently need to be treated before the results are available. For patients unable to produce sputum, samples for microscopy and culture are obtained by induced sputum or bronchoscopy.
- Nucleic acid amplification tests: a positive result suggests active tuberculosis and confirms that the acid-fast bacilli in a positive sample are *M. tuberculosis* rather than an NTM species. These tests also rapidly identify rifampicin resistance.
- Mantoux tests and interferon-γ release blood tests: these tests identify a cell-mediated immune response to *M. tuberculosis* antigens. The results are usually positive if a patient has latent tuberculosis. A positive result does not necessarily mean that a patient has active disease. The Mantoux test is also positive after BCG vaccination and, conversely, is often negative in miliary tuberculosis.
- Lung biopsy (CT-guided or video-assisted thoracoscopic surgery): biopsy is occasionally necessary, especially to exclude other diagnoses. Histology shows caseating granulomas and acid-fast bacilli–positive organisms.

Methods used to confirm the diagnosis of extrapulmonary tuberculosis depend on the site of disease (**Table 8.21**).

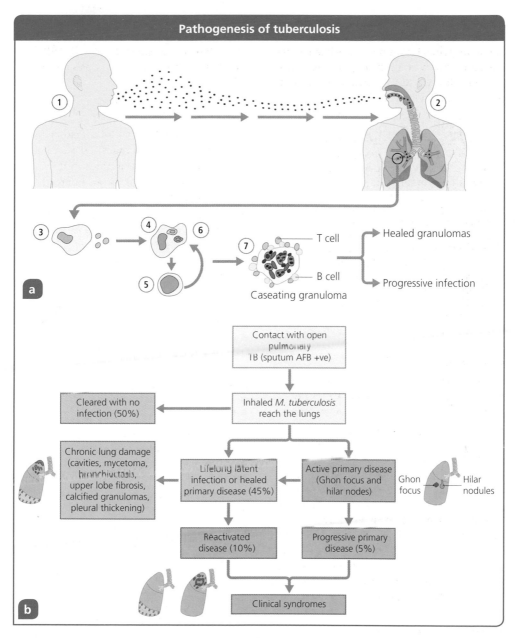

Pathogenesis of tuberculosis

T cell

B cell

Caseating granuloma

Healed granulomas

Progressive infection

a

Contact with open pulmonary TB (sputum AFB +ve)

Inhaled *M. tuberculosis* reach the lungs

Cleared with no infection (50%)

Chronic lung damage (cavities, mycetoma, bronchiectasis, upper lobe fibrosis, calcified granulomas, pleural thickening)

Lifelong latent infection or healed primary disease (45%)

Active primary disease (Ghon focus and hilar nodes)

Ghon focus — Hilar nodules

Reactivated disease (10%)

Progressive primary disease (5%)

Clinical syndromes

b

Figure 8.13 (a) Pathogenesis of tuberculosis part 1. ① Person infected with pulmonary TB coughs creating droplets containing *M. tuberculosis*. ② Droplets are inhaled and reach the lungs. ③ and ④ *M. tuberculosis* invades resident alveolar macrophages preventing normal phagolysomal function and it survives inside the cell. ⑤ and ⑥ Macrophage cytokine signalling to T cells causes cytokine response that boosts macrophage killing of *M. tuberculosis*. ⑦ Granuloma forms containing infected macrophages, surrounding macrophages, T cells and B cells. Balance between immune system and *M. tuberculosis* dictates whether primary infection is controlled or progresses. If controlled, *M. tuberculosis* lies dormant within the macrophages, but it can reactivate and either remain local or spread (via macrophage migration) to local lymph nodes or throughout the body. (b) Potential outcomes from inhaling *M. tuberculosis*.

Extrapulmonary tuberculosis

Site (% of cases)	Presentation	Diagnosis
Lymph node (30+) (**Figure 8.15**)	Smooth firm enlargement of cervical, mediastinal, axillary, or abdominal nodes; can form sinuses	Lymph node biopsy for histology, acid-fast bacilli and culture ■ 15% acid-fast bacilli smear–positive ■ 65% acid-fast bacilli culture–positive
Pleura (10)	Unilateral lymphocytic exudate effusion	Pleural biopsy for: ■ histology (granulomas in 85%) ■ acid-fast bacilli (10% positive) ■ culture (50% positive)
Bone and joint (vertebral, large joint and paravertebral abscess) (5–10) (**Figure 8.14**)	Swelling of affected bone or joint with underlying tissue destruction	Biopsy or aspiration for histology, acid-fast bacilli and culture
Brain: meningitis (5)	Headache, focal neurological signs and coma	Lumbar puncture and MRI ■ Cerebrospinal fluid (collected by lumbar puncture): high protein and white cell count, and low glucose ■ MRI: enhancement of meninges
Brain: tuberculoma (<5)	Headache and focal neurological signs	Radiology and brain biopsy ■ CT and MRI: ring-enhancing focal intracerebral lesions ■ Brain biopsy for histology
Abdominal (terminal ileum and mesenteric) (5–10)	Abdominal pain and ascites	Ultrasound, CT, ascitic fluid analysis and biopsy ■ Ultrasound and CT: appearances of tissue infiltration and ascites ■ Acid-fast bacilli and culture of ascitic fluid ■ Percutaneous or surgical biopsies
Genitourinary (kidneys, fallopian tubes and ureters) (10–15)	Pain, haematuria and ureteric obstruction	Ultrasound, CT, urinary analysis and biopsy ■ Ultrasound and CT: appearances of tissue infiltration ■ Early morning urine acid-fast bacilli and culture ■ Percutaneous or surgical biopsies
Pericardium (<5)	Pericardial effusions and constrictive pericarditis	Radiology, ECG, echocardiography, pericardial fluid analysis and biopsy ■ Chest X-ray, CT, ECG or echocardiogram: identifies effusion ■ Pericardial fluid: lymphocytic; acid-fast bacilli–or culture-positive in 50% ■ Pericardial biopsy: granulomas
Miliary disease (blood-borne spread to lungs, marrow, central nervous system, liver, etc.) (<5) (**Figure 8.12**)	Insidious malaise, weight loss, fever and cough	Radiology, blood tests, sputum analysis and biopsy ■ Micronodular infiltrate on chest X-ray and CT scan of the lung ■ Abnormal liver function tests ■ Sputum acid-fast bacilli–positive in 25%, culture-positive in 65% ■ Transbronchial biopsy or liver and bone marrow biopsy ■ Blood cultures for acid-fast bacilli

CT, computerised tomography; ECG, electrocardiogram; MRI, magnetic resonance imaging.

Table 8.21 Sites, presentation and diagnosis of the most common sites of extrapulmonary tuberculosis

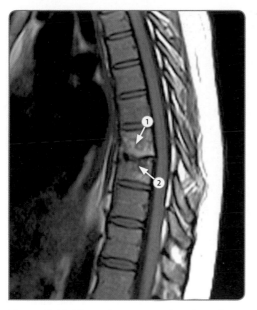

Figure 8.14 Magnetic resonance imaging of the spine, showing extrapulmonary tuberculosis infection of the thoracic vertebrae (Pott's disease). ① Increased signal of infected vertebrae. ② Vertebral collapse causing angulation of the spine.

Management

The standard tuberculosis treatment regimen is:

- rifampicin, isoniazid, ethambutol and pyrazinamide for 2 months
- then rifampicin and isoniazid alone for 4 months

Adherence is improved by directly observed therapy given by health care workers 3 times weekly. Central nervous system tuberculosis and drug-resistant disease require extended treatment for ≥ 12 months. Multidrug resistant tuberculosis is very difficult to treat, and requires prolonged treatment with complex and often toxic combinations of four or five second or third-line antimycobacterial agents. The results of liver function tests should be monitored to identify drug-induced hepatitis, which occurs in 5% of patients. Oral corticosteroids are used in patients with tuberculosis of the pericardium, ureter and central nervous system to prevent organ damage as the disease heals and causes fibrosis of the affected tissues.

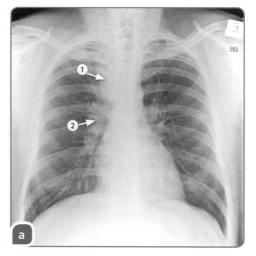

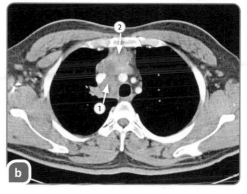

Figure 8.15 Extrapulmonary tuberculosis: mediastinal nodes. (a) Chest X-ray. ① Paratracheal lymphadenopathy ② and right hilar lymphadenopathy. (b) Computerised tomography scan of the same patient enlarged ① paratracheal and ② anterior mediastinal lymph nodes with a characteristic low attenuation centre due to necrosis.

Before antibiotics, tuberculosis treatments aimed to collapse the affected lobe by therapeutic pneumothorax, thoracoplasty (removal of ribs, **Figure 8.16**) or plombage. Plombage was the insertion of inert material, such as olive oil, paraffin wax or Lucite balls, into the pleural space. Some patients who underwent these treatments are still alive today.

Prognosis

The cure rate for properly treated tuberculosis is 95%. Failure to improve is usually the

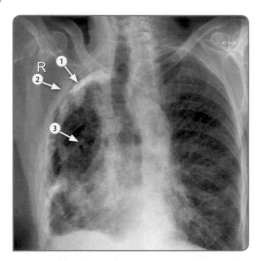

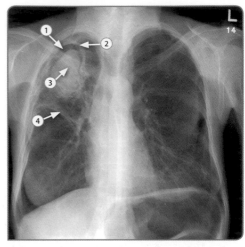

Figure 8.16 Chest X-ray showing the changes of a right-sided thoracoplasty, a preantibotic era treatment for pulmonary tuberculosis. ① Plate-like patches of pleural calcification caused by previous pleural tuberculosis. ② Upper ribs angled inwards. ③ Loss of volume of the right hemithorax, with tracheal and mediastinal deviation to the right.

Figure 8.17 Chest X-ray showing a pulmonary mycetoma. (1) Air crescent above the mycetoma. (2) Upper wall of the cavity. (3) Rounded mass of the mycetoma inside the cavity. (4) Horizontal fissure angled upwards, showing loss of volume of the right upper lobe due damage from the previous tuberculosis.

result of poor adherence or drug-resistant disease, or else the patient's condition was misdiagnosed. Multidrug resistance disease is frequently fatal.

Healed primary or pulmonary tuberculosis commonly causes chest X-ray abnormalities such as granulomas, apical scarring and pleural thickening. Extensive damage is often complicated by bronchiectasis, mycetomas in tuberculosis cavities (**Figure 8.17**), chronic non-progressive lung fibrosis, extensive pleural thickening, restrictive or obstructive lung function defects.

> **Resistant *M. tuberculosis* is common in some countries (e.g. Russia, China and India) and develops when patients receive inadequate or poorly supervised treatment**. The use of a single therapy against tuberculosis is likely to create drug resistance. Therefore treatment regimens include multiple agents and should be carefully supervised.

Non-tuberculous mycobacteria

Lung infections can be caused by environmental mycobacteria that reside in soil or water. These are termed nontuberculous mycobacteria (NTM) infections.

Aetiology

Common environmental mycobacterial species that cause NTM infections include *M. kansasii, xenopi, avium, intracellulare* and *fortuitum*.

Clinical features

NTM infections are uncommon. They usually affect only patients with pre-existing lung disease or those who are immunosuppressed (e.g. by HIV infection). The major presentations are:

- macronodular or cavitating lung infection similar to pulmonary tuberculosis
- multiple small cavities, nodules and progressive bronchiectasis

- disseminated disease causing lung infiltrates, lymph node and bone marrow involvement (usually only in immunosuppressed patients, for example those who are HIV-positive with low CD4 counts)

Management

A positive sputum culture for an NTM often represents colonisation, and a diagnosis of NTM disease requires two or more positive cultures combined with clinical and radiological evidence of active infection. Antibiotic treatment varies with the NTM species. It requires prolonged combinations of antimycobacterial drugs, macrolides, and/or aminoglycosides. Treatment response is often poor, and many patients die of progressive infection.

Answers to starter questions

1. The abbreviations are expanded as follows: CAP: community-acquired pneumonia, HAP: hospital-acquired pneumonia, VAP: ventilator-acquired pneumonia, CPE: complicated parapneumonic effusion, NTM: non-tuberculous mycobacteria. Each describes a form of lung infection with a different microbial cause and therefore requires a different type of antibiotic treatment. Accurately defining which type of lung infection is affecting the patient is essential in order to use the correct treatment.

2. A positive sputum culture for M. tuberculosis and L. pneumophila means the patient is infected with those organisms, as does a positive nasopharyngeal aspirate for a respiratory virus.

    In contrast, a sputum culture that is positive for S. pneumoniae, H. influenzae, M. catarrhalis, P. aeruginosa and S. aureus could reflect asymptomatic colonisation, which is common in patients with chronic lung disease (e.g. bronchiectasis or COPD). However, in a patient with pneumonia, a positive sputum culture for one of these organisms means that it is the likely cause of the infection.

3. No. In the past, atypical pneumonia was the term used for patients presenting with interstitial pneumonia caused by M. pneumoniae or C. pneumoniae infection. Classically, these organisms cause mild disease that persists for 2–3 weeks, and the chest X-ray shows bilateral indistinct infiltrates. However, these bacteria also cause lobar pneumonia, so the term is not clinically useful.

    However, M. pneumoniae, C. pneumoniae and L. pneumophila are sometimes described as atypical organisms, because they:

    - are difficult to culture using conventional microbiological techniques
    - are not sensitive to β lactam antibiotics
    - have bacteriological features that differentiate them from 'pyogenic', highly proinflammatory bacteria such as S. pneumoniae and S. aureus.

4. Only half of patients with pulmonary tuberculosis have visible mycobacteria in their sputum (smear-positive disease). Therefore in many patients with suspected tuberculosis, diagnosis is not confirmed until the sputum cultures become positive after 3–4 weeks.

    Patients with a clinical presentation that strongly suggests tuberculosis and who are at high risk of the disease (e.g. born in a country with a high incidence of tuberculosis) should probably be started on antituberculous therapy without delay – before sputum culture results are available. The recent increasing use of nucleic acid amplification tests to rapidly identify active infection in smear-negative cases will help reduce this uncertainty.

Answers to starter questions

5. CURB-65 is used to assess severity in cases of CAP; a score of ≥ 3 indicates severe disease. In addition, bilateral consolidation; marked hypoxia; positive blood cultures; infection with *S. aureus*, *P. aeruginosa* or gram-negative bacilli; and high C-reactive protein (>250 mg/L) are all markers for more severe infection. Mortality of CAP increases with age and coexisting comorbidities.

6. Seasonal influenza infection only rarely causes severe disease in young or previously well patients. However, it often causes fatal exacerbations of pre-existing chronic diseases (e.g. COPD and cardiac failure) in the elderly.

    In contrast, intermittent worldwide epidemics of new influenza variants (e.g. the 1918 flu pandemic and swine flu in 2009) infect a high proportion of the population over a short time. These organisms frequently cause primary influenza pneumonia or secondary bacterial pneumonias, which result in large numbers of deaths of previously healthy people.

    Rare cases of 'bird flu' occur. The cause is an avian influenza virus caught directly from infected birds. The disease results in a primary influenza pneumonia with a very high mortality. Fortunately, bird flu viruses have not yet evolved to spread from human to human.

Chapter 9
Bronchiectasis and cystic fibrosis

Starter questions

Answers to the following questions are on page 284

1. What mechanisms cause bronchiectasis to develop?
2. What common pathogens are found in the sputum of patients with bronchiectasis?
3. Why does bronchiectasis cause respiratory failure?

Introduction

Bronchiectasis is abnormal dilation of the bronchi. The disease is easily detected by computerised tomography (CT). Areas of bronchiectasis readily develop chronic infection with pathogenic bacteria. These infections result in persisting symptoms and potentially progressive lung disease. Cystic fibrosis is a genetic disease that causes a frequently severe bronchiectasis, mainly in young people, and is associated with a range of additional clinical problems. Consequently, patients are often treated separately to those with bronchiectasis.

Case 12 Chronic cough with sputum production

Presentation

Mrs Connors is a non-smoking 56-year-old who had previously been well. She has been referred by her general practitioner to the respiratory outpatient department with a chronic cough and daily sputum production.

Initial interpretation

There are many possible differential diagnoses for chronic cough. However, most do not produce much phlegm. In a non-smoker a history of daily sputum production is unusual and raises the possibility of bronchiectasis.

Case 12 *continued*

History

Mrs Connors has had chest infections every winter for over 10 years. These infections resolved quickly with antibiotic treatment. However, for the past 18 months she has had a daily cough and is now producing two tablespoons of light green phlegm each day. She feels generally tired and has intermittent left-sided chest pain. She has had three episodes of minor haemoptysis. The cough and phlegm resolved after 5 days of amoxicillin but returned within 2 weeks.

Interpretation of history

In a non-smoker, a persisting cough with discoloured phlegm that improves only temporarily with antibiotic treatment suggests bronchiectasis. In a smoker, chronic bronchitis is more likely. Asthma can cause daily cough with phlegm, which is usually yellow. However, phlegm production by patients with chronic bronchitis or asthma does not resolve with antibiotics.

Musculoskeletal chest pain and fatigue are common in patients with bronchiectasis.

Further history

Mrs Connors has no history of severe childhood chest infections, tuberculosis, asthma, rheumatological conditions, ulcerative colitis or non-pulmonary infections. She is on no regular medication and has no upper respiratory tract symptoms.

Examination

Examination findings are normal except for coarse crepitations heard on auscultation over both lung bases posteriorly.

Interpretation of findings

The persisting crepitations indicate chronic lung damage and strongly support a possible diagnosis of bronchiectasis.

In this case, the history does not suggest an obvious cause for bronchiectasis, such as previous lung infection, tuberculosis, rheumatoid arthritis or immune defects. A chest X-ray and CT scan are necessary to identify whether she has bronchiectasis and spirometry is required to assess whether there is any associated airway obstruction.

Investigations

The chest X-ray is normal. However, the spirometry results show a mild obstructive defect with a forced expiratory volume (FEV_1) of 1.8 L/sec and forced vital capacity of 2.8 L. Because of the strong clinical suspicion for bronchiectasis, a CT scan is arranged. CT identifies widespread bilateral basal cylindrical bronchiectasis **(Figure 9.1)**.

Diagnosis

Daily purulent phlegm suggested bronchiectasis, a diagnosis confirmed by the CT. Additional tests are now required to identify specific causes and associated conditions, for example total immunoglobulin (Ig)G and IgE, *Aspergillus*-specific IgG and IgE, protein electrophoresis and sputum culture for mycobacteria and other bacteria.

However, in 50% of patients no cause is identified.

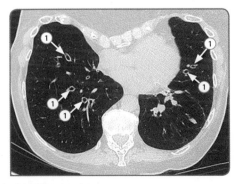

Figure 9.1 Computerised tomography showing cylindrical bronchiectasis. ① Dilated thick walled bronchi

Non–cystic fibrosis bronchiectasis

Bronchiectasis is the result of many different causes of bronchial injury and is commonly asymptomatic. However, bronchiectasis is often associated with chronic bronchial infection; pathogenic bacteria (**Table 9.1**) cause persisting symptoms that greatly decrease patients' quality of life and are associated with a significant mortality.

There are several anatomical types of bronchiectasis (**Table 9.2**). The most common is cylindrical bronchiectasis.

Epidemiology

Median age at diagnosis is 50 years. However, patients have often had symptoms for 10-20 years before diagnosis. Most cases (60%) occur in women. The estimated prevalence in industrialised countries is 1 in 1000 adults; the figure is much higher in developing countries.

Widespread use of CT scans mean that bronchiectasis is now increasingly identified as a complication of other chronic lung diseases, especially chronic obstructive pulmonary disease (COPD) and asthma.

Aetiology

Bronchiectasis has a wide range of causes (**Table 9.3**). The most common identifiable cause is a previous severe lung infection. However, 30-50% of cases have no obvious cause and are termed idiopathic bronchiectasis.

Pathogens that cause bronchiectasis	
Disease severity	Infection type(s)
Mild	Colonisation with common respiratory pathogens, for example *Haemophilus influenzae*, *Streptococcus pneumoniae*, *Moraxella catarrhalis* and *Staphylococcus aureus*
Moderate	Intermittent *Pseudomonas aeruginosa* colonisation
Severe	Chronic *P. aeruginosa* colonisation or infection with unusual pathogens, for example *Burkholderia* and *Stenotrophomonas* Superinfection with non-tuberculous mycobacteria

Table 9.1 Common bacterial pathogens found in the sputum of patients with bronchiectasis

Types of bronchiectasis	
Type of bronchiectasis	Features
Cylindrical (**Figure 9.1**)	Smooth bronchial dilatation (ratio > 1.1 of accompanying blood vessel)
Saccular or cystic (**Figure 9.4**)	Severe disease Grossly dilated and irregular bronchi Can extend to pleura
Traction	Caused by bronchial walls being pulled outwards in areas of lung fibrosis Asymptomatic
Diffuse	Widespread disease More prominent in lower lobes Upper lobe disease more common in allergic bronchopulmonary aspergillosis and cystic fibrosis
Localised	Localised to specific areas of the lung Caused by previous localised infection or bronchial obstruction of affected areas

Table 9.2 Types of bronchiectasis and their features

Causes of bronchiectasis		
Category (% of cases)	Causes (% of cases)	Specific diagnostic tests
Idiopathic (30–50%)		None (diagnosed by excluding known causes)
Immune defects of the respiratory tract		
Physical immune defects (<5%)	Cystic fibrosis	Sweat, nasal potential difference and CFTR genetic tests
	Ciliary dyskinesia	Saccharin test, electron microscopy and genetic tests
Immunodeficiency (10%)	Primary immunoglobulin deficiency (e.g. common variable immunodeficiency)	Total IgG, A and M concentration, IgG subclasses and antibody response to vaccines
	Secondary Ig deficiency (e.g. myeloma and bone marrow transplantation)	Total IgG concentration and protein electrophoresis
	HIV infection	HIV test
Inflammatory bronchial wall damage		
Post-infective (30%)	Previous whooping cough, pneumonia or measles	None (diagnosis suggested by history)
	Active non-tuberculous mycobacteria infection	Sputum and bronchial washings for acid-fast bacilli, and computerised tomography appearances (cavities and nodules)
Airways inflammation (25%)	Chronic obstructive pulmonary disease (variable)	Spirometry with reversibility testing
	Allergic bronchopulmonary aspergillosis (5–10%)	Total IgE, *Aspergillus*-specific IgG and IgE, *Aspergillus* skin test, sputum culture and cytological investigations
	Recurrent pulmonary aspiration (5%)	Barium swallow and 24-h oesophageal pH manometry
	Rheumatoid arthritis (10%)	Rheumatoid factor
	Ulcerative colitis (rare)	Colonoscopy and biopsy
	Bronchiolitis obliterans (rare)	Spirometry with reversibility testing
Bronchial obstruction (<5%)		
	Post-tuberculosis stricture, inhaled foreign body and benign bronchial tumours	Bronchoscopy
	Congenital bronchial wall defects	Bronchoscopy

CFTR, cystic fibrosis transmembrane conductance regulator. Ig, immunoglobulin.

Table 9.3 Causes of bronchiectasis and diagnostic tests

Pathology

Bronchial wall damage is initially caused by inflammation which is either a response to infection or due to an inflammatory disease affecting the bronchi. The damage causes bronchial dilatation (and therefore bronchiectasis) and epithelial damage, which disrupts mucociliary clearance and allows colonisation of the bronchi by pathogenic bacteria. This chronic bronchial infection stimulates a neutrophilic inflammatory response and increased mucous production, resulting in purulent phlegm and also further damages the bronchial wall. The increased damage to the bronchial wall makes it even more difficult to eradicate pathogenic bacteria from the bronchi, leading to further inflammation and damage. This is the vicious circle hypothesis of the pathogenesis of bronchiectasis (**Figure 9.2**).

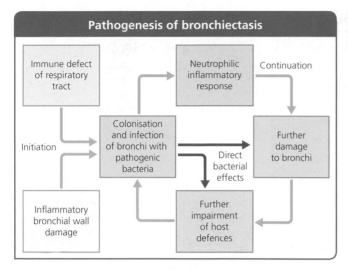

Figure 9.2 The pathogenesis of bronchiectasis: the vicious circle hypothesis.

In more severe bronchiectasis, the inflammation in the bronchi also spreads to affect the small airways, causing an obliterative bronchiolitis (small airways obstruction) and the physiological effects of airways obstruction.

> Patients with bronchiectasis may find the constant production of phlegm with cough socially embarrassing. These symptoms limit their social interactions and reduce their quality of life.

Clinical features

The cardinal symptom of bronchiectasis is cough with chronic daily sputum production. The sputum is mucoid, mucopurulent or frankly purulent; the daily volume varies from one or two teaspoons to 300 mL or more in severe cases. Infective exacerbations are common and increase sputum volume, viscosity and purulence. Other common symptoms, especially during exacerbations, include:

- minor haemoptysis
- malodorous breath
- malaise
- fatigue
- dyspnoea on exertion
- wheeze
- musculoskeletal type chest pain

Bronchiectasis, whether idiopathic or bronchiectasis caused by ciliary dyskinesia, cystic fibrosis, allergic bronchopulmonary aspergillosis or immune defects, often coexists with chronic rhinitis and sinusitis. Poorly controlled disease causes progressive small airways obstruction, which eventually results in type 2 respiratory failure and death. Major haemoptysis and amyloidosis are other complications.

On examination, the fingers of patients with bronchiectasis are clubbed in 10% of cases. Focal crepitations are audible over the affected lobes, usually bibasally over lower lobes. Patients with severe disease also have signs of airway obstruction.

> Recurrent positive sputum cultures for common respiratory pathogens (e.g. *H. influenzae*) in a young person or an older non-smoker suggests bronchiectasis. It is unusual for these pathogens to be repeatedly found in the sputa unless there is a structural lung disease present.

Diagnostic approach

Bronchiectasis is an anatomical diagnosis made when radiological evidence of dilated bronchi is found. Chest X-rays sometimes show bronchial wall thickening, ring shadows and tramlines (**Figure 9.3**) but are normal in half of cases.

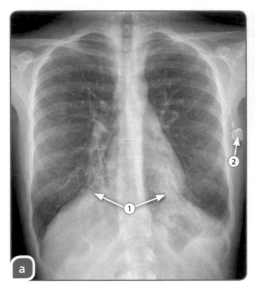

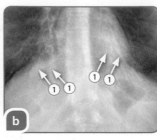

Figure 9.3 (a) Chest X ray changes in bronchiectasis with crowding of lung markings, bronchial wall thickening and 'tramlines' in the lower lobes (indicated by the arrows, ①). There is also a portacath ② visible in the left axilla, which is a permanent placed subcutaneous port connected to a large central vein that is often used in patients with cystic fibrosis and severe bronchiectasis for frequent administration of intravenous antibiotics. (b) Close up of ① bronchial wall thickening and crowding with tramlines.

Because of the limitations of chest X-rays, the diagnosis of bronchiectasis is usually confirmed or excluded by CT findings. These include the following:

- Bronchial dilatation (to a width greater than that of the accompanying blood vessel) and non-tapering bronchi. The dilated bronchi are usually present in both lungs and are most evident in the lower lobes. However, bronchial obstruction or post-infective bronchiectasis is frequently be localised to a single lobe. Furthermore, cystic fibrosis affects mainly the upper lobes, and allergic bronchopulmonary aspergillosis the central and upper lobes.
- Bronchial wall thickening
- Tree-in-bud changes, which suggest small airways inflammation and active disease
- Mosaicism and areas of gas trapping on expiration, caused by small airways obstruction

Once the diagnosis of bronchiectasis is confirmed by CT, the following tests are necessary.

- Pulmonary function tests, with reversibility testing, to assess the degree of associated obstructive lung disease; the results are used as a baseline for monitoring disease progression

- Sputum culture for bacterial pathogens and mycobacteria to identify potential infecting pathogens and their drug sensitivities
- Specific tests for potential causes (**Table 9.3**); which tests are used depends on the clinical scenario. For example, most patients should have their IgG measured to exclude Ig deficiencies, but tests for cystic fibrosis are usually limited to younger patients or those with predominantly upper lobe disease and no obvious other cause of bronchiectasis.

Management

The three principles of managing bronchiectasis are as follows.

1. Identify, and when possible treat, the cause, e.g. intravenous immunoglobulin replacement therapy for IgG deficiency (**Tables 9.3** and **9.4**).
2. Improve quality of life by minimising daily sputum production and reducing the frequency of exacerbations.
3. Maintain or improve pulmonary function by:

- minimising active chronic infection
- reducing the frequency and severity of exacerbations

Treatment for bronchiectasis	
Cause	**Treatment**
Cystic fibrosis	Ivacaftor therapy for some less common specific CFTR mutations
Immunoglobulin deficiency	Intravenous immunoglobulin therapy every 3–4 weeks
Allergic bronchopulmonary aspergillosis	Inhaled or oral corticosteroids, and long-term itraconazole
Recurrent pulmonary aspiration	Proton pump inhibitors, domperidone, surgery and percutaneous endoscopic gastrostomy feeding
Ulcerative colitis	High-dose inhaled corticosteroids
Obstructive causes	Endobronchial interventions and surgical resection
HIV infection	Antiretroviral therapy
Non-tuberculous mycobacteria	Antimycobacterial antibiotic therapy
CFTR, cystic fibrosis transmembrane conductance regulator.	

Table 9.4 Treatments for specific causes of bronchiectasis

- using bronchodilators (β-agonist and possibly steroid inhalers) regularly

Daily sputum production and the frequency of exacerbations are reduced by the following.

- Regular use of self-administered lung clearance techniques to reduce bacterial build-up in the lungs; these techniques require patient education by a respiratory physiotherapist.
- Effective treatment of exacerbations with prolonged courses of appropriate antibiotics (e.g. 10–14 days) (**Table 9.5**).

- Severe disease frequently requires oral or nebulised prophylactic antibiotic therapy (**Table 9.5**)
- Long-term azithromycin therapy (250–500 mg, three times per week) has anti-inflammatory effects that frequently are very effective at reducing daily sputum production and exacerbation frequency.

Antibiotic resistance and patient intolerance of antibiotics are the most significant factors limiting effective therapy. Frequent sputum cultures are necessary to ensure the correct antibiotic therapy is being used. The common

Antibiotics for bronchiectasis		
Disease severity	**Treatment of exacerbations (10–14 days)**	**Prophylactic antibiotics***
Mild	Amoxicillin Doxycycline Macrolides (e.g. clarithromycin)	Usually unnecessary
Moderate	Co-amoxiclav Doxycycline	Low-dose daily amoxicillin, doxycycline or co-amoxiclav Azithromycin three times per week
Severe	Co-amoxiclav Ciprofloxacin Intravenous antipseudomonal antibiotics (e.g. piperacillin, ceftazadine or meropenem)	Low-dose daily doxycycline or co-amoxiclav Azithromycin three times a week Nebulised colomycin or aminoglycoside (e.g. gentamicin)
*Consider if more than 3 exacerbations annually or in cases with progressive reduction in lung function.		

Table 9.5 Antibiotic treatments for bronchiectasis

infecting organisms for mild disease are *H. influenzae, S. pneumoniae, M. catarrhalis* and *S. aureus*, which are usually treated with amoxicillin, co-amoxiclav, doxycycline or macrolides.

In severe disease (**Figure 9.4**), *P. aeruginosa* is a significant problem and responds only to oral ciprofloxacin. However, *P. aeruginosa* readily becomes resistant to ciprofloxacin. In such cases, intravenous antipseudomonal antibiotics are often necessary.

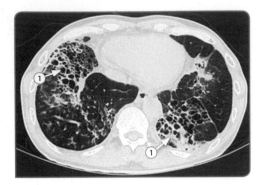

Figure 9.4 Computerised tomography showing ① focal areas of severe saccular bronchiectasis.

Prognosis

Non-cystic fibrosis bronchiectasis usually progresses slowly. However, about one in five patients have more severe, progressive disease with reductions in FEV_1 of $>50\,mL/$ year; this is more common in patients with bronchiectasis caused by allergic bronchopulmonary aspergillosis, ciliary dyskinesia, or infection with non-tuberculous mycobacteria. Progressive disease eventually causes respiratory failure, and 15% of patients die from their bronchiectasis.

In patients with progressive bronchiectasis, repeated sputum cultures are needed. These exclude infection with organisms that are difficult to treat such as *P. aeruginosa* or non-tuberculous mycobacteria. They are also used to assess the results of aggressive antibiotic therapy used to control infections and therefore to slow or reverse any decline in lung function.

Cystic fibrosis

Cystic fibrosis is an inherited cause of severe bronchiectasis. The disease affects young people and has significant additional extrapulmonary features. Therefore it needs to be considered separately from non–cystic fibrosis bronchiectasis.

Epidemiology

Cystic fibrosis is the most common fatal genetic disorder in western countries; in Europe, it affects 1 in 2000–3000 newborn infants.

Aetiology

Cystic fibrosis is caused by autosomal recessive mutations of the gene encoding the cystic fibrosis transmembrane conductance regulator (CFTR). CFTR is a transmembrane chloride channel found in the respiratory epithelium, exocrine glands (including the pancreas) and sweat ducts. By transporting chloride ions across cell membranes (**Figure 9.5**), CTFR controls the movement of sodium and water out of the cell and into the mucous layer. This movement of water is necessary for the production of thin, freeflowing mucus.

Over 1500 CFTR mutations are recognised. These mutations are categorised into five groups depending on their effect on the synthesis or function of CFTR (**Figure 9.6**). If CFTR is not synthesised, or if it functions poorly, chloride flow across cell membranes is impaired, the mucous is inadequately hydrated, and becomes thick and sticky.

Over 70% of cases of cystic fibrosis are caused by a mutation affecting amino acid 508. Homozygous or compound heterozygous

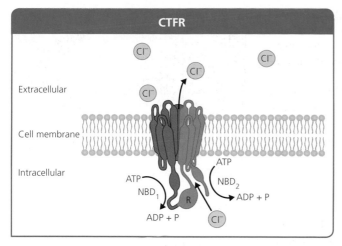

Figure 9.5 The cystic fibrosis transmembrane conductance regulator (CFTR). The regulatory domain has a phosphorylation site. When a phosphate ion binds, the regulatory domain causes the channel to open. NBD, nucleotide-binding domain; R, regulatory domain.

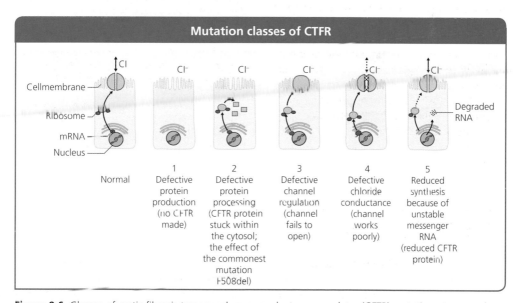

Figure 9.6 Classes of cystic fibrosis transmembrane conductance regulator (CFTR) mutations. In normal cells, CFTR is produced from the DNA in the nucleus and modified by the endoplasmic reticulum. It then travels to the apical cell membrane.

(two different mutations, one on each chromosome) mutations of CFTR (**Figure 9.7**) result in cells producing mucus with a high sodium and chloride content and viscosity, which impairs mucociliary clearance and the innate immunity of the respiratory epithelium (**Figure 9.8**). Mucus blockages of the pancreatic ducts cause pancreatic damage and failure.

Clinical features

Patients with cystic fibrosis have chronic bronchial colonisation with pathogenic bacteria and progressive bronchiectasis with small airways obstruction. Therefore they present similarly to patients with non–cystic fibrosis bronchiectasis, with chronic phlegm

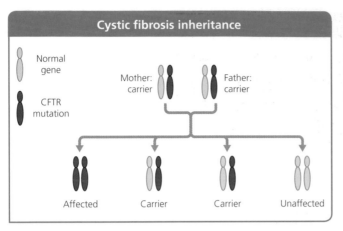

Cystic fibrosis inheritance

Normal gene

CFTR mutation

Mother: carrier

Father: carrier

Affected   Carrier   Carrier   Unaffected

Figure 9.7 Inheritance of cystic fibrosis. If both parents carry a cystic fibrosis transmembrane conductance regulator (CFTR) mutation, their child has a 25% chance of being born with the condition.

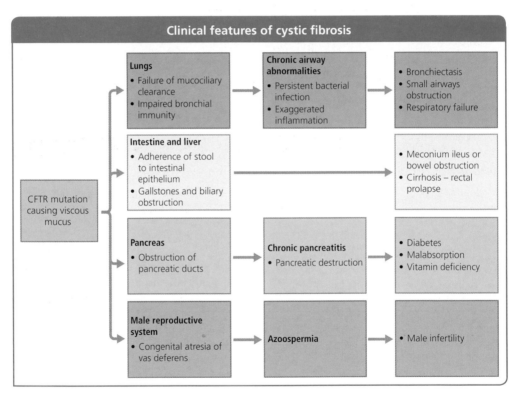

Clinical features of cystic fibrosis

CFTR mutation causing viscous mucus

Lungs
- Failure of mucociliary clearance
- Impaired bronchial immunity

Chronic airway abnormalities
- Persistent bacterial infection
- Exaggerated inflammation

- Bronchiectasis
- Small airways obstruction
- Respiratory failure

Intestine and liver
- Adherence of stool to intestinal epithelium
- Gallstones and biliary obstruction

- Meconium ileus or bowel obstruction
- Cirrhosis – rectal prolapse

Pancreas
- Obstruction of pancreatic ducts

Chronic pancreatitis
- Pancreatic destruction

- Diabetes
- Malabsorption
- Vitamin deficiency

Male reproductive system
- Congenital atresia of vas deferens

Azoospermia

- Male infertility

Figure 9.8 Pathophysiology of common clinical features of cystic fibrosis. CFTR, cystic fibrosis transmembrane conductance regulator.

production and recurrent infective exacerbations. However, unlike non–cystic fibrosis bronchiectasis, the disease

- usually starts in early childhood
- is usually worse in the lung apices
- almost always results in fatal respiratory failure due to severe airways obstruction

Most patients with severe disease have marked clubbing, low body mass index, extensive crepitations in both lungs and obvious signs of airways obstruction with poor respiratory function (**Figure 9.9**). Cystic fibrosis is also associated with a wide range of extrapulmonary complications (**Table 9.6**

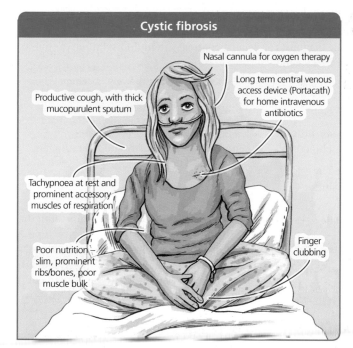

Figure 9.9 Typical clinical features of severe cystic fibrosis.

Cystic fibrosis

Nasal cannula for oxygen therapy

Long term central venous access device (Portacath) for home intravenous antibiotics

Productive cough, with thick mucopurulent sputum

Tachypnoea at rest and prominent accessory muscles of respiration

Poor nutrition – slim, prominent ribs/bones, poor muscle bulk

Finger clubbing

Complications of cystic fibrosis

Pulmonary (% of patients affected)	Extrapulmonary (% of patients affected)
Bronchiectasis (>95%)	Glucose intolerance and diabetes (25% require insulin)
Respiratory failure (small airways obstruction) (>95%)	Pancreatic insufficiency with malabsorption and deficiency of vitamins A, D and K (95%)
Lobar collapse (common)	Chronic sinusitis (95%)
Allergic bronchopulmonary aspergillosis (5%)	Meconium ileus (intestinal obstruction in neonates) (10%)
Major haemoptysis (<5%)	Meconium ileus equivalent (small bowel obstruction) (<5%)
Pneumothorax (<5%)	Infertility (male, 99%; female, partial)
Non-tuberculous mycobacteria infection (5%)	Digital clubbing (>90%) or hypertrophic osteoarthropathy (<5%)
Chronic invasive aspergillosis (<5%)	Abnormal liver function tests (30%) and cirrhosis (<5%)
	Vasculitic rashes (1–2%)
	Gallstones (10%)
	Osteoporosis (50%)
	Nasal polyps (20%)
	Heat stroke (very rare)
	Reactive arthritis (5–10%)

Table 9.6 Pulmonary and extrapulmonary complications of cystic fibrosis

and **Figure 9.8**). The most common of these is pancreatic insufficiency, which results in malabsorption and glucose intolerance or diabetes.

Less common mutations can cause milder disease that does not present until adulthood.

Diagnostic approach

Postnatal testing is routine in several European countries to identify cases before symptoms appear. The main diagnostic test is measurement of sweat chloride concentration, which is increased in patients with cystic fibrosis. The nasal potential difference test also identifies patients with cystic fibrosis. The diagnosis is confirmed by genetic testing for CFTR gene mutations.

Management

The management principles for cystic fibrosis are similar to those for severe bronchiectasis:

- regular physiotherapy supported by a chest clearance device (e.g. the flutter valve or chest cuirass)
- frequent antibiotics for bronchial infections
- regular use of inhaled β-agonists

Most patients have prophylactic therapy with flucloxacillin against chronic *S. aureus* colonisation, as well as azithromycin. Nebulised DNase and hypertonic saline slow the decline in lung function. Extrapulmonary manifestations need specific treatment, and nutrition and psychological support is vital. Patients with cystic fibrosis due to the unusual G551D mutation that affects the opening of the chloride channel are treated with ivacaftor which increases chloride secretion via CFTR and improves lung function.

Because of the severity and complexity of cystic fibrosis, patients are best treated in specialist centres with multidisciplinary input.

> **Gene replacement therapy is being investigated as a treatment for cystic fibrosis.** The CFTR gene could be given by nebuliser, targeting delivery to the main affected organ. However, it is difficult to maintain gene stability and to ensure it is integrated into a high number of cells.

Prognosis

Cystic fibrosis is almost universally fatal; the cause of death is slowly progressive type 2 respiratory failure. Improvements in treatment have increased the median age of death from the mid twenties in the 1970s to the mid forties now. Lung transplantation is curative for some patients.

> **A diagnosis of cystic fibrosis affects the whole family.** The burden of physiotherapy and administration of treatments falls to the parents of the affected child. As the child becomes an adult, the parents have to witness the functional decline and eventual death of their child.

Answers to starter questions

1. Bronchiectasis develops when inflammation damages the bronchial wall. A single episode of a common infections (e.g. tuberculosis or measles) can damage the bronchi directly. Patients with a physical immune defect (e.g. cystic fibrosis or an obstructed bronchus), low levels of immunoglobulins or a condition that causes airways inflammation (e.g. COPD) are also common causes of bronchiectasis.

2. Common pathogens detected in the sputum of patients with non–cystic fibrosis bronchiectasis are *H. influenzae* (40%), *P. aeruginosa* (30%), *S. pneumoniae* (15–20%), *M. catarrhalis* (10–15%) and *S. aureus* (5%). Bronchiectasis can be complicated by non-tuberculous mycobacteria infection, which is one cause of deteriorating disease.

3. Inflammation and infection in medium-sized bronchi spreads to smaller airways. This process causes bronchoconstriction with fixed airways obstruction, which can progress to respiratory failure. Controlling the infection in the bronchi and reducing the frequency of exacerbations reduces bronchiolar inflammation. These measures prevent progressive small airways obstruction and the subsequent development of respiratory failure.

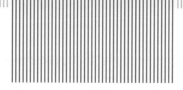

Chapter 10
Circulatory disorders

Starter questions

Answers to the following questions are on page 299

1. What is pleurisy?
2. When is a D-dimer test useful, and when is it not?
3. Which patients need investigations for a possible predisposition to thromboembolism?
4. How are patients with pulmonary hypertension identified?

Introduction

Pulmonary vascular disease refers to disorders affecting the pulmonary veins or arteries. The entire blood volume passes from the heart to the lungs and back to the heart and any obstruction to this flow has serious, and even life-threatening, consequences. The severity of these disorders depends on whether the underlying cause is treatable or reversible, and how quickly the disorder develops. A sudden obstruction to blood flow due to a large pulmonary embolus can cause sudden death, whereas multiple small pulmonary emboli accumulating over time will affect the pressures within the pulmonary circulation, but over a period of time in which adaptations can occur. Pulmonary vascular disorders are often difficult to diagnose as they produce non-specific symptoms and few clinical signs. Initial investigations such as a chest X ray are usually normal. Specialist investigations and clinical assessments are usually needed.

Case 13 Four days of chest pain on breathing

Presentation

Mrs Lepard, aged 52 years, attends the emergency department with a 4-day history of sharp right-sided chest pain that worsens when taking deep breaths.

Initial interpretation

Mrs Lepard has pleuritic chest pain. This is usually caused by pleurisy (inflammation of the pleura, often as a result of underlying pneumonia) or by pulmonary embolism. However, other, less common causes are possible (see Table 2.8).

History

The pain started suddenly and has been associated with shortness of breath for the past 2 days. Mrs Lepard has not had a fever or coughed up any blood or sputum.

Interpretation of history

Dyspnoea occurs with both pneumonia and pulmonary embolism. However, the absence of fever or cough makes pneumonia less likely. Assessment of risk factors for pulmonary embolism is necessary (Table 10.1).

Further history

Mrs Lepard was previously well and has no family history of blood clots or clotting disorders. She returned from a holiday in Australia 5 days ago. She has had no calf pain or swelling.

Examination

Mrs Lepard is in pain when taking deep breaths but is apyrexial. She has a regular heart rate of 115 beats/min, blood pressure of 135/70 mmHg and respiratory rate of 18 breaths/min. She is not cya-nosed, and her oxygen saturation is 94%. Heart sounds are normal. Chest examination is normal except for a quiet pleural rub heard over the right lateral chest wall. The calves are soft and non-tender to palpation; they are not swollen.

Interpretation of findings

The pleural rub confirms inflammation of the pleura. The lack of fever makes infection unlikely. Therefore, even without clinical evidence of deep vein thrombosis, pulmonary embolism is the most likely diagnosis, especially as the recent flight is a major risk factor for pulmonary embolism. Saturations in the normal range do not rule out pulmonary embolism. A raised heart rate > 100 beats/min suggests significant physiological derangement. Mrs Lepard's Wells score (Table 10.2) is 4.5, which suggests PE is a likely diagnosis. The seriousness of the probable diagnosis mandates immediate further investigation.

Investigations

The electrocardiogram (ECG) shows sinus tachycardia but does not show right heart strain, making a massive PE unlikely. The chest X-ray does not show evidence of alternative diagnoses such as a pneumothorax but it does show a small wedge-shaped patch of peripheral consolidation in the right lung, consistent with a pulmonary infarct caused by a pulmonary embolus. Computerised tomography pulmonary angiography (CTPA) can identify pulmonary emboli as a filling defect in contrast-enhanced pulmonary arteries and confirmed pulmonary embolism in Mrs Lepard, with emboli visible on both sides (Figure 10.1).

Case 13 *continued*

Risk factors for deep vein thrombosis and pulmonary embolism	
Category	Risk factors*
Altered blood constituents (acquired)	Malignancy (commonly lung, pancreatic or colon cancer) Trauma Pregnancy Congestive cardiac failure Myeloproliferative disorders (e.g. polycythaemia rubra vera) Inflammatory bowel disease Antiphospholipid syndrome Use of oral contraceptives, hormone replacement therapy or tamoxifen Cigarette smoking
Altered blood constituents (inherited)	Factor V Leiden mutation Protein S deficiency Protein C deficiency Antithrombin deficiency Dysfibrinogenaemia
Endothelial wall damage	Central venous catheter in situ Trauma Intravenous drug use Surgery (particularly pelvic and orthopaedic)
Altered blood flow	Prolonged immobility of any cause Surgery (particularly pelvic and orthopaedic) Pregnancy

*Patients often have multiple risk factors.

Table 10.1 Risk factors for deep vein thrombosis and pulmonary embolism

Wells score for pulmonary embolism	
Clinical features	Score*
Deep vein thrombosis symptoms and signs	3 each
Pulmonary embolism is the most likely diagnosis	
High heart rate (> 100 beats/min)	1.5 each
Immobility or recent surgery	
History of deep vein thrombosis, pulmonary embolism or both	
Coughing blood from the lungs	1 each
Malignancy	

*A combined score of >4 means that pulmonary embolism is likely

Table 10.2 The two-level Wells score for pulmonary embolism

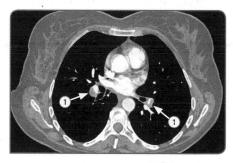

Figure 10.1 Computerised tomography pulmonary angiogram showing ① bilateral pulmonary emboli in the central pulmonary arteries.

Case 13 *continued*

Diagnosis

With pulmonary embolism confirmed by CTPA, anticoagulation with subcutaneous low-molecular-weight heparin (LMWH) is started immediately. Warfarin is then started for long term anticoagulation although LMWH is continued until the international normalised ratio (INR) is in the therapeutic range. Warfarin treatment continues for 3 months, and the INR is monitored regularly at the anticoagulation clinic.

Patients on warfarin need regular blood tests to monitor INR for dose adjustment. Testing is more frequent during the initiation of treatment and when patients are on drugs which interact with warfarin. Patients carry a yellow book to record INRs and doses. Newer anticoagulants such as rivaroxiban require less monitoring but are not suitable for all patients.

Case 14 Leg swelling in a patient with COPD

Presentation

Mr Nowak is a 74-year-old man with severe chronic obstructive pulmonary disease (COPD). He has been referred to the respiratory outpatient clinic with significant swelling of both legs.

Initial interpretation

Swelling of both legs is common in older patients and has several possible causes. The use of drugs such as oral corticosteroids and calcium channel blockers cause swollen legs, as does congestive cardiac failure, chronic venous insufficiency and cor pulmonale. A more detailed history is required to determine the most likely cause.

Further history

Mr Nowak has had COPD for 20 years. He stopped smoking 15 years ago. Over the past 2 years, he has had increasing shortness of breath on exertion and is now breathless after walking 10–20 m. His legs became swollen over the past 2 months.

He has no previous history of hypertension, ischaemic heart disease, deep vein thrombosis or diabetes. His only regular medications are salbutamol, ipratropium and beclomethasone inhalers.

Examination

Mr Nowak is short of breath on minimal exertion. He has central cyanosis and pitting oedema up to both knees. Jugular venous pressure is increased, and a prominent V wave is present. He has a loud P2, and a right-sided parasternal heave is felt. Respiratory examination shows the typical features of COPD (see Chapter 2).

Interpretation of findings

This combination of examination findings indicates pulmonary hypertension with right ventricular hypertrophy and failure complicating COPD. The combination of pulmonary hypertension with right ventricular hypertrophy is termed cor pulmonale (**Table 10.5**). The history suggests no other likely causes of leg swelling.

Case 14 *continued*

Cor pulmonale: presentation in a patient with COPD

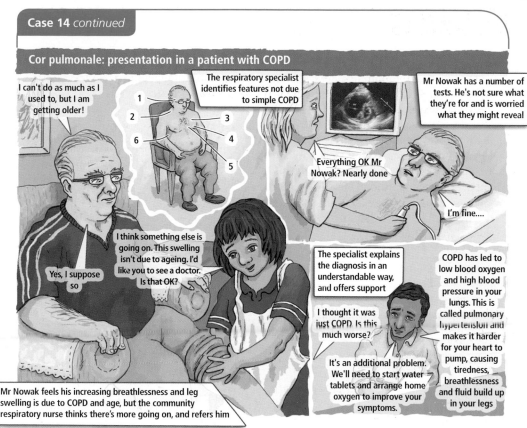

1. Plethoric face, 2. Elevated jugular venous pressure, 3. Loud P2 second heart sound, 4. Left parasternal heave, 5. Palpable thrill, 6. Hepatomegaly.

Investigations

The ECG shows P pulmonale, right axis deviation and partial right bundle branch block and therefore confirms right heart strain. The chest X-ray excludes other diagnoses and shows hyperinflated lungs with no focal abnormalities.

An echocardiogram identifies right ventricular hypertrophy and poor right ventricular function. However, the left ventricle and heart valves are normal. This confirms that the right heart failure is due to chronic respiratory failure and not a primary cardiac problem.

Pulmonary artery systolic pressure is estimated to be 60 mmHg. Arterial blood gas analysis shows hypoxaemia, with a Pao_2 of 7.1 kPa on air.

Diagnosis

There is clinical, ECG and echocardiogram evidence of pulmonary hypertension and right ventricular failure. When this is due to chronic hypoxia it is called cor pulmonale.

Diuretics are prescribed to reduce the oedema. Home oxygen therapy is prescribed to decrease pulmonary artery systolic pressure and improve long-term survival. A referral is made for pulmonary rehabilitation, and Mr Nowak's inhaler treatments are optimised.

Pulmonary embolism

Pulmonary embolism is the most common disorder affecting the pulmonary vessels. It is potentially life threatening and requires prompt investigation and treatment.

Usually, pulmonary embolism is the result of obstruction of a pulmonary artery or arterioles by a thrombus. Rarely, it is caused by tumour, infected thrombus, fat (after fracture of a long bone) or amniotic fluid emboli.

Types

Acute pulmonary embolism

This type of pulmonary embolism causes symptoms and signs in a few hours or days. When associated with cardiac arrest or life-threatening shock, it is called massive or submassive pulmonary embolism (see Chapter 11).

Chronic pulmonary embolism

In this type of pulmonary embolism, multiple small pulmonary emboli cause dyspnoea and pulmonary hypertension that progress slowly over weeks or months.

Epidemiology

The annual incidence of pulmonary embolism is about 110 cases per 100,000 people in the UK and USA, with slightly lower estimated incidences in Europe. Autopsy studies show that the diagnosis is often missed, and that pulmonary emboli are a major cause of sudden death.

Aetiology

Risk factors for pulmonary embolism are similar to those for deep vein thrombosis (**Table 10.1**). Most pulmonary emboli arise from thrombi in a deep vein of a lower limb. Thrombi become detached and travel through the venous circulation and the right ventricle before lodging in a pulmonary artery. Thrombi also originate in the inferior vena cava, the upper limb veins or the right atrium or ventricle, especially if indwelling intravascular devices (e.g. central lines and pacing wires) are present.

Prevention

Prevention of deep vein thrombosis prevents pulmonary embolism. On admission, all hospital in-patients must be assessed for risk of deep vein thrombosis. Antithromboembolism stockings and prophylactic LMWH are prescribed to all patients at risk, unless contraindicated.

Pathogenesis

The three factors contributing to venous thromboembolism are referred to as Virchow's triad (**Table 10.1**) and are:

- alterations to the constituents of blood (inherited or acquired)
- injury to the vascular endothelium
- changes in blood flow

Clinical features

Acute pulmonary embolism

Acute pulmonary embolism presents with dyspnoea, pleuritic chest pain, cough and haemoptysis. These symptoms appear suddenly or develop insidiously, over days or weeks. The most common signs are central cyanosis, tachypnoea, tachycardia, a pleural rub, signs of a small effusion and a loud P2 on auscultation of the heart. However, respiratory examination is often normal. Signs of deep vein thrombosis in a lower limb (i.e. unilateral firm calf swelling with tenderness) is sometimes present.

Massive pulmonary emboli present with sudden onset of syncope, hypotension and severe dyspnoea; they can cause cardiac arrest. As well as signs of acute pulmonary embolism, the patient sometimes develops acute right ventricular failure, with increased jugular venous pressure, a parasternal heave and a right ventricular S3 added heart sound.

Chronic pulmonary embolism

Chronic pulmonary embolism presents with progressive dyspnoea developing over weeks or months, sometimes associated with episodes of chest pain and haemoptysis. In severe disease, patients are centrally cyanosed. As for acute pulmonary embolism, the results of respiratory examination are usually normal. Signs of pulmonary hypertension (i.e. a loud P2, raised jugular venous pressure with prominent V waves, right parasternal heave and peripheral oedema) are present in some patients.

Diagnostic approach

Pulmonary embolism is difficult to diagnose clinically: often, the symptoms are non-specific, the signs are subtle or non-existent, and the chest X ray is normal. The diagnosis of pulmonary embolism must be confirmed by CTPA showing a clot in one or more pulmonary arteries, or by a ventilation–perfusion scan (VQ scan) showing reduced perfusion to a ventilated area of lung. Both investigations expose the patient to significant radiation.

Clinical assessment of the patient's risk for pulmonary embolism (e.g. using the modified Wells score, **Table 10.2**) is necessary to interpret equivocal scans (**Figure 10.2**).

> **Unexplained decreases in oxygenation** and sudden onset of dyspnoea suggest acute pulmonary embolism. Suspect chronic pulmonary embolism in patients with chronic dyspnoea and decreased transfer factor whose lung function is otherwise normal.

Investigations

Blood tests

D-dimer is a degradation product of fibrin, the end product of the coagulation cascade and principal component of blood clots. The serum concentration of D-dimer is increased in >90% of patients with acute pulmonary embolism as a result of clot breakdown. However, this finding is non-specific, because D-dimer concentration is increased for many reasons, including malignancy, recent surgery, pregnancy, renal failure and advanced age.

Troponin T and brain natriuretic peptide or NT-proBNP are often high in patients with acute and massive pulmonary embolism. The results of other routine blood tests are usually normal. Arterial blood gas results show type 1 respiratory failure and respiratory alkalosis.

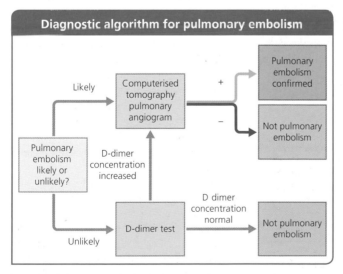

Diagnostic algorithm for pulmonary embolism

Figure 10.2 Diagnostic algorithm for pulmonary embolism.

Electrocardiography

Non-specific ECG abnormalities are common in patients with pulmonary embolism due to right atrial and ventricle dilatation and right ventricle ischaemia. Findings include sinus tachycardia and T-wave inversions in right ventricular leads. The classic ECG findings for pulmonary embolism are S1Q3T3, right ventricular strain and new right bundle branch block, although these are rare in practice (**Figure 10.3**).

Imaging

Chest X-ray

A chest X-ray excludes other diseases (e.g. pneumonia) but cannot show the emboli themselves and is therefore frequently normal. However, the lung damage caused by pulmonary emboli is visible as areas of atelectasis and wedge-shaped peripheral consolidation. They also cause reduced blood vessel markings and small pleural effusions.

Ventilation–perfusion scan

This type of scan shows which areas of the lung are ventilated and which are perfused. Mismatched perfusion defects indicate pulmonary embolism. A normal VQ scan virtually excludes pulmonary embolism. However, the results are often indeterminate, meaning that the diagnosis cannot be confirmed or excluded. Furthermore, the scan is difficult to interpret in patients with chronic lung disease due to the presence of ventilation defects.

Computerised tomography pulmonary angiography

The technique of CTPA is highly sensitive and specific, making it the first-line test for pulmonary embolism (Figure 10.1). The lung tissue is shown as well as the blood vessels, therefore CTPA detects other lung diseases that could be causing the patient's symptoms.

Venous ultrasound and echocardiography

Deep vein thrombosis is detected on ultrasound of the lower limb and is used to identify patients at risk of pulmonary embolism.

In patients with massive or submassive pulmonary embolism, echocardiography shows right ventricular dilatation, decreased right ventricular function or tricuspid regurgitation. This allows the diagnosis to be confirmed rapidly by a bedside test.

Angiography

The gold standard test for pulmonary embolism is pulmonary angiography. However, this procedure is rarely used as it requires insertion of a catheter into the femoral vein, which is then threaded up to the right atrium, so contrast can be injected into the pulmonary arteries. It is therefore an invasive procedure that requires a trained operator.

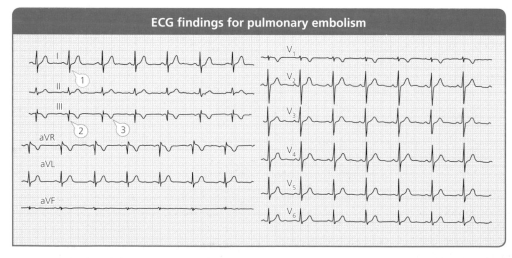

ECG findings for pulmonary embolism

Figure 10.3 Electrocardiographic findings for pulmonary embolism: S1Q3T3 (1) S wave in lead I, (2) Q wave in lead III, (3) inverted T waves in lead III.

Management

Patients with acute pulmonary embolism receive supportive oxygen therapy, analgesics for pleuritic chest pain and fluid for hypotension. Patients with massive pulmonary embolism require urgent stabilisation. They must be admitted to intensive care and considered for thrombolysis (see Chapter 11).

Medication

Patients with pulmonary embolism require anticoagulation to speed clot resolution and prevent further emboli. Patients are first treated for 5–7 days with subcutaneous injections of LMWH. Long-term oral anticoagulation with warfarin starts at the same time. The aim is to achieve a therapeutic INR of 2.0–4.0. LMWH is continued until this target INR is achieved.

Patients with a known reversible cause for their condition (e.g. recent surgery) continue warfarin therapy for 3 months. Patients with recurrent pulmonary embolism or a permanent risk factor (e.g. cancer) usually require lifelong treatment with anticoagulation.

> **Because pulmonary embolism is life threatening**, initial treatment is empirical. LMWH is started before CTPA confirmation of the diagnosis unless there is a high bleeding risk.

Mechanical treatments

Surgical or interventional radiological embolectomy is considered for patients who have massive pulmonary embolism and are at high risk of bleeding. Inferior vena cava filters are implanted devices that prevent recurrent pulmonary embolism in patients who have persisting deep vein thrombi and repeated emboli despite anticoagulation therapy. The filters are also used for patients at unacceptably high risk of bleeding.

> **Less severely affected patients (those with pulmonary embolism in the absence of significant comorbidities) are increasingly treated on ambulatory pathways rather than being admitted to hospital.** These patients inject LMWH themselves or attend hospital daily for the injection while waiting for their INR to be in range on warfarin.

Prognosis

For untreated pulmonary embolism, mortality is as high as 30%, but this figure is significantly reduced by appropriate treatment. Massive pulmonary embolism has higher mortality; up to half of patients die, even with treatment.

Factors associated with higher mortality are listed in **Table 10.3**. Less than 5% of patients with acute pulmonary embolism develop the long-term complication of chronic thromboembolic pulmonary hypertension.

Factors associated with increased mortality in pulmonary embolism
Increased concentration of brain natriuretic peptide, NT-proBNP
Right ventricular dysfunction on echocardiography
Right ventricular thrombus
Advanced age
History of cancer

Table 10.3 Factors associated with increased mortality from pulmonary embolism

Pulmonary hypertension

Pulmonary hypertension is present when mean systolic pressure in the pulmonary artery is over 25 mmHg at rest or 30 mmHg during exercise. The condition is either primary or secondary.

■ **Primary pulmonary hypertension** is caused by pathological processes that directly affect the pulmonary circulation, e.g. narrowing of pulmonary vessels as a result of pulmonary embolism (the most common cause).

■ **Secondary pulmonary hypertension** is caused by gradual changes in the pulmonary circulation, arising as result of chronic diseases of the lung (e.g. COPD) or heart (e.g. congestive cardiac failure) (**Table 10.4**).

When chronic hypoxic lung disease causes pulmonary hypertension and right heart failure (right ventricular failure), the condition is termed cor pulmonale (**Table 10.5**).

> **Pulmonary hypertension is sometimes known by the abbreviation PAH, which stands for pulmonary arterial hypertension.**

Epidemiology

Most patients with chronic hypoxic lung disease develop secondary pulmonary hypertension. Primary pulmonary hypertension is rare and although there are many causes,...in most cases caused by pulmonary embolism. Idiopathic pulmonary arterial hypertension has an incidence of only 1 or 2 cases per million people.

Aetiology

Pulmonary hypertension arises as a result of pathological processes that increase pulmonary vascular resistance, pulmonary venous pressure or pulmonary vascular flow, including:

Cor pulmonale	
Factor	Description
Definition	Right heart failure secondary to chronic hypoxic lung disease
Characteristics	Pulmonary hypertension
	Right ventricular hypertrophy (right heart failure) and dilatation
Signs	Central cyanosis
	Ankle oedema
	Raised jugular venous pressure
	Atrial gallop rhythm
	Loud pulmonary second sound
	Tricuspid regurgitation

Table 10.5 Cor pulmonale: a major complication of pulmonary hypertension

Causes of pulmonary hypertension	
Category	Causes and associations
Pulmonary arterial disease	Idiopathic HIV infection Connective tissue disease (e.g. systemic sclerosis) Toxins (e.g. aminorex, fenfluramine, rapeseed oil and cocaine) Sickle cell disease
Right-to-left shunts	Congenital cardiac disease Hepatopulmonary syndrome Pulmonary arteriovenous malformation
Chronic hypoxic lung disease	Chronic obstructive pulmonary disease* Interstitial lung disease Respiratory hypoventilation (e.g. caused by obesity hypoventilation syndrome)* Living at high altitude
Pulmonary venous disease	Left-sided atrial or ventricular heart disease* Left-sided valvular heart disease* Pulmonary venous occlusive disease
Thromboembolic disease	Chronic pulmonary emboli* Poorly resolved acute pulmonary emboli Schistosomiasis
Other	Sarcoidosis
*The more common causes.	

Table 10.4 Causes of pulmonary hypertension

- primary thickening of pulmonary arterial walls due to cellular proliferation (rare, e.g. primary pulmonary hypertension)
- increased left atrial pressure (common, e.g. valvular heart disease, congestive cardiac failure)
- chronic pulmonary vasoconstriction in response to hypoxia and acidosis (common, e.g. severe COPD, ILD)
- loss of pulmonary vessels by scarring or destruction of alveolar walls (common, e.g. emphysema)
- occlusion of pulmonary vessels, usually by thrombus (fairly common, e.g. pulmonary emboli)
- increased pulmonary vascular flow caused by a left-to-right shunt (rare, e.g. congenital cardiac disease)

Clinical features

The main symptoms of pulmonary hypertension are progressive dyspnoea on exercise and fatigue. In secondary pulmonary hypertension, it is difficult to recognise that the patient's exercise tolerance is decreasing because of the developing pulmonary hypertension rather than the underlying pulmonary or cardiac disease.

Some patients also complain of chest pain on exertion. The pain is caused by right ventricular hypertrophy, which increases myocardial oxygen demand. Patients occasionally have syncope on exertion, caused by the inability to increase cardiac output during exercise.

As well as signs of the cause, with severe pulmonary hypertension the patient should be cyanosed and have signs of raised pulmonary artery pressure, i.e.:

- a loud P2 (the sound of forceful closure of the pulmonary valve as a result of high pressure in the pulmonary artery)
- raised jugular venous pressure with prominent V wave

And right ventricular hypertrophy i.e.:
- parasternal heave (caused by right ventricular hypertrophy)
- an additional S3 (the mid-diastolic gallop caused by right ventricular failure) or S4 heart sound (the presystolic gallop caused

by a poorly compliant hypertrophied right ventricle)

Eventually, right-sided cardiac failure occurs, with:

- peripheral oedema
- pleural effusions and ascites
- signs of tricuspid regurgitation (left parasternal pansystolic murmur, visible S waves in the jugular venous pressure and, rarely, pulsatile hepatomegaly) due to right ventricular dilatation

> **Worsening pulmonary hypertension is a potentially treatable cause of decreasing exercise tolerance in chronic lung disease such as interstitial lung disease.** Investigate deterioration with ECG and echocardiography.

Diagnostic approach

Pulmonary hypertension is not easy to recognise, but is considered patients with unexplained shortness of breath or deterioration of an existing lung disease with no other explanation. Investigations are necessary to confirm pulmonary hypertension, determine the severity and identify its cause if it is not obvious)

Investigations

Echocardiography

The essential screening test for identifying pulmonary hypertension is echocardiography; it is the only non-invasive test that can measure pulmonary artery pressure. The echocardiogram also shows right ventricular hypertrophy and tricuspid regurgitation caused by the pulmonary hypertension. In addition, it identifies any coexisting left-sided or valvular cardiac disease that might be the cause of pulmonary hypertension.

Chest X-ray

The chest X-ray is often normal in pulmonary hypertension. However, the central pulmonary arteries are sometimes enlarged and the peripheral blood vessels less prominent, with oligaemic lung fields. The cardiac silhouette is sometimes bigger because of right ventricular hypertrophy. Chest X-rays also demonstrate evidence of lung and cardiac diseases that might be the cause of pulmonary hypertension.

Electrocardiography

In established pulmonary hypertension ECGs show signs of right ventricular hypertrophy and strain: right axis deviation, a lead V1 R wave:S wave ratio > 1, right bundle branch block and P pulmonale (i.e. an increased P wave amplitude in lead 2).

Pulmonary function tests

Pulmonary hypertension decreases the transfer factor and this test identifies patients who might have pulmonary hypertension as a cause of unexplained dyspnoea. Six-minute walk tests are used to monitor the severity of the condition. Spirometry, lung volumes, oxygen saturations and PaO_2 will be very abnormal if the pulmonary hypertension is secondary to lung disease (cor pulmonale).

Ventilation–perfusion scan or computerised tomography pulmonary angiogram

These scans can identify whether pulmonary emboli are the cause of pulmonary hypertension. CTPA also shows whether the patient has lung disease and will show enlarged pulmonary arteries if there is significant pulmonary hypertension.

Right heart catheterisation

Echocardiography provides a provisional measurement of pulmonary artery pressure, but an accurate value requires right heart catheterisation, which is also used to identify potential causes and determine disease severity. However, it is an invasive procedure generally reserved for patients being considered for advanced treatments or those with no obvious cause such as idiopathic pulmonary hypertension.

Management

For all patients with pulmonary hypertension, the following are considered:

- diuretics to reduce oedema due to right heart failure
- domiciliary oxygen therapy to help reduce pulmonary artery pressures by reversing hypoxia-driven vasoconstriction
- anticoagulation to prevent pulmonary emboli
- pulmonary rehabilitation

The cause must be treated, for example valvular heart disease or chronic lung disease.

Medication

Pulmonary hypertension caused by chronic pulmonary embolism is treated with anticoagulation. Severe pulmonary hypertension is treated with pulmonary artery vasodilators. These include sildenafil, oral calcium channel blockers, bosentan, nitric oxide and epoprostenol; these treatments are usually only given by specialist centres.

Surgery

For patients with pulmonary hypertension caused by chronic pulmonary embolism, surgical thromboembolectomy is considered. The procedure often produces marked clinical improvement.

Combined heart–lung transplantation is sometimes necessary for younger patients with pulmonary hypertension that is idiopathic or severe.

Prognosis

The prognosis for idiopathic or severe pulmonary hypertension is poor. Most patients die within 5 years of diagnosis.

Pulmonary vasculitis

The vasculitides are a mixed group of mostly immune-mediated diseases causing inflammation of blood vessel walls. Lung vasculitis is rare and usually caused by:

- granulomatosis with polyangiitis (GPA, previously called Wegener's granulomatosis)
- eosinophilic granulomatosis with polyangiitis (EGPA, previously called Churg–Strauss syndrome)

- anti–glomerular basement membrane antibody disease (previously called Goodpasture's syndrome)

Epidemiology

All pulmonary vasculitides are very rare; their main importance is as a potential differential diagnosis for much more common lung diseases such as cavitating infections, pneumoniae or cancer.

Aetiology

Vasculitides are caused by dysregulation of the immune system. Immune dysregulation can result in a targeted autoimmune attack on blood vessel tissue. Blood vessels are also damaged indirectly by the deposition of immune complexes in the vessel wall.

Pathological findings include infiltration of inflammatory cells and necrosis of the blood vessel wall, with alveolar damage and haemorrhage.

Clinical features

Patients with pulmonary vasculitis often have marked systemic symptoms. They present with cough, haemoptysis and dyspnoea. GPA produces lung nodules that frequently cavitate, as well as alveolar haemorrhage. EGPA causes asthma, sometimes with lung infiltrates. Anti-glomerular basement membrane antibody disease results in alveolar haemorrhage (**Table 10.6**).

A significant clue to the diagnosis is evidence of disease in other organs, for example:

- upper airways disease (GPA and EGPA)

- mononeuritis multiplex and peripheral neuropathy (GPA and EGPA)
- kidney damage (anti–glomerular basement membrane antibody disease and GPA)
- skin nodules and cardiac involvement (EGPA)

The severity of the vasculitis varies unpredictably over time.

Diagnostic approach

The presentations of vasculitis mimic those of other, much commoner conditions, such as cancer, tuberculosis and pneumonia. Radiological appearances are highly variable but include:

- nodules, which cavitate (GPA) (**Figure 10.4**)

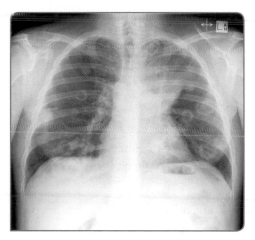

Figure 10.4 Chest X-ray showing multiple cavitating nodules, a characteristic finding in pulmonary vasculitis, in this case granulomatosis with polyangiitis.

Type of pulmonary vasculitis			
Associated disease	Granulomatosis with polyangiitis (GPA)	Eosinophilic granulomatosis with polyangiitis (EGPA)	Anti-glomerular basement membrane antibody disease
Upper airway disease	✓	✓	
Mononeuritis multiplex and peripheral neuropathy	✓	✓	
Kidney damage	✓		✓
Skin nodules and cardiac involvement		✓	

Table 10.6 Association of pulmonary vasculitis with other disease

- stenosis of the upper airways, and nasal or sinus involvement (GPA)
- so-called 'ground glass' (alveolar) infiltrates

Patients often have positive autoantibodies: anti-neutrophilic cytoplasmic antibodies for GPA, and anti–glomerular basement membrane for anti–glomerular basement membrane antibody disease. Eosinophilia is common in EGPA. Haematuria, proteinuria or increased creatinine concentration suggest that the kidneys are affected.

The diagnosis of vasculitis should be confirmed histologically, by biopsy of the lung or other affected organs.

Management

Without treatment, the prognosis for vasculitis is poor. However, most patients go into remission after intense immunosuppression with systemic corticosteroids and cyclophosphamide. Plasma exchange is considered for severe cases.

Arteriovenous malformation

Arteriovenous malformations are abnormal connections between the pulmonary veins and arteries. In the lung, these connections cause a right-to-left shunt of deoxygenated blood into the arterial circulation.

Arteriovenous malformations can be idiopathic, congenital, due to hereditary haemorrhagic telangiectasia, or associated with liver cirrhosis.

Clinical features

Pulmonary arteriovenous malformations are usually asymptomatic. However, they sometimes cause dyspnoea, haemoptysis, platypnoea (increased dyspnoea in the upright position) and hypoxia. Strokes or cerebral abscesses can be caused by paradoxical embolisation through the malformation.

Patients with hereditary haemorrhagic telangiectasia may have visible telangiectasia of the tongue and lips. Rarely, large arteriovenous malformations cause an audible bruit. On chest X-rays and computerised tomography scans, arteriovenous malformations are visible as well-demarcated nodules with feeding blood vessels.

Management

Management is aimed at closure of the arteriovenous connection. This is effected by embolisation of the feeding vessel with metallic coils during pulmonary angiography.

Answers to starter questions

1. Pleurisy is inflammation of the parietal pleura. Any pathological process that causes inflammation causes pleurisy, but the commonest are pneumonia and pulmonary embolism. Patients have sharp lateral chest pain that is worse when taking a deep breath.

2. The D-dimer test is a sensitive but non-specific test for pulmonary embolism. It is useful when deep vein thrombosis or pulmonary embolism is unlikely; a low D-dimer concentration negates the need for further tests. If deep vein thrombosis or pulmonary embolism are suspected imaging studies are necessary and the D-dimer result adds nothing to diagnostic decision making.

3. Patients who require investigations for predisposition to thromboembolism are those who have had multiple pulmonary emboli or deep vein thrombi but have no identifiable risk factors, and those with a family history of pulmonary embolism, deep vein thrombosis and recurrent miscarriage. Testing is done when the patient is not receiving anticoagulants, so is deferred until 3–6 months after treatment.

4. Diagnosis of pulmonary hypertension is challenging; the signs are difficult to detect, lung volumes are unaffected by raised pulmonary artery pressures and the chest X-ray is often normal. However, patients with unexplained breathlessness should have their transfer factor measured, an ECG and an echocardiogram to check for evidence of pulmonary hypertension.

Chapter 11
Respiratory emergencies

Introduction

Respiratory emergencies usually present with severe shortness of breath (dyspnoea) and are rapidly fatal if untreated.

In an emergency, the patient must be assessed and treated simultaneously. Use a structured approach to ensure that the most life-threatening features are treated first. Being unable to breathe is frightening, so keep the patient as calm as possible.

Managing a medical emergency is stressful. Remember the following:

- Treat the most life-threatening features first. Detailed, methodical clinical assessment is done when the patient's condition is more stable.

- Memorise the doses of essential drugs, as well as the anatomical landmarks for key procedures.

- Seek support from senior colleagues early.

Massive pulmonary embolism

Case 15

Presentation

Mrs Gallagher, a 60-year-old inpatient on a gynaecological ward, has suddenly developed breathlessness and pleuritic chest pain. Eight days ago, she had pelvic surgery for cervical cancer. Her observations show a heart rate of 120 beats/min, a blood pressure of 80/40 mmHg and an oxygen saturation of 90% on air.

Initial interpretation

Sudden onset of breathlessness and hypotension in a post-operative patient is probably caused by pulmonary embolism;

Case 15 *continued*

patients who have recently had pelvic surgery are at particularly high risk due to pressure on large veins during the operation. Another likely cause is a large haemorrhage.

History and examination

Mrs Gallagher has been immobile since surgery, because of scar pain and vomiting. She had no respiratory symptoms before the sudden breathlessness. She also feels dizzy and faint. She has no regular medications and no personal or family history of thromboembolism.

On examination, Mrs Gallagher has cool peripheries and a prolonged capillary refill time. Her heart rate is regular but fast (120 beats/min). Her blood pressure is 80/40 mmHg. She has a parasternal gallop rhythm, an increased respiratory rate (30 breaths/min) and a localised pleural rub over the right chest laterally but no other respiratory signs. Her calves are soft, non-tender and equal in size. Oxygen saturation is 90% on air.

Immediate intervention

Sudden dyspnoea, pleuritic chest pain, tachypnoea, tachycardia and a pleural rub support a diagnosis of pulmonary embolism. Her hypotension shows she is in shock and that this is a massive, life-threatening pulmonary embolism.

- Oxygen is given to achieve 94–98% saturation.
- A large-bore cannula is inserted and blood samples are taken for full blood count, urea and electrolytes, D-dimer test, clotting screen and group and save.
- Intravenous fluids are given to increase blood pressure.
- Clinical suspicion of life-threatening pulmonary embolism is strong. Therefore treatment with low-molecular-weight heparin is started immediately, before confirmation of the diagnosis by radiological or echocardiographic findings.

Pulmonary embolism is common and life-threatening. It has few specific clinical signs, and bedside investigations are often normal. A suspected pulmonary embolism is usually treated by rapid anticoagulation with heparin before the diagnosis is confirmed by the results of the following investigations.

- Electrocardiography (ECG): tachycardia and right ventricular strain, possibly with a classic S1Q3T3 pattern (Figure 10.3)
- Chest X-ray: this is often normal but can show reduction in visible blood vessel markings, small effusions or wedge-shaped peripheral areas of consolidation
- Bedside echocardiogram: isolated right ventricular strain and dysfunction suggest massive or submassive pulmonary embolism
- Troponin T or I level – indicates myocardial damage, and suggests a massive or submassive PE

- Computerised tomography pulmonary angiogram: this is the definitive diagnostic investigation; patients need to have a scan as soon as their condition is stable enough

Transfer patients with continuing hypotension, hypoxia or both to an intensive care unit; they often need inotropes or ventilation.

Thrombolysis (e.g. with altepase) is sometimes considered. In Mrs Gallagher's case, the surgical team must decide if the risk of postoperative bleeding is too high for this. The alternative is interventional radiological or surgical embolectomy. However, this is a high-risk intervention reserved for life-threatening situations that are not responding to conventional anticoagulation, or when thrombolysis is contraindicated.

Type 2 respiratory failure

Case 16

Presentation

Mr Williams, a 69-year-old man, is brought by ambulance to the accident and emergency department. He is drowsy and short of breath. His wife says that he has chronic obstructive pulmonary disease (COPD), and that he has been coughing more than usual for 1 week. He became confused this morning. Initial observations show that he is barely rousable and has an oxygen saturation of 81% on 4 L/min oxygen through a simple face mask.

Initial interpretation

Confusion and drowsiness in someone with chronic lung disease suggests type 2 (hypercapnoeic) respiratory failure. The cough suggests a preceding infective exacerbation of COPD.

History and examination

Mr Williams has had COPD for 10 years, with five exacerbations requiring admission to hospital. One of these hospital stays was 2 years ago; he was intubated and spent 20 days in the intensive care unit. During another admission this year, he was treated with non-invasive ventilation. Since then, he has used home oxygen and regular nebulised salbutamol and ipratropium bromide.

On examination, Mr Williams has a Glasgow Coma Scale score of 9, central cyanosis, a regular heart rate of 66 beats/min and normal blood pressure. His breathing rate is irregular and laboured, at 20 breaths/min. Bilateral chest expansion is poor. The percussion note is resonant throughout, and breath sounds are quiet but with no added noises.

Immediate intervention

Mr Williams is drowsy. Therefore immediate assessment is needed to determine whether he is able to maintain his own airway (usually possible with a Glasgow Coma Scale score >8) or requires emergency intubation.

- The airway is safe, so controlled oxygen therapy is given through a Venturi mask to achieve saturation of 88–92%.
- Salbutamol 5 mg plus ipratropium bromide 500 µg are given through nebulisers driven by air.

Arterial blood gases are measured to confirm and assess the suspected type 2 respiratory failure; pH is 7.28, $Paco_2$ is 12 kPa, Pao_2 is 7.6 kPa and HCO_3^- is 32 mmol/L. These results indicate severe type 2 respiratory failure with acidosis. The increased HCO_3^- shows it is partly compensated. Chest X-ray excludes a pneumothorax and he is immediately started on non-invasive ventilation.

With non-invasive ventilation established, Mr Williams's level of consciousness, respiratory rate and arterial blood gases are monitored closely to ensure that $Paco_2$ is decreasing, pH is normalising and a safe level of oxygenation is being maintained.

Type 2 respiratory failure is common in advanced COPD. The acidosis should be treated by non-invasive ventilation, which is often given in the accident and emergency department or on a respiratory ward. An alternative temporary treatment for patients unable to tolerate non-invasive ventilation is intravenous doxapram, a respiratory stimulant.

Further investigations are necessary to exclude life-threatening complications. These investigations include ECG to look for dysrhythmia and a chest X-ray to rule out pneumothorax or pneumonia. Routine blood tests are done to exclude metabolic causes of an altered level of consciousness. Sputum culture is also necessary.

Infective exacerbations of COPD are treated with antibiotics, nebulised (sometimes intravenous) bronchodilators and systemic corticosteroids. Intravenous administration of corticosteroids is needed if the patient is drowsy and therefore unable to swallow safely.

If the patient has no clear history of established COPD as the cause of hypercapnoeic respiratory failure, and their level of consciousness is decreased, other diagnoses (**Table 11.1**) must be considered.

Escalation decisions

Every patient with COPD who is started on non-invasive ventilation must have a decision made about the maximum level of ventilatory support they will receive. Failure of the patient's condition to improve with non-invasive ventilation is an indication for mechanical ventilation, but only if this aggressive procedure is judged appropriate.

The following factors influence intubation decisions in chronic lung disease.

- The wishes of the patient and their family (an advance directive helps)
- The severity of the underlying chronic lung disease when not exacerbated, judged by spirometry results, exercise tolerance and whether or not long-term oxygen is used
- The response to previous treatment with non-invasive ventilation or intubation and mechanical ventilation

Causes of type 2 respiratory failure	
Type	Examples
Obstructive lung disease	Exacerbation of chronic obstructive pulmonary disease
	Acute asthma (life-threatening attack)
	Bronchiectasis or cystic fibrosis (advanced disease)
	Severe obstructive sleep apnoea (repeated upper airways obstruction)
Decreased central ventilatory drive	Opiates, benzodiazepines and other sedatives or narcotics
	Obesity hypoventilation syndrome
	Brain stem cerebrovascular accident
	Encephalitis
Neuromuscular weakness	Duchenne muscular dystrophy
	Motorneurone disease
	Cervical cord lesion or damage
	Myasthenia gravis
	Guillain–Barré syndrome
	Diaphragmatic paralysis
Chest wall disease	Thoracoplasty
	Kyphoscoliosis
	Obesity

Table 11.1 Causes of acute type 2 (hypercapnoeic) respiratory failure

- The reversibility of the acute illness (e.g. acute pneumonia is a readily reversible cause of deterioration in COPD, but slow deterioration of COPD itself over weeks is not)

In severe airways disease (COPD or severe asthma), breath sounds are quiet, making it difficult to identify an underlying pneumothorax, lobar collapse or pneumonia by clinical examination. Chest X-ray is essential to clarify the diagnosis for patients presenting with a clinical deterioration.

Acute severe asthma

Case 17

Presentation

Emma, a 19-year-old student, presents to the accident and emergency department unable to breathe. She is too short of breath to speak. She has an irregular breathing pattern, with a respiratory rate of 28 breaths/min, a heart rate of 45 beats/min and blood pressure of 80/50 mmHg. Her oxygen saturation is 92% despite 8 L/min oxygen through a non-rebreathe mask. In her pocket is an empty salbutamol inhaler.

Initial interpretation

Asthma is the most common cause of severe dyspnoea in younger patients. The inhaler supports this diagnosis. The observations suggest that this is an acute life-threatening attack (**Table 11.2**), and that Emma is close to cardiorespiratory arrest.

History and examination

On examination, Emma's airway is clear. However, she is cyanotic and taking shallow breaths. Her chest is quiet on auscultation. She is afebrile. No further history is possible at this point.

Immediate intervention

The inability to speak, irregular breathing pattern, bradycardia, quiet chest and hypoxia despite high-flow oxygen are worrying signs. Treatment must be immediate, before any investigations.

- Emma is sat up and continues to receive high-flow oxygen through the non-rebreathe mask.
- Salbutamol 5 mg plus ipratropium bromide 500 µg are given through

Clinical assessment of asthma severity	
Asthma severity	Clinical findings
Severe	Peak expiratory flow < 50% of predicted or previous best
	Unable to complete sentences in one breath
	Respiratory rate > 25 breaths/min
	Heart rate > 110 beats/min
Life-threatening	Peak expiratory flow < 30% of predicted or previous best
	Silent chest, cyanosis or feeble respiratory effort
	Bradycardia or hypotension
	Exhaustion, confusion or coma
	Normal or high P_{CO_2} and low P_{O_2} (< 8 kPa) despite oxygen therapy, and acidosis

Table 11.2 Clinical assessment of asthma severity

nebulisers driven by oxygen; this treatment is repeated until her condition improves.
- An intravenous cannula is inserted and blood samples are taken for full blood count, urea and electrolytes, and C-reactive protein.

The results of the arterial blood gases test are pH, 7.35; P_{aO_2}, 7.8 kPa; and P_{aCO_2}, 6.5 kPa. The mild respiratory acidosis confirms a life-threatening asthma attack (Table 11.2). Intravenous hydrocortisone 200 mg and intravenous magnesium sulphate 2 g over 20 min are given. A portable chest X-ray is done, which excludes a pneumothorax.

The intensive care unit is contacted, to arrange intubation and ventilation if Emma's condition fails to respond rapidly to treatment.

When treating acute severe asthma, the priorities are to:

- rapidly assess its severity (**Table 11.2**)
- start treatment immediately
- frequently review progress to judge whether to continue medical treatment or to intubate and mechanically ventilate the patient

> **Patients with mild to moderate exacerbation of asthma usually have low $Paco_2$. Their $Paco_2$ is low because their tachypnoea blows off carbon dioxide. Normal or high $Paco_2$ is a major cause for concern.**

Patients having a severe acute asthma attack are often unable to give a history. However, essential components of the history that need to be obtained later include:

- the duration of asthma
- usual and current treatment
- the frequency and severity of previous attacks (including those warranting admission to hospital and intubation)
- best peak expiratory flow
- any recent exposure to known triggers (e.g. a recent upper respiratory tract infection, exposure to smoke or stress)
- the level of asthma control in the period leading up to the latest attack (frequency of salbutamol inhaler use, changes in dyspnoea, wheeze, cough and nocturnal symptoms)

Many of these details will be obtained from the patient's previous notes and from discussion with one of their friends or relatives.

If the initial treatment with oxygen, nebulisers and steroids is ineffective, consider intravenous magnesium or theophylline. Cardiac monitoring for arrhythmia is necessary.

If the patient's condition remains unstable, they require monitoring on the intensive care ward in case intubation becomes necessary.

> **Intravenous hydrocortisone is often used to treat life-threatening asthma attacks or type 2 respiratory failure due to COPD.** Hydrocortisone has no pharmacological advantage over prednisolone, but it can be administered intravenously when drowsiness or tachypnoea leaves patients unable to safely swallow oral prednisolone.·

Acute respiratory distress syndrome

Case 18

Presentation and initial interpretation

Mr Johns is a 37-year-old man. He has breathlessness, cough productive of green sputum and fever for 2 days. His condition worsens and he is brought to A&E by his partner. His initial observations show oxygen saturations of 83% on 15L oxygen via non-rebreathe mask, a respiratory rate of 36 breaths/min, a fever of 40 degrees, a pulse rate of 125 bpm and a blood pressure of 80/50mmHg. The history suggests a chest infection, and the observations indicate severe sepsis. The degree of hypoxia is concerning as it suggests either extensive pneumonia or acute respiratory distress syndrome. A PE should be considered, but the fever is more in keeping with an infectious cause.

History and examination

Mr Johns was previously well with no chronic medical problems. He works as an investment banker and has had no recent travel. He is peripherally vasodilated with a bounding pulse which is regular. He is

Case 18 *continued*

unable to speak due to breathlessness and he is drowsy. He is centrally cyanosed. His trachea is central and chest expansion is equal. He has bilateral course crackles throughout the chest. Heart sounds are normal, although there is a flow murmur. He has no peripheral oedema.

Immediate intervention

Mr Johns is hypoxaemic despite high flow oxygen. An ABG confirms that he is in type I respiratory failure. Blood tests are sent for FBC, U+Es, LFTs, CRP, a HIV test and blood cultures. Broad spectrum antibiotics are given immediately following the blood cultures. A portable chest X-ray shows widespread bilateral alveolar infiltrates (**Figure 11.1**) and a diagnosis of acute respiratory distress syndrome due to severe pneumonia is made. The ICU team is called immediately to assess him

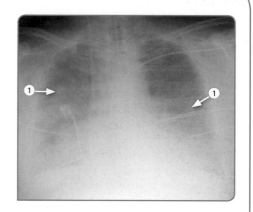

Figure 11.1 Chest X-ray showing ① bilateral alveolar infiltrates in acute respiratory distress syndrome.

and he is intubated and mechanically ventilated. Fluid resuscitation is given but his blood pressure does not respond so he is given inotropes, in this case noradrenaline. He is moved to the intensive care unit.

Acute respiratory distress syndrome (ARDS) is a severe, life-threatening form of microvascular lung injury. The lung injury is triggered by a number of pulmonary or extrapulmonary exposures (**Table 11.3**). Whatever the initial cause, the result is severe inflammation causing endothelial and epithelial damage. Traditionally ARDS was thought to have three phases:

- exudative: protein rich fluid leaks out of the circulation and into the interstitium and alveolar space. Cells such as neutrophils also migrate out and release inflammatory cytokines
- proliferative: fibroblasts and type II pneumocytes proliferate. These secrete extracellular matrix proteins such as collagen
- fibrotic: deposition of collagen and other substances leads to interstitial and inter-alveolar fibrosis

Causes of acute respiratory distress syndrome	
Category	Causes and associations
Pulmonary (direct lung injury)	Aspiration of gastric contents
	Severe pneumonia
	Near-drowning
	Inhalation of chlorine or smoke
Extrapulmonary (indirect lung injury)	Sepsis
	Severe trauma (e.g. extensive surgery, gunshot wounds or injuries from a road traffic accident)
	Massive blood transfusion
	Drug overdose (e.g. of aspirin, cocaine, opioids or tricyclic antidepressants)
	Acute pancreatitis
	Idiosyncratic drug reaction (e.g. to intravenous contrast agent)

Table 11.3 Causes of acute respiratory distress syndrome

There is now evidence that many of these processes occur in parallel. This provides targets for possible future treatments. The causes of ARDS can produce milder forms of ARDS-like disease called acute lung injury.

Patients with ARDS present as emergencies with rapidly worsening dyspnoea and severe hypoxaemia. On auscultation, widespread crackles are heard throughout the lung fields. Chest X-ray shows widespread bilateral alveolar infiltrates (**Figure 11.2**).

Management is supportive; the aim is to maintain adequate oxygenation whilst the patient recovers from the initial insult. All patients require high-concentration oxygen therapy. Most require intubation and mechanical ventilation. Management strategies for patients with ARDS include:

- low tidal volume ventilation as the lungs become stiff and are at risk of barotrauma and pneumothorax
- intermittent high levels of continuous positive airway pressure

- prone positioning to recruit areas of the lung less affected by oedema
- conservative fluid management to reduce oedema

No specific therapy has proved effective. Some patients are given steroids, but there is little evidence for their use. Mortality of ARDS is high, between 40 and 60%. Patients die from the underlying cause of the ARDS, the direct effects of inflammation and fibrosis in the alveoli and the resultant hypoxaemia, or from a secondary infection or organ failure.

Patients who survive are generally those who show improvement within a week on the ventilator. Even those with a good outcome often spend a prolonged period on intensive care. As they wean from the ventilator they usually need a tracheostomy. They require intensive rehabilitation as their muscles weaken considerably. Other long-term complications include pulmonary fibrosis with reduced lung function and memory, cognitive and emotional problems due to the effects of prolonged low oxygen levels.

Stridor

Case 19

Presentation

Mrs Rayne is 63 years old and has locally invasive lung cancer of the upper trachea. She presents with difficulty breathing; her breathlessness has been increasing over a few weeks and has suddenly deteriorated. Her inhalers have been ineffective.

She has audible stridor, a respiratory rate of 30 breaths/min, a heart rate of 110 beats/min, blood pressure of 130/80 mmHg and an oxygen saturation of 92% on high-flow oxygen.

Initial interpretation

Stridor (inspiratory wheeze) indicates potentially fatal upper airways obstruction. In this case, the cause is extension of the known cancer now blocking most

of the trachea. Other causes of stridor are listed in Table 3.1.

History and examination

Mrs Rayne's cancer was diagnosed 9 months ago. She is receiving palliative radiotherapy. She is distressed, and widespread inspiratory and expiratory wheezes are heard on auscultation of the upper chest.

Immediate intervention

The history of progressive dyspnoea suggests that the tumour has advanced, slowly blocking the trachea; the acute deterioration could be caused by additional mucus plugging or tissue swelling.

Case 19 *continued*

- Oxygen therapy is given to maintain 94–98% saturation. If available, use heliox (oxygen mixed with helium), because it has a lower viscosity and is more readily inhaled than mixtures of oxygen and air.
- Nebulised salbutamol 5 mg (driven by oxygen) and nebulised adrenaline (epinephrine) (3–5 mL at 1:1000 strength) are given.
- An intravenous cannula is inserted and blood samples are taken for full blood count, urea and electrolytes, liver function tests, C-reactive protein and clotting screen.
- Hydrocortisone 200 mg is given intravenously to reduce any oedema surrounding the cancer.
- Intravenous fluids are given, because dehydration is common.

Upper airways obstruction is fatal if untreated. If simple measures are ineffective and the patient's condition is deteriorating, intubation or tracheotomy is required, as appropriate. Intubation of a patient with upper airways obstruction is technically difficult. The procedure is best done in a semiplanned manner with support from an ear, nose and throat surgeon in case an immediate tracheotomy is needed.

Once the patient's condition is stable enough, identify the location of the airways obstruction by:

- X-rays of the chest, neck or both (these are sometimes normal)
- computerised tomography of the chest and neck
- nasendoscopy (shows obstruction at or above the level of the vocal cords)
- bronchoscopy (shows obstruction below the level of the vocal cords)

Bronchoscopy carries a high risk, because the anaesthetic and the procedure itself can further reduce the diameter of an already critically narrowed airway. However, depending on the site and nature of the obstruction, therapeutic interventions to relieve the obstruction can be done through bronchoscopy. These interventions include laser ablation, stent insertion and balloon dilatation.

Major haemoptysis

Case 20

Presentation

Mr Kapur, aged 52 years, has a known aspergilloma. He presents to the accident and emergency department with a large-volume haemoptysis, estimated as 400 mL (1.5 cups) in the past 6 h. He is still coughing up blood on arrival, and has a heart rate of 115 beats/min, blood pressure of 110/75 mmHg and an oxygen saturation of 94% on 8 L/min oxygen through a non-rebreathe mask.

Initial interpretation

Mr Kapur has major haemoptysis (defined as >200 mL of blood produced in 24 h). The likely cause is the known aspergilloma, and his airway is at risk from the volume of blood being produced.

Case 20 *continued*

History and examination

Twenty years ago, Mr Kapur had tuberculosis. After a minor haemoptysis 5 years ago, a chest X-ray showed an aspergilloma in a post-tuberculosis right upper lobe cavity. The finding was confirmed by computerised tomography scan and positive sputum culture for an *Aspergillus* species.

Mr Kapur is not taking any anticoagulants. His trachea is deviated to the right. Expansion of the right hemithorax is poor. The percussion note is normal, but breath sounds are decreased over the right mid and lower zones anteriorly.

Immediate intervention

The aims of immediate management of major haemoptysis are to protect the airway, identify the source of bleeding, slow or stop the bleeding (if possible), and decide which additional therapeutic interventions are possible.

- The airway is cleared by suction of the mouth.
- Oxygen is continued to maintain > 94% saturation.
- A large-bore intravenous cannula is inserted and blood samples are taken for full blood count, urea and electrolytes, clotting screen and cross-matching.
- Intravenous fluids are given.
- The blood bank is called to request an urgent cross-match in case blood transfusion is necessary.
- A portable chest X-ray and ECG are done.
- Tranexamic acid is given to promote clotting.
- Mr Kapur is positioned on his right, the side of the bleeding, to prevent aspiration of the blood into the non-bleeding lung.

There are many causes of minor haemoptysis, but only a few common causes of major haemoptysis (**Table 11.4**).

Once the results of the clotting screen are available, any identified coagulopathy must be reversed (e.g. platelet transfusion for thrombocytopenia). If the bleeding is blocking the airway, urgent intubation and mechanical ventilation is necessary; use a double-lumen endotracheal tube to selectively ventilate the unaffected lung.

Following immediate stabilisation, the following options must be considered in discussion with cardiothoracic surgeons and interventional radiologists:

- flexible bronchoscopy to identify the source of the bleeding
- arteriography and embolization of the bleeding vessel
- surgery to resect the source of the bleeding (adequate lung function reserve is needed for this option, and knowing the stable spirometry values is vital)

Sometimes, for example in cases of advanced lung cancer, it is not possible or appropriate to intervene in massive haemoptysis. The patient is treated palliatively with intravenous diamorphine 10 mg and intravenous midazolam 10 mg to reduce anxiety and distress. Death occurs rapidly.

Major haemoptysis causes	
Common	Rare
Primary lung cancer (particularly squamous cell carcinoma)	Pulmonary lung metastases
Aspergilloma	Arteriovenous malformations
Bronchiectasis and cystic fibrosis	Vasculitis
Tuberculosis	Clotting disorders

Table 11.4 Causes of major haemoptysis

Massive haemoptysis resulting from erosion of the pulmonary artery is an uncommon cause of sudden death in patients with lung cancer. Witnessing such a dramatic death is very distressing for the family and staff; support from the team, for the family and staff is necessary to address this.

Tension pneumothorax

Case 21

Presentation

Mr Singh, a 32-year-old salesman, has been in a road traffic accident. He has significant blunt trauma to the chest but no other injuries. In the ambulance, he becomes increasingly short of breath. In the accident and emergency department, he has a respiratory rate of 38 breaths/min, a heart rate of 150 beats/min, blood pressure of 80/55 mmHg and an oxygen saturation of 89% on 4 L/min oxygen through a simple face mask.

Initial interpretation

Blunt chest trauma has a high risk of causing a pneumothorax. Rapid deterioration, tachycardia and hypotension suggest a tension pneumothorax.

History and examination

Mr Singh feels faint on sitting up. His trachea is deviated to the right. A hyper-resonant percussion note is audible over the left lung, but no breath sounds. He has localised tenderness and bruising over the left lateral chest wall, suggesting rib fractures.

Immediate intervention

The signs confirm a pneumothorax, and the symptoms of presyncope plus hypo-

tension mean that immediate action is needed.

- High-flow oxygen is given through a non-rebreathe mask.
- Needle decompression of the pneumothorax is done by inserting a large-bore cannula into the second intercostal space in the mid-clavicular line on the left (**Figure 11.2**)

A hiss is audible as air is expelled from the thoracic cavity. Heart rate and respiratory rate decrease, and blood pressure increases

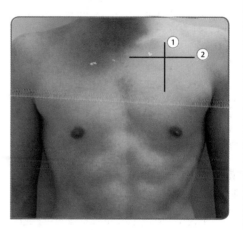

Figure 11.2 Location of needle decompression of a left-sided pneumothorax. ① Mid-clavicular line. ② 2nd intercostal space.

Tension pneumothorax is an uncommon but life-threatening complication of spontaneous or traumatic pneumothorax. A tension pneumothorax is recognised by hypotension, tachycardia, and clinical or chest X-ray evidence of major mediastinal shift (deviated trachea, flattened or even inverted diaphragm, and cardiac shift across the midline) (**Figure 11.3**).

In this case, the pneumothorax was caused by trauma. Therefore treatment follows the Advanced Trauma Life Support protocol to identify and treat any other injuries.

After immediate decompression of the pneumothorax, a portable chest X-ray is done and a chest drain inserted to drain the residual pneumothorax and prevent recurrence during healing of the hole in the visceral pleura caused by the rib fractures.

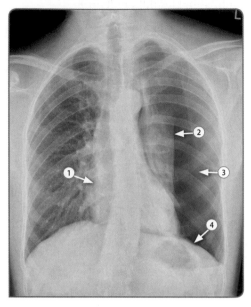

Figure 11.3 Chest X-ray of a tension pneumothorax. (1) Mediastinal shift to the other side. (2) Lung edge. (3) Large pneumothorax. (4) Flattened diaphragm.

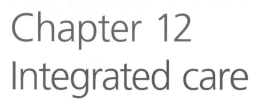

Chapter 12
Integrated care

Starter questions

Answers to the following questions are on page 321.

1. When is the right time to discuss advance care planning with patients?
2. Why is a holistic approach to patient care so important?
3. Do disease prevention interventions work?

Introduction

A particular patient's problems are often managed by both a primary care physician (the general practitioner, GP) in the community and a specialist secondary care physician. This is an artificial division in care, and good communication between GP and specialist is required for patients to be treated safely and effectively.

Secondary care is often provided by individual specialists, so the approach is very disease-oriented. In contrast, in primary care the approach is more patient-centred.

Secondary care specialists have traditionally been based in hospitals. However, the situation is changing, with more specialists employed by primary care organisations and working in the community. Various models have been proposed for this approach, but no standard has been agreed.

General practitioners are usually the first point of contact for patients. GPs need to have extensive knowledge of medical conditions to assess patients and decide whether referral to a specialist is appropriate. GPs also play an essential role in disease prevention, patient education and the promotion of healthy lifestyles.

Case 22 Poorly controlled asthma

Presentation

Claire, aged 19 years, has had asthma since childhood. Her symptoms have been well controlled by budesonide–formoterol inhaler for some time. However, she now complains to her GP of sleeping badly; most nights of the week, she wakes coughing and feeling tight-chested. She has been wheezy during the day and is using her salbutamol inhaler up to 8 times daily.

> **A quick way to assess whether a patient's asthma is well controlled is to ask how many times a day they need to use their rescue bronchodilator.** Daily use suggests that the preventive therapy needs to be increased, unless clinical assessment identifies an obvious reason for the poor control, such as an inability to use inhalers effectively. Using a salbutamol inhaler several times a day indicates poor asthma control.

Initial interpretation

Claire's asthma has become poorly controlled. The GP needs to identify potential reasons why **(Table 12.1)**.

Further history

Claire has recently started university. Her room is damp, and the bathroom wall is mouldy. Claire's inhaler ran out, and she has not had time to get a new one until now. She has also started smoking and has noticed that she is more breathless than her friends when out clubbing.

Examination

Claire looks well. On auscultation, a polyphonic end expiratory wheeze is heard throughout the chest. Peak expiratory flow rate is 250 L/min; it had been stable at 400 L/min. Oxygen saturation is 96% on room air.

Interpretation of findings

The wheeze on auscultation and low peak expiratory flow rate confirm that the asthma is poorly controlled. The history suggests several reasons for poor asthma control, including stress from starting university, exposure to environmental allergens (in this case, damp accommodation), medication non-adherence and smoking.

Investigations

At this stage, no additional investigations are needed. A chest X-ray and blood tests to identify allergic bronchopulmonary aspergillosis may be necessary if Claire's asthma remains poorly controlled despite the identified potential reasons for poor control being addressed.

Management

In management of asthma, the aim is to make patients symptom-free both at night and during the day (see Chapter 3). For Claire, this aim may be achieved by represcribing her budesonide-formoterol inhaler. However, it should also be discussed with her why she let her inhaler run out. It is also important to ensure that she fully understands the reasons for asthma treatment, so that she is able to manage her condition more effectively herself. Claire could learn more about asthma from patient information leaflets and websites, as well as discussions with her GP or the community asthma nurse.

Claire's damp living conditions may be worsening her asthma symptoms. By writing a letter of support, the GP could help her improve her housing environment. The GP visit is also a key opportunity to discuss

Case 22 *continued*

Causes of poorly controlled asthma

Cause	Solution
Medication non-adherence	Educate patient about the need for regular use of inhaled steroids even when asymptomatic
Poor inhaler technique	Educate patient about inhaler technique
Smoking or use of recreational drugs	Advise patient to stop smoking or using recreational drugs
Increased exposure to triggers: ■ stress ■ damp or poorly ventilated housing ■ occupational causes (see Table 2.12) ■ pollution ■ pets (e.g. cats, dogs and rodents) ■ poorly controlled hay fever	Identify potential triggers by taking a careful history and help the patient limit exposure to them
Gastro-oesophageal reflux	Identify through history, possibly with gastrointestinal investigations, and treat
Drugs (β-blockers, non-steroidal anti-inflammatory drugs)	Take a drug history and modify medication as appropriate
Premenstrual period or pregnancy	Identify through history, with pregnancy test (if appropriate), and increase treatment as necessary
Upper respiratory tract disease (sinusitis or chronic rhinitis)	Identify through history followed by radiology, and treat accordingly
Development of allergic bronchopulmonary aspergillosis	Diagnosis (usually by secondary care physician through blood and skin tests)

Table 12.1 Causes of poorly controlled asthma

the importance of both good asthma control and smoking cessation.

Ideally, Claire would be able to manage her asthma by herself, following a self-management plan drawn up after discussion with the GP or community asthma nurse. If her asthma remains poorly controlled despite the above measures, she should be referred to a secondary care physician. Their expertise could confirm that the diagnosis is accurate. It would also exclude other significant causes of poorly controlled asthma, such as allergic bronchopulmonary aspergillosis and occupational asthma.

Smoking exacerbates asthma directly by increasing airways inflammation and bronchospasm. Smoking also seems to lessen the beneficial effects of inhaled corticosteroids.

Case 23 Repeated admissions for COPD

Presentation

Mr Barnes, aged 68 years, is seen in the community COPD clinic by a consultant and nurse. He has had chronic obstructive pulmonary disease (COPD) for the past 10 years. He has severe disease, with a forced expiratory volume (in 1 s) of 0.9 L and chronic hypoxia requiring long-term oxygen therapy.

Mr Barnes repeatedly phones for an ambulance when he feels breathless and anxious. He has been admitted to hospital six times in the past 2 months. Most admissions lasted 3–4 days, and he has not been home for more than 7 days at a time before readmission.

Initial interpretation

Mr Barnes's admissions are probably too frequent to be caused by true exacerbations of his COPD. The admissions are probably precipitated by his feelings of helplessness during temporary episodes of worsening dyspnoea. Such episodes are common in severe COPD. They last from minutes to a few hours, but could be managed safely at home.

It is crucial to establish Mr Barnes's expectations and understanding of the disease. It is also necessary to ensure that he has a clear plan for managing the episodes of dyspnoea, so that he phones for an ambulance less frequently.

Further history

Mr Barnes's wife died a year ago. Since then, he has lived alone. He describes becoming very anxious, particularly at night. He has started smoking again, and his COPD has worsened.

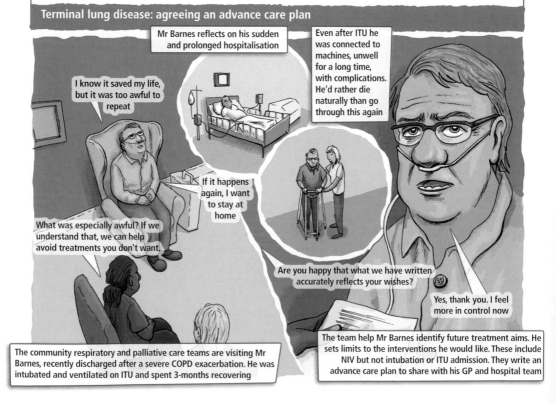

Terminal lung disease: agreeing an advance care plan

Mr Barnes reflects on his sudden and prolonged hospitalisation

I know it saved my life, but it was too awful to repeat

Even after ITU he was connected to machines, unwell for a long time, with complications. He'd rather die naturally than go through this again

If it happens again, I want to stay at home

What was especially awful? If we understand that, we can help avoid treatments you don't want.

The community respiratory and palliative care teams are visiting Mr Barnes, recently discharged after a severe COPD exacerbation. He was intubated and ventilated on ITU and spent 3-months recovering

Are you happy that what we have written accurately reflects your wishes?

Yes, thank you. I feel more in control now

The team help Mr Barnes identify future treatment aims. He sets limits to the interventions he would like. These include NIV but not intubation or ITU admission. They write an advance care plan to share with his GP and hospital team

Case 23 *continued*

He receives inhaler therapy and adheres to the optimal treatment regimen. He also uses nebulised ipratropium and salbutamol at home three or four times daily.

Interpretation of findings

Several issues are relevant.

- Mr Barnes's condition is deteriorating despite seemingly optimal treatment.
- He has severe COPD, so his life expectancy is poor.
- He has started smoking, and this could be contributing to the deterioration in his COPD.
- His recent bereavement, anxiety and social isolation could be impairing his ability to cope with his severe disability.

Management

Mr Barnes requires coordinated care from both primary and secondary care physicians, supported by various other health care professionals.

- Mr Barnes's COPD is worsening. Review by a secondary care physician could identify possible reasons for this, and his treatment may need to be changed.
- Smoking is exacerbating his symptoms, so he should be given advice on smoking cessation.
- A multidisciplinary case conference including the GP and secondary care physician, as well as the palliative care, community nursing and physiotherapy teams, could decide a plan for dealing with his episodes of dyspnoea.
- A psychologist could suggest coping strategies for both his physical and psychological problems.
- Mr Barnes's views on admission to an intensive therapy unit and 'Do not attempt resuscitation' orders should be elicited and discussed with him.
- Mr Barnes needs support at home to help with daily activities. He needs to consider moving to sheltered accommodation or living with his family instead of on his own.

End-stage respiratory disease

Several long-term respiratory conditions are progressive and eventually cause death. Therefore advance care planning (i.e. about end-of-life care) is a critical part of treatment for patients with respiratory disease.

End-of-life care needs to be considered carefully. The GP, secondary care physician, and palliative care services (both community- and hospital-based) are involved, as well as the patient and their immediate family members or carers. An important question is whether the patient would prefer to die at home, in a hospice or in a hospital.

Common symptoms that affect patients with severe chronic respiratory conditions, and the management of these symptoms, are shown in **Table 12.2**. Fatigue, pain, cough and breathlessness are common physical symptoms. Patients also have psychological difficulties, including emotional distress, social isolation, insomnia, anxiety and depression. These problems necessitate specialist help from palliative care teams.

Unlike diseases (e.g. cancer) with a clear downward trajectory, with some long-term respiratory diseases (e.g. COPD and interstitial lung disease) it is difficult to estimate the pace and timescale of a patient's decline. This complicates timing any referral to palliative care. Criteria for palliative care referral include:

- severe incurable chronic respiratory disease

Management of non-specific symptoms in respiratory disease

Symptom	Management
Depression	Antidepressants
	Anxiolytics
	Counselling
Dyspnoea	Opioids
	Oxygen (if hypoxic)
	Benzodiazepine (e.g. lorazepam), as required
	Anxiety management
	Lifestyle changes
Cough	Opioids
	Cough suppressants (but poor efficacy)
Tenacious sputum	Physiotherapy
	Mucolytics
	Nebulised saline
Weight loss	Oral nutritional support
	Percutaneous endoscopic gastrostomy (for a minority of patients)
Fatigue	Ensure optimal treatment and nutritional support
	Support for activities of daily living
Anxiety	Benzodiazepine and opioids, as required
	Long-term anxiolytics
	Psychological support

Table 12.2 Management of common non-specific symptoms of chronic respiratory diseases

- an expected life expectancy of 6–12 months
- physical symptoms (e.g. breathlessness) or psychological symptoms uncontrolled by optimal therapy
- increasing number of emergency admissions

Prognostic factors for each disease help identify patients whose condition is likely to have a poor outcome. **Table 12.3** lists factors associated with a poor prognosis in COPD. Similar

Poor prognostic indicators in COPD

Cor pulmonale

Low body mass index (< 20 kg/m^2)

Depression

Previous admission to an intensive care unit

Use of corticosteroids for > 6 weeks in the past 12 months

Use of long-term oxygen therapy

More than three admissions to hospital in the past 12 months

Table 12.3 Indicators of poor prognosis in patients with chronic obstructive pulmonary disease

factors are probably relevant for other chronic lung diseases, such as interstitial lung disease.

Good documentation of care planning across primary and secondary care is essential. The sharing of such documentation is facilitated by palliative care registers accessible by all health care providers.

Communication between health care professionals and the patient and their family is key to effective advance care. Some health care professionals find these conversations difficult. Open-ended questions help broach the subject and thus allow patients to begin discussing the issues.

Patients presenting to the emergency department at the point of death may be unable to communicate the existence of an advance directive stating their desire not to be treated by intubation or cardiopulmonary resuscitation. Copies of the directive must be attached to the electronic and physical notes and given to the local ambulance service. The patient's wishes must also be reiterated in letters from members of medical teams involved in their care. Patients' relatives should also be aware of the contents of the directives.

Disease prevention

Public health measures for disease prevention help improve population health. Disease prevention interventions are usually the responsibility of GPs, sometimes supported by advice from secondary care physicians.

Several disease prevention interventions are relevant for respiratory disease. The most obvious and commonest of these is smoking cessation.

Smoking cessation

Cigarette smoking is highly addictive, and quitting is difficult. Smokers often make multiple attempts to stop smoking and need encouragement from family and health care professionals.

Psychological support is helpful, but nicotine replacement therapy and medications (Chapter 2) are useful adjuncts. Patients need to be supported in their attempts to stop smoking by health care professionals trained in providing individually tailored advice.

Respiratory health benefits of smoking cessation include:

- decreased risk of lung cancer
- decreased risk of developing COPD and slower progression in confirmed cases
- improved control of asthma
- decreased risk of pulmonary fibrosis, pneumonia and pneumothorax
- slower decline in lung function
- improvement in respiratory symptoms (cough and breathlessness)

Stopping smoking also improves non-respiratory health. These benefits include a decreased risk of coronary artery and cerebrovascular disease, and of oral, urological and gastrointestinal cancers.

Occupational lung disease

Common occupational exposures resulting in lung disease are listed in Table 2.12. Disease severity is often related to the duration and intensity of exposure. GPs need to be aware of important occupational lung diseases, such as asbestosis, to identify patients whose symptoms are related to their current or previous job and to refer them to a specialist.

Pollution

High levels of atmospheric pollution, which are associated with urban centres, cause deteriorations in airways diseases such as asthma and COPD. Prevention of atmospheric pollution is a matter of public health care policy.

Vaccination and antimicrobial prophylaxis

Vaccination against influenza is one of the most effective health care interventions. All suitable patients should be vaccinated (Table 11.17). Vaccines are available for some respiratory microbial pathogens.

Antimicrobial prophylaxis is also used against specific infections. For example, anti-tuberculosis therapy is offered to patients with latent disease who are immunosuppressed, as well as to their close contacts; and co-trimoxazole therapy for HIV-positive patients to prevent *Pneumocystis jirovecii* pneumonia.

Many patients are convinced that influenza vaccination exacerbates their chest symptoms temporarily. The results of large studies suggest that this belief is based on coincidence: the influenza vaccine is given at the time of year when viral infections are common. The results also show that influenza vaccination is an effective intervention to reduce the increased mortality caused by influenza infection in the elderly.

Exposure to environmental allergens

The symptoms of airways diseases often seem to increase when patients are exposed to damp environments and fungal spores. Conversely, symptoms may be relieved by dry and well-ventilated housing or work environments.

Pregnancy and respiratory disease

Pregnancy entails multiple physiological and anatomical changes.

- As the uterus expands, the diaphragm is pushed up by about 4 cm. This change in position decreases functional residual capacity by about 20% at term.
- Oxygen demand increases to fuel fetal metabolism.
- Tidal volume and minute ventilation increase throughout pregnancy. These changes are the result of an increase in respiratory drive in response to higher concentrations of progesterone. Consequently, respiratory alkalosis develops; $PaCO_2$ falls to 3.7–4.3 kPa, and HCO_3^- to 18–21 mmol/L.
- Cardiac output increases by about 40%, and relaxation of the cardiac sphincter causes heartburn.

Specific respiratory problems during pregnancy include dyspnoea, infections, asthma, pulmonary embolism, pulmonary oedema and acute respiratory distress syndrome. Pre-existing lung diseases can also complicate pregnancy.

Dyspnoea

Breathlessness is common in pregnancy. The feeling is caused by awareness of the increased tidal volume.

Infections

Pneumonia is a rare but important cause of maternal mortality. The risk of death from other infections, such as chickenpox pneumonitis, is also increased by pregnancy.

- Most commonly used antibiotics, including penicillin, cephalosporins and erythromycin, are safe in pregnancy.
- Antibiotics contraindicated in pregnancy include tetracyclines, antituberculous drugs, quinolones and aminoglycosides.

Asthma

About a third of women with asthma report an improvement in symptoms in pregnancy; another third, deterioration; and the final third, no change. It is not possible to predict who will fall into which of these groups.

Poorly controlled asthma increases the risk of preterm delivery, low birth weight and prenatal mortality. Treatment of asthma in pregnant women is the same as that for non-pregnant women.

Pulmonary embolism

Pregnancy is a procoagulant state, and the gravid uterus inhibits flow through the inferior vena cava. Pulmonary embolism is about 5 times more likely during pregnancy. The disorder occurs in perhaps 1% of patients.

- If pulmonary embolism is suspected, treat patients with heparin rather than warfarin; warfarin is teratogenic, especially in the first trimester.
- Decisions about imaging are difficult. Weigh the radiation risk of a ventilation–perfusion scan or computerised tomography pulmonary angiogram against the likelihood of diagnosis.

Amniotic fluid embolism occurs if amniotic fluid or fetal material enters the pulmonary circulation. This is a rare but life-threatening complication of delivery.

Pulmonary oedema and acute respiratory distress syndrome

Causes of cardiogenic or non-cardiogenic pulmonary oedema in pregnancy include:

- β-agonist therapy (used to delay contractions)
- eclampsia
- peripartum cardiomyopathy
- aspiration

Pre-existing lung disease

Diseases that cause persisting chronic impairment of lung function are rare in women of child-bearing age. The exceptions are cystic fibrosis, post-tuberculosis lung damage, and (more rarely) systemic lupus erythematosus and lymphangioleiomyomatosis.

In patients whose lung function is severely impaired by these disorders, changes in respiratory physiology during pregnancy can be life-threatening. These patients require careful assessment and monitoring by a multidisciplinary team including their GP, chest specialist and obstetrician.

Answers to starter questions

1. Decisions about the care of patients at the end of their lives take into account their preferences, as well as their general health. There is often no ideal time to discuss advance care planning, and a single discussion may be insufficient. Patients may need a series of discussions, as well as time for further consideration, before reaching decisions about the type of care they wish to receive.

2. Patients benefit from a holistic approach, because they rarely have just one disease; it is important to consider the influence of comorbidities and medications alongside the presenting condition. Furthermore, patients' mental health often affects their physical symptoms.

   Each person is unique. A management plan that works for one patient does not necessarily work for another.

3. Disease prevention interventions work. Multiple public health measures are helping to prevent respiratory disease. Examples include vaccination against respiratory tract infections and smoking cessation advice. Health can also be improved by lifestyle changes such as improving diet, increasing physical activity, and reducing alcohol intake.

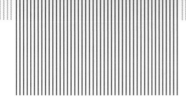

Chapter 13
Self-assessment

SBA questions

Airways disease

1. A 24-year-old man known to have asthma has had a cough, myalgia and fever for 7 days. He is wheezy and has been using his usual inhalers every half hour. He feels that the inhalers are not having any effect on his symptoms. Which single finding is not an indication of a life-threatening attack of asthma?

- **A** Blood pressure of 90/60 mmHg
- **B** Inability to complete sentences
- **C** Inaudible air entry bilaterally
- **D** Peak expiratory flow rate < 33% of predicted
- **E** Saturations < 88% on air

2. A 22-year-old woman with asthma has been using her salbutamol 100 µg inhaler with increasing frequency over the past 4 weeks. Her observations are normal. However, her peak expiratory flow rate is 76% of predicted, and her symptoms are not well controlled. What is the single most appropriate next step in management?

- **A** Add aminophylline tablets to her treatment
- **B** Add inhaled long-acting β_2 agonist to her treatment
- **C** Prescribe 10 days of oral prednisolone 40 mg once per day
- **D** Provide a home nebuliser
- **E** Start an inhaled steroid

3. A 62-year-old man has chronic obstructive pulmonary disease (COPD) and uses long-term oxygen therapy at home. He has not left his house for a week, and his wife says that he has been confused today. She has brought him to hospital, where he has been given nebulized salbutamol and ipratropium bromide. The patient's observations are temperature, 37.1°C; heart rate, 95 beats/min; respiratory rate, 10 breaths/min; blood pressure, 138/85 mmHg; and oxygen saturation, 88% on 2 L/min[4] oxygen through nasal cannula. Arterial blood gases on 2 L/min oxygen are pH, 7.1; $PaCO_2$, 7.1 kPa; PaO_2, 8.2 kPa; base excess, 5.4 mmol/L; and HCO_3^-, 34mmol/L Which is the single most appropriate next step?

- **A** Increase oxygen to 4 L/min
- **B** Give intravenous aminophylline
- **C** Give oxygen at 15 L/min through a non-rebreathe mask
- **D** Trial non-invasive ventilation
- **E** Trial continuous positive airway pressure

4. A 58-year-old woman has become gradually breathless over 4 months. She is now unable to complete her normal cycle ride to work. She has no cough or fever but has had a single episode of haemoptysis. Which is the single most useful associated feature that indicates large airways obstruction?

- **A** Bronchiectasis on a computerised tomography scan of the chest
- **B** High Empey index (forced expiratory volume in 1 s, FEV_1:peak flow ratio) score
- **C** Polyphonic wheeze on auscultation
- **D** Reduced exercise tolerance
- **E** Reduced FEV_1

5. A 71-year-old woman has become increasingly breathless over several years. She gets breathless with strenuous walking. She has had an average of one chest infection a year in each of the past 3 years. She is a smoker, and her general practitioner suspects COPD. He sends her for pulmonary function tests. The results show that FEV_1/forced vital capacity is 0.68; her FEV1 is 65% of the predicted value. What is the single best description of the severity of her COPD?

- **A** Stage 1 (mild) and Global Initiative for Chronic Obstructive Lung Disease (GOLD) classification A
- **B** Stage 2 (moderate) and GOLD classification A
- **C** Stage 3 (severe) and GOLD classification C
- **D** Stage 4, (very severe) and GOLD classification D
- **E** These results do not confirm COPD

6. A 20-year-old woman has had episodes of cough and dyspnoea lasting a few hours for the past 4 months. She works in an office and occasionally smokes socially.
What is the single most likely cause of her breathlessness?

   A Asthma
   B Cardiac failure
   C COPD
   D Ischaemic heart disease
   E Pneumothorax

7. A previously well 60-year-old man has worsening shortness of breath over 2 weeks. He has a non-productive cough and no chest pain. He has a 30 pack-year history of smoking and works as a factory foreman. He has a history of diabetes and hypertension. On examination he is afebrile, has a tachycardia of 100 beats/min and has oxygen saturations of 91% on air. On auscultation there are fine crepitations bibasally.
What is the single most likely cause of these findings?

   A Bronchiectasis
   B COPD
   C Idiopathic pulmonary fibrosis
   D Pneumonia
   E Pulmonary oedema

8. A 68-year-old man has stridor when lying flat, a persistent hoarse voice and weight loss. He is diagnosed with laryngeal cancer. A CT scan shows that the cancer has metastasised to the lungs with a large mass at the left upper hilum partially obstructing the trachea.
Which is the single most likely blood vessel through which the cancer has spread?

   A Bronchial veins into the hemiazygous vein
   B Directly into the superior vena cava
   C Pharyngeal venous plexus into the internal jugular vein
   D Pterygoid venous plexus which becomes the maxillary vein
   E Superior thyroid vein into the internal jugular vein

9. A 63-year-old man has a persistent cough but is only breathless when he rides his bike uphill. He has had no chest infections in the last year but has smoked 20 cigarettes a day for 35 years. He works as a train driver. He has obstructive spirometry without reversibility. His FEV1 is 72% predicted.
What is the single most appropriate treatment?

   A Long-acting β2-agonist and inhaled corticosteroid combination inhaler
   B Long-acting muscarinic antagonist inhaler
   C Non-invasive ventilation
   D Oral prednisolone 30mg for 5 days
   E Smoking cessation therapy

Interstitial lung disease

1. A 67-year-old woman has become progressively breathless over the last 6 months with no chest pain, haemoptysis, weight loss or sputum production. She smokes 15 cigarettes a day and is a retired air hostess. She lives with her grandson who has been helping with the weekly shop. Her doctor suspects she may have idiopathic pulmonary fibrosis (IPF). Which is the single feature found on examination that makes the doctor suspect IPF?

   A Coarse upper zone crepitations
   B Deviated trachea
   C Finger clubbing
   D Central cyanosis
   E Unilateral reduced chest expansion

2. An 80-year-old man has a CT urogram for investigation of haematuria. The scan includes the bases of the lungs and shows a number of features suggestive of idiopathic pulmonary fibrosis. He undergoes a dedicated HRCT.
What is the single most likely pattern of findings on HRCT?

   A Bilateral hilar lymphadenopathy
   B Lower lobe subpleural honeycombing
   C Nodular infiltrates with areas of coalescence and cavitation
   D Patchy peripheral consolidation
   E Upper lobe predominant ground glass opacification with cysts

3. A 28-year-old man has episodic breathlessness, wheeze and a cough. His symptoms seem to improve when he is on holiday rather than at work. Spirometry shows a mixed obstructive–restrictive pattern. Computerised tomography (CT) of the chest during a period of severe symptoms shows patchy diffuse infiltrates, as well as nodules in the middle and upper zones bilaterally.
What is the single most likely diagnosis?

   A Asbestosis
   B Hypersensitivity pneumonitis
   C Idiopathic pulmonary fibrosis
   D Occupational asthma
   E Sarcoidosis

4. A 40-year-old man from Nigeria attends the accident and emergency department complaining of chest pain. The pain is considered most likely to be musculoskeletal. Therefore

the plan is to prescribe analgesic medication and discharge him. However, chest X ray shows bilateral symmetrical smooth hilar lymphadenopathy. Blood tests results are haemoglobin, 14 g/dL; white cell count, 4.6 10^9/L; and calcium, 3.1 mmol/L (high).
What is the single most likely diagnosis?

A Lymphoma
B Tuberculosis
C Sarcoidosis
D Silicosis
E Bronchogenic carcinoma

5. A 72-year-old man has become increasingly breathless over 8 months. He has a persistent non-productive cough but has not had any chest infections. He has no chest pain or haemoptysis. He is a non-smoker and keeps no pets. On examination he has fine basal inspiratory crackles bilaterally.
What is the single most likely associated investigation finding?

A Eosinophilia on full blood count
D Hypercapnoea on arterial blood gas analysis
C Pleural effusion on chest X-ray
D Positive Mantoux test
E Restrictive pattern on pulmonary function tests

6. A 68-year-old man is investigated for shortness of breath. High-resolution CT finds evidence of pulmonary fibrosis. He has never been exposed to asbestosis, and he does not have rheumatological or autoimmune disease. Pulmonary function tests show a restrictive pattern and decreased transfer factor.
What is the single most likely drug to be the cause?

A Amiodarone
B Amitriptyline
C Amoxicillin
D Aspirin
E Azathioprine

7. A 60-year-old woman had idiopathic pulmonary fibrosis diagnosed 6 years ago. It has progressed over this time despite treatment with pirfenidone.
What is the single feature which should trigger referral for lung transplantation?

A A fall in TLCO of 5% over 24 months
B A TLCO of less than 40% of expected
C Extensive honeycombing on HRCT
D Reduction in FVC of 5% over 9 months
E Resection of a colonic cancer 2 years previously

Sleep and ventilatory disorders

1. A 58-year-old woman with a BMI of 45kg/m2 is semi-comatose. Her husband says she has gained 13Kg over the past year and that her legs have been more swollen for 3 months. She does not snore and there are no localising neurological or respiratory signs. Her pulse oximetry shows an oxygen saturation of 88% on air.
What is the single most appropriate investigation to perform?

A Arterial blood gas
B CT scan of the brain
C High resolution CT scan of the lungs
D Spirometry
E Transfer factor

2. A 62-year-old woman is found unwell at home by a neighbour. She is coughing and has a fever. The paramedics suspect a severe chest infection. On the way to hospital, she receives oxygen at 15 L/min through a non-rebreathe mask. On arrival, her Glasgow Coma Scale score is 10, and she is drowsy but rousable. Her neighbour says that the patient has a neurological condition, but he is unsure which one. The patient's arterial blood gases show type 2 respiratory failure.
What is the single most likely neurological condition to lead to this presentation?

A Friedrich's ataxia
B Guillain–Barré syndrome
C Huntingdon's disease
D Lewy body disease
E Motor neurone disease

3. A 51-year-old lorry driver has been snoring and feeling tired during the day. He is assessed in the sleep clinic and is found to have a body mass index of 31 kg/m$_2$ and an Epworth Sleepiness Scale score of 15. He has a sleep study, which gives an apnoea–hypopnoea index of 35 events/h. Continuous positive airway pressure (CPAP) treatment is offered.
What is the single best advice to give him?

A He can continue to drive his car but must not drive lorries until treatment has started
B He must inform the national driver-licensing authority (in the UK, this is the Driver and Vehicle Licensing Agency, DVLA) and cannot drive at all until successfully treated
C He must inform the DVLA but can continue to drive both cars and lorries
D You will inform the DVLA on his behalf, and he must not drive until 2 weeks after the start of treatment

E No restrictions on driving are necessary, as long as he does not feel too tired to drive

4. A 58 year-old-man with a BMI of 42kg/m2 has been irritable and excessively sleepy. His wife is worried that he stops breathing during the night and has encouraged him to have investigations for obstructive sleep apnoea.
What single investigation result will confirm a diagnosis of obstructive sleep apnoea?

A Apnoea/hypopnoea index of 18 on polysomnography
B Electrocardiogram showing right heart strain
C Hyperexpanded lung fields with flattened diaphragms on chest x-ray
D Mallampati score of 3
E Sawtooth pattern on overnight oximetry

Pleural disease

1. A 26-year-old man has a sudden pain around his left upper chest. He feels breathless.
His trachea is central. There is no wheeze, but there is decreased air entry at the left apex. The patient's temperature is 36.8°C; heart rate, 110 beats/min; respiratory rate, 20 breaths/min; and blood pressure, 130/70 mmHg. Oxygen saturation is 96% on air.
Which is the single most appropriate next action?

A Give high-dose low-molecular-weight heparin (LMWH)
B Give ibuprofen 400 mg
C Insert a cannula into the 5th intercostal space mid-clavicular line
D Do a chest X-ray
E Request a computerised tomography pulmonary angiogram (CTPA)

2. A 70-year-old woman has become progressively breathless over 4 months. She has a history of a previous myocardial infarction (with coronary stents inserted 2 years ago), breast cancer treated by mastectomy 6 years ago, alcohol dependence and diabetes. Examination finds dullness to percussion and reduced air entry in the left mid and lower zone. The chest X-ray is consistent with a pleural effusion. This diagnosis is confirmed on bedside ultrasound when a pleural tap is done. The results of pleural fluid analysis are protein, 39 g/L; glucose, 3.1 mmol/L; pH, 7.3; and no organisms seen on Gram stain. The results of culture and cytological investigations are awaited. The lactate dehydrogenase (LDH) pleura:serum ratio is 0.8.
What is the single most likely cause of the pleural effusion?

A Cardiac failure
B Liver cirrhosis
C Nephrotic syndrome
D Malignancy
E Tuberculosis

3. A 57-year-old man has been feeling unwell with fevers, fatigue and chest pain for a week. He is febrile and has tachycardia. Chest X-ray shows a unilateral pleural effusion. Ultrasound of the chest shows that the effusion has loculations.
A sample of the fluid is taken. Pleural fluid results are protein, 42 g/L; glucose, 2.3 mmol/L; pH, 7.0; LDH pleura:serum ratio, 1.1. Results from microscopy, culture and cytology are awaited.
What is the single most appropriate next step in management?

A Ask the microbiology team for advice on antibiotic choice
B Insert a chest drain under ultrasound guidance
C Prescribe intravenous furosemide 40 mg
D Request a CT scan of the chest
E Refer the patient to a cardiothoracic surgeon

4. A 78-year-old man has sudden-onset breathlessness. On arrival at the accident and emergency department, he has a heart rate of 110 beats/min (regular), respiratory rate of 32 breaths/min and blood pressure of 155/75 mmHg. Oxygen saturation is 84% on air. He is too breathless to provide a history, but computerised records show that pulmonary function tests this year gave a forced expiratory volume (in 1 s) (FEV_1) of 0.8 L (35% of predicted) and a forced vital capacity (FVC) of 1.6 L, giving a FEV_1/FVC ratio of 0.5.
On examination, expansion is decreased on the left, and breath sounds are absent in the upper zone. Controlled supplementary oxygen is given through a Venturi mask. Blood samples are sent for tests. A chest X-ray is requested. It shows an apical left-sided pneumothorax of 4 cm.
What is the single most appropriate management?

A Aspirate the pneumothorax using an 18-gauge cannula
B Insert a chest drain with underwater seal
C Observe the patient, and consider discharge with an outpatient review in 2 weeks
D Observe but admit for observation for 48 h
E Refer the patient to cardiothoracic surgeons

5. A 70-year-old man with a history of ischaemic heart disease, aortic stenosis, hypertension and hypothyroidism is increasingly short of breath. He has no cough or haemoptysis and has not lost any weight. He has decreased breath sounds in the right mid and lower zones, with a dull percussion note and reduced tactile vocal fremitus. He has pitting oedema of both calves. Chest X-ray and ultrasound show a moderate right-sided and a small left-sided pleural effusion. A sample of fluid is taken.

What is the single most likely result of the pleural fluid aspiration?

A Protein, 22 g/L; glucose, 3.7 mmol/L; pH, 7.4; LDH pleura:serum ratio, 0.4
B Protein, 22 g/L: glucose, 1.2 mmol/L; pH, 7.4; LDH pleura:serum ratio, 0.4
C Protein, 22 g/L; glucose, 3.7 mmol/L; pH, 7.4; LDH pleura/serum ratio, 1.0
D Protein, 36 g/L; glucose, 3.7 mmol/L; pH, 7.4; LDH pleura/serum ratio, 0.4
E Protein, 36 g/L; glucose, 3.7 mmol/L; pH, 7.4; LDH pleura/serum ratio, 1.0

6. A 58-year-old man has been breathless for 2 months. He is afebrile. There is no lymphadenopathy or scars. The trachea is central. He has reduced expansion and dullness to percussion in the right base.

What is the single most likely cause of the clinical findings?

A Large bullae
B Obesity
C Pleural effusion
D Pneumothorax
E Pneumonectomy

7. A 71-year-old man has a pre-operative chest X-ray before undergoing a total knee replacement. It shows bilateral pleural plaques and left mid-zone pleural thickening. A chest X-ray done 2 years ago had a similar appearance. He is not breathless and has not suffered any chest pain. His weight is stable. He is an ex-smoker with a 35 pack year history and is a retired heating engineer.

Which is the single most likely cause of the X-ray appearances?

A Benign asbestos-related thickening
B Chronic aspergillosis
C Lung adenocarcinoma
D Mesothelioma
E Non-tuberculous mycobacteria

8. A 70-year-old woman has hypertension for which she takes ramipril, bisoprolol and bendroflumethiazide. She has rheumatoid arthritis which is under good control on an anti-TNF biologic agent. She smokes 30 cigarettes a day. She is become progressively breathless on exertion over 4 months but has no cough or chest pain. She has a chest X-ray which shows a unilateral pleural effusion. She has an ultrasound guided pleural aspiration. The pleural fluid analysis results are protein 27g/L, protein content of pleural fluid 0.4 of serum protein, glucose 3.4mmol/L, pH 7.34 and no organisms seen on Gram stain.

Which is the single most likely cause of the pleural effusion?

A Benign asbestos effusion
B Cardiac failure
C Hypothyroidism
D Pulmonary embolism
E Rheumatoid arthritis

9. A 53-year-old woman has a chest drain inserted to drain a secondary spontaneous pneumothorax in association with emphysema. On the ward round the doctor asks the patient to take a deep breath, and to cough, and examines the drain which is swinging but not bubbling.

Which is the single best explanation for the chest drain appearance?

A The drain is correctly sited in the pleural space and there is a large effusion
B The drain is correctly sited in the pleural space and there is still a pneumothorax
C The drain is correctly sited in the pleural space and the pneumothorax has resolved
D The drain is incorrectly sited in the thoracic wall
E The drain is incorrectly sited in the abdominal cavity

10. A 17-year-old man becomes suddenly short of breath while training for an athletics competition. His chest X-ray shows a large primary spontaneous pneumothorax with complete collapse of the left lung. An aspiration is performed using an 16 gauge cannula and aspirates 2.4L of air. A repeat chest X-ray shows that the pneumothorax has decreased in size but is still >2.5cm at the hilum. His symptoms are improved but he is still breathless on walking to the bathroom.

Which is the single most appropriate next step in management?

A Admit to hospital and observe for 24 hours
B Discharge home and ask him to return for another chest X-ray in 24 hours
C Discharge home and book a clinic appointment in 2 weeks
D Insert a chest drain and admit to hospital
E Repeat the pleural aspiration using an 18 gauge cannula

Malignancy

1. An 80-year-old man has abdominal pain and is found to be constipated. He has general aches, feels low in mood and has lost 7 kg in weight in the past 6 months. He is a former smoker and has had a persistent cough over this time too. Chest X-ray shows a 4-cm opacity.
    What is the single most likely diagnosis?

    A Bronchial carcinoid tumour secreting serotonin
    B Bronchial carcinoma with metastases to the liver and brain
    C Colonic carcinoma with metastasis to the lung
    D Small-cell lung cancer secreting voltage-gated calcium channel antibodies
    E Squamous cell lung cancer secreting parathyroid hormone

2. A 65-year-old man who is known to have chronic obstructive pulmonary disease feels non-specifically unwell. He has a friend who was recently diagnosed with lung cancer and is worried that he may have this too. His general practitioner takes a full history and does a thorough examination to determine whether urgent referral to a chest physician is required to investigate this possibility.
    What is the single best reason for urgent referral to a chest physician?

    A Cough lasting 2 weeks
    B Bilateral end expiratory wheeze on auscultation of the chest
    C Hoarseness of the voice
    D Nausea with decreased appetite but no associated weight loss
    E Two infective exacerbations of COPD in the past month

3. A 45-year-old woman has palpitations and is assessed in the accident and emergency department. She is found to have a supraventricular tachycardia, which subsequently resolves. She is referred for outpatient follow-up with a cardiologist. Chest X-ray shows an incidental peripheral 3-cm mass in the right midzone, but the mediastinum and hila appear normal. The patient has no pre-existing medical conditions and is a non-smoker. The mass is found to be cancer.
    What is the single most likely pathological type?

    A Adenocarcinoma
    B Bronchoalveolar carcinoma
    C Lymphoma
    D Small-cell lung cancer
    E Squamous cell carcinoma

4. A 57-year-old man is seen in the chest clinic for urgent assessment of a possible lung cancer. He is a smoker with unintentional weight loss of 8 kg in the past month. He has also had three episodes of haemoptysis. He has already had a chest X-ray, which he has been told shows a shadow. He goes on to have a computerised tomography (CT) scan of the chest. The findings are reported as follows.
    'There is a 4-cm spiculated mass in the left upper lobe at the apex, with a small 1-cm nodule in the same lobe. There are enlarged ipsilateral mediastinal nodes, including the subcarinal node.'
    What is the single best investigation to obtain a pathological diagnosis?

    A Bronchoscopy with bronchoalveolar lavage
    B Bronchoscopy and endobronchial biopsy
    C Bronchoscopy with endobronchial ultrasound and mediastinal lymph node biopsy
    D Sputum cytology
    E Video-assisted thorascopic surgery biopsy

5. A 76-year-old man has an incidental mass on chest X-ray. He has now also had a CT scan of the chest, as well as positron emission tomography (PET), and the radiologist is asked to stage the tumour. She describes the findings on imaging as follows: 'There is a 2.5-cm, well-defined mass in the anterior segment of the right upper lobe, which is strongly FDG [fluorodeoxyglucose]-avid on PET. There are no enlarged hilar or mediastinal nodes, and no abnormalities of the remaining lung, the liver or the adrenals. There are no other FDG-avid lesions.'
    What is the single best description of the stage of this tumour?

    A T1a N0 M0
    B T1a N1 M0
    C T1b N2 M0
    D T1b N1 M1a
    E T1b N2 M1a

6. A 61-year-old man has a T1b N0 M0 squamous cell carcinoma of the lung in the right upper lobe. He has diabetes and hypertension. He is otherwise generally well and continues to work as a bricklayer. His pulmonary function tests show a forced expiratory volume (in 1 s) 3.3 L (94% of predicted) and a forced vital capacity of 4.3 L.
    What single most appropriate treatment should the multidisciplinary team recommend?

    A Chemoradiotherapy
    B Combination chemotherapy
    C Radical radiotherapy
    D Surgical resection: right upper lobectomy
    E Surgical resection: right pneumonectomy

7. A 67-year-old man has a T4 N3 M1a non–small-cell lung cancer. The primary mass encases the right main bronchus and invades the mediastinum; he has an enlarged supraclavicular node and a moderate right pleural effusion. He has ongoing frequent haemoptysis and is short of breath. He is mobile only within his house. Therefore he spends most of the day in his chair, reading and listening to the radio. What is the single most appropriate treatment that the multidisciplinary team should recommend?

A Combination chemotherapy
B No active treatment
C Palliative radiotherapy
D Radical radiotherapy
E Surgical resection: pneumonectomy

8. An 80-year-old man has become increasingly fatigued and short of breath over the past 2 months. He has constant right-sided chest pain. He has a 10 pack-year smoking history. He has had various jobs. He worked for many years as a painter and decorator. He also worked as a navy cook and on a production line in an automobile factory when he was younger. He has a chest X-ray, which shows a pleural effusion but no parenchymal mass. A sample of fluid is taken; it is blood-stained. The results of analysis are protein, 40 g/L; glucose, 3.2 mmol/L; pH, 7.3; and lactate dehydrogenase (LDH) pleura:serum ratio, 0.55. Numerous red blood cells and lymphocytes are visible but no organisms. The results of cytological investigations are awaited. What is the single most likely cause of the pleural effusion?

A Benign asbestos effusion
B Lymphoma
C Mesothelioma
D Metastatic lung cancer
E Metastatic prostate cancer

9. A 56-year-old man has had a cough for 3 months. He is an ex-smoker with a 40 pack year history and works as an estate agent. A chest X-ray reveals a left upper lobe mass. He is awaiting further investigations including a CT of the chest. His doctor thinks the cancer has spread beyond the primary mass. Which is the single best evidence that the cancer has spread to the left hilar nodes?

A Chest wall pain
B Dilated veins over the chest wall
C Hoarse voice
D Stridor
E Weight loss of 2kg in 4 months

10. A 55-year-old man has lethargy, nausea, polyuria and abdominal pain. He has lost 13Kg over 1 month and has a poor appetite. He smokes 40 cigarettes a day and works as a landscape gardener. An abdominal X-ray shows faecal loading. A chest X-ray shows a mass in the right lower lobe with central cavitation. His corrected calcium is 3.2mmol/L. Which is the single most likely cause of these findings?

A Adenocarcinoma
B Lymphoma
C Small cell carcinoma
D Squamous cell carcinoma
E Large cell carcinoma

11. A 62-year-old female librarian has an adenocarcinoma of the lung. A staging CT and PET scan stage her disease as T1b N1 M0. She is independent with activities of daily living and continues to do her own shopping but has had to reduce her hours at work due to fatigue and has stopped attending her kickboxing class. Which is the single most accurate WHO performance scale grade for this patient?

A 0
B 1
C 2
D 3
E 4

Lung infections

1. A 75-year-old man who currently smokes 20 cigarettes daily develops a productive cough, fever, fatigue and shortness of breath. His symptoms have been worsening for 4 days. He has focal coarse crepitations at the left base. His temperature is 38.1°C; heart rate, 115 beats/min; respiratory rate, 22 breaths/min; and blood pressure, 140/60 mmHg. Oxygen saturation is 91% on air. Which is the single most likely causative organism?

A *Haemophilus influenzae*
B *Legionella pneumophila*
C *Mycoplasma pneumoniae*
D *Staphylococcus aureus*
E *Streptococcus pneumoniae*

2. A 41-year-old woman is admitted to hospital with fever, shortness of breath and a productive cough. Chest X-ray reveals left lower lobe consolidation. Her observations are temperature, 38.3°C; heart rate, 120 beats/min; respiratory rate, 24 breaths/min; blood pressure, 120/65 mmHg; and oxygen saturation, 91% on air.

What is the single most appropriate initial management?

A Start high-flow oxygen at 15 L/min through a non-rebreathe mask

B Start oxygen through nasal cannulae at 6 L/min

C Start oxygen through a non-invasive ventilation mask at 4 L/min

D Start 35% oxygen through a Venturi mask

E Take samples for analysis of arterial blood gases before administering oxygen

3. A 64-year-old woman has been an in-patient in hospital for 3 weeks after a road traffic accident. The accident fractured her hip, humerus and ribs. She was doing well with rehabilitation, but her oxygen requirements have been increasing over the past 24 h. Observations are now temperature, 38.1°C; heart rate, 115 beats/min; respiratory rate, 31 breaths/min; blood pressure, 95/52 mmHg; and oxygen saturation, 94% on 40% oxygen through a Venturi mask. Crepitations are audible in the right mid and lower zone. Chest X-ray shows multifocal cavitating consolidation.
What is the single most likely organism to be causing her infection?

A Influenza A
B *L. pneumophila*
C *Mycobacterium tuberculosis*
D *S. aureus*
E *S. pneumoniae*

4. A 26-year-old woman is in intensive care following a road traffic accident. She is intubated and ventilated, and on day 5 develops fevers and increasing peak ventilation pressures. A chest X-ray shows extensive consolidation bibasally. Copious thick yellow secretions are suctioned through her endotracheal tube and sent for microscopy, culture and sensitivities. Gram negative bacilli are seen on gram stain.
What is the single most likely organism to be isolated?

A *Coxiella burnetti*
B *Escherichia coli*
C *Moraxella catarrhalis*
D *M. tuberculosis*
E *S. pneumoniae*

5. A 26-year-old man has a 3-day history of cough (which produces white sputum), nasal discharge, frequent sneezing, headache, fever and fatigue. He has lost his appetite and is worried because he feels so unwell. On examination, his chest is clear. His temperature is 37.8°C; heart rate, 110 beats/min; respiratory rate, 18 breaths/min; and blood pressure 120/75 mmHg. His oxygen saturation is 98% on air.

What is the single most appropriate next step?

A Advise fluids, rest and analgesia

B Prescribe a 7-day course of amoxicillin 500 mg three times daily

C Send the patient to hospital for urgent assessment including chest X-ray and blood tests

D Take nasopharyngeal aspirate and throat swab for respiratory viruses

E Take blood tests and arrange to see him again in 2 days

6. A 71-year-old man with known bullous emphysema has a 3-day history of increased shortness of breath. His observations are temperature, 37.7°C; heart rate, 95 beats/min; respiratory rate, 26 breaths/min; blood pressure, 140/70 mmHg; and oxygen saturation, 94% on 3 L/min oxygen through nasal cannula. Chest X-ray shows hyperexpanded lungs, flattened diaphragms, decreased lung markings in the right apex, left apex and left midzone, and patchy shadowing over an indistinct right heart border.
What is the single most likely cause of these findings?

A Right lower lobe malignancy
B Right middle lobe pneumonia
C Right upper lobe collapse
D Right pulmonary embolus
E Right pneumothorax

7. An 82-year-old woman has had right-sided chest pain and fever for 2 days. She has right lower lobe consolidation on chest X-ray. Her observations are temperature, 37.4°C; heart rate, 110 beats/min; respiratory rate, 26 breaths/min; blood pressure, 100/65 mmHg; and oxygen saturation, 92% on air. Her abbreviated mental test score is 9/10. Blood test results are haemoglobin, 11.5 g/dL; white cell count, 2.1×10^9/L; platelets, 160×10^9/L; sodium, 136 mmol/L; potassium, 3.7 mmol/L; urea, 8.1 mmol/L; creatinine 130 µmol/L; and C-reactive protein, 105 mg/L.
What is the single best assessment of her CURB-65 score?

A 1
B 2
C 3
D 4
E 5

8. A 42-year-old man has a 3-week history of shortness of breath. He usually attends the gym daily. However, today he is breathless on climbing one flight of stairs. He has HIV and is on antiretroviral therapy, but he has been troubled by adverse effects and has missed many doses in the past few months. His observations

are temperature, 37.6°C; heart rate, 90 beats/min; respiratory rate, 16 breaths/min; blood pressure, 110/75 mmHg; and oxygen saturation, 98% on air at rest but 89% on climbing stairs. On examination, no added sounds are audible on auscultation.
What is the single most likely cause?

A Aspergillus fumigatus
B Cytomegalovirus
C Pneumocystis jirovecii
D Pseudomonas aeuruginosa
E Mycobacterium pneumoniae

9. A 26-year-old man has lost 12 kg over 4 months, unintentionally. He feels weak and tired, and has had night sweats on and off. His chest is clear on examination. Chest X-ray shows left upper lobe patchy consolidation with cavitation. He lives in London and works as a computer programmer. Originally from Pakistan, he moved to the UK 3 years ago.
What is the single most likely causative organism?

A Aspergillus fumigatus
B Klebsiella pneumoniae
C Mycobacterium bovis
D M. tuberculosis
E M. pneumoniae

10. A 50-year-old woman has a 4-month history of cough, weight loss and intermittent fevers. She has no permanent address, because she was recently released from prison and now resides in a homeless shelter. Her chest X-ray shows patchy shadowing in the right upper lobe. She has provided three sputum samples, which are negative for acid-fast bacilli. The samples have been sent for culture, but nothing is growing at week 2. A Mantoux test is positive.
What is the single most appropriate management?

A Admit the patient to hospital, with isolation in a negative-pressure room for at least 2 weeks while treatment is initiated with rifampicin and isoniazid
B Await the results of sputum culture before initiating any treatment
C Treat with a once daily regimen of rifampicin, ethambutol, pyrazinamide and isoniazid
D Treat with a once-daily regimen of rifampicin, ethambutol, pyrazinamide and moxifloxacin
E Treat with three times weekly directly observed therapy including rifampicin, ethambutol, pyrazinamide and isoniazid

11. A 16–year-old man lives with a relative with active pulmonary TB and inhales droplets containing M. tuberculosis. These reach the lungs and invade resident alveolar macrophages. Granulomas are formed and the infection is controlled leading to scarring in the right upper lobe with calcification. The man is not aware of this process and he does not receive treatment for latent TB.
Which is the single most accurate chance of reactivation of M. tuberculosis in later life?

A 0.5%
B 1%
C 5%
D 15%
E 50%

Chronic suppurative lung disease

1. A 55-year-old woman has had chronic daily sputum production for several years. She has recently had two episodes of haemoptysis, which prompted her to seek medical help. Computerised tomography (CT) shows marked cylindrical bronchiectasis localised to the left lower lobe. The rest of the lungs are normal. The patient is a non-smoker and does not remember any childhood respiratory infections. However, she did have an episode of severe pneumonia 8 years ago, which required admission to hospital for 10 days. She has no other medical problems other than osteoarthritis.
What is the single most likely cause of the bronchiectasis?

A Common variable immune deficiency
B Cystic fibrosis
C HIV infection
D Post-infective
E Primary ciliary dyskinesia

2. A couple have one child with cystic fibrosis and are planning a second pregnancy. The couple themselves are well and do not suffer from the disease. They seek advice and wish to know what the chances are of their next child also having cystic fibrosis.
What is the single best estimate of the likelihood of their next child having cystic fibrosis?

A 1 in 20
B 1 in 5
C 1 in 4
D 1 in 3
E 1 in 2

3. A 12-year-old girl has recurrent chest infections and chronic sputum production. She is underweight and has had significant amounts of time off school. Her doctor suspects she has cystic fibrosis.
What is the single best investigation to confirm the diagnosis?

A Arterial blood gas analysis
B CFTR gene mutation
C High resolution CT scan of the chest
D Sputum microscopy and culture
E Sweat chloride concentration

4. A 31-year-old man with primary ciliary dyskinesia has diffuse bronchiectasis with frequent exacerbations. He has severe disease and takes azithromycin 3 times weekly. He has an increase in sputum volume and change in colour, with fatigue.
Which is the single most likely organism to be isolated on sputum microscopy?

A *Candida albicans*
B *Haemophilus influenzae*
C *Legionella pneumophila*
D *Moraxella catarrhalis*
E *Pseudomonas aeruginosa*

Circulatory disorders

1. A 51-year-old woman has recently been on a transatlantic flight. She has a swollen left calf which is painful. She is a smoker of 30 pack years and previously had lung cancer which was resected with left upper lobectomy. Her observations are T: 36.9°C, HR: 110bpm, BP: 130/65, RR: 16 breaths/min, sats: 95% on air. Her Well's score is 7.5.
What is the single best investigation to perform?

A Coronary angiogram
B CTPA
C Echocardiogram
D HRCT
E *V/Q* scan

2. A 35-year-old woman with vitiligo and systemic sclerosis has become progressively breathless over 6 months. She is tired all the time and gets breathless on walking to work as a pastry chef. On examination she has a raised JVP and a parasternal heave but normal vesicular breath sounds with no added sounds. Initial investigations including a chest X-ray and ECG have not identified a cause.
What is the single best investigation to perform?

A Bubble echocardiogram
B CTPA
C Right heart catheterisation

D Myocardial perfusion scan
E Spirometry including lung volume

3. A 42-year-old woman has had a cough for 3 months and feels breathless when carrying her children or doing housework. She has been treated with two courses of antibiotics but symptoms persist. She is a non-smoker and works at home caring for triplets. A chest X-ray shows patchy consolidation of the right mid and lower zone. Blood tests show: Hb 10.5g/dL, WCC 5.7 x 10^9/L, neutrophils 3.8 x 10^9.L, urea 6.2mmol/L creatine 80 µmol/L, CRP 35mg/L. Urine dip shows: leucocytes +, nitrites - , blood ++, protein ++.
What is the single most likely diagnosis?

A Anti-glomerular basement membrane antibody disease
B Eosinophilic granulomatosis with polyangiitis
C Granulomatosis with polyangiitis
D Mixed connective tissue disease
E Systemic lupus erythematosus

4. A 70-year-old man has progressive breathlessness over several months on a background of severe chronic obstructive pulmonary disease (COPD). He has a non-productive cough. Chest X-ray shows oligaemic lung fields and cardiomegaly. No pulmonary emboli are visible on a computerised tomography pulmonary angiogram (CTPA). However, it does show enlarged pulmonary arteries and right ventricular hypertrophy.
What is the single most likely cause for the progressive breathlessness?

A Chronic thromboembolism
B Cor pulmonale
C Dilated cardiomyopathy
D Progression of COPD
E Pulmonary fibrosis

5. A 44-year-old woman has had a non-productive cough, fatigue, nasal congestion, nosebleeds and weight loss of 4 kg. She has had three episodes of small-volume haemoptysis in the past month. Examination is unremarkable. A urine dipstick shows microscopic haematuria and proteinuria. Computerised tomography of the chest shows multiple small nodules in both upper lobes, some of which show cavitation.
What is the single best diagnostic test for this condition?

A 24-h urine collection for protein
B Blood test for antineutrophil cytoplasmic antibody
C Full blood count to identify eosinophilia
D Positron emission tomography (PET) scan
E Renal biopsy

Respiratory emergencies

1. A 27-year-old woman has given birth to a healthy baby. However, 5 h later she has sudden onset of shortness of breath and left-sided sharp chest pain. Her observations are temperature, 37.4°C; heart rate, 130 beats/min; respiratory rate, 30 breaths/min; blood pressure, 85/45 mmHg; and oxygen saturation, 89% on air. There is no evidence of postpartum haemorrhage. She is given supplemental oxygen, and the medical and obstetric teams are called.
   What is the single clearest symptom or sign that this may be a massive pumonary embolism?

   A Breathlessness
   B Hypotension
   C Localised pleural rub on auscultation
   D Pleuritic chest pain
   E Tachycardia

2. A 67-year-old man with obesity hypoventilation syndrome is brought to hospital because of increasing confusion, drowsiness and some breathlessness. He was hypoxic when the ambulance arrived, and has been given 28% supplemental oxygen on his way to hospital. Chest X-ray shows right lower lobe consolidation and a small effusion. His Glasgow Coma Scale score is 14/15. Blood gases results are pH, 7.27; Pa_{O_2}, 7.1 kPa; Pa_{CO_2}, 12.5 kPa; and HCO_3^-, 32 mmol/L.
   What is the single most appropriate next step in management?

   A Bilevel positive airway pressure
   B Continuous positive airway pressure (CPAP)
   C Intravenous doxopram
   D Insertion of a chest drain
   E Intubation and invasive ventilation

3. A 17-year-old man with known asthma is brought to hospital by ambulance after becoming wheezy at college. He is unable to talk because of his breathlessness. His condition is deteriorating despite treatment with 15 L/min oxygen through a non-rebreathe mask, back-to-back salbutamol nebulisers, intravenous hydrocortisone and magnesium sulphate. His observations are temperature, 37.3°C; heart rate, 47 beats/min; respiratory rate, 10 breaths/min; blood pressure, 100/60 mmHg; and oxygen saturation, 94%. His Glasgow Coma Scale score is 9. Arterial blood gases results are pH, 7.32; pO_2, 9.7 kPa; pCO_2, 6.3 kPa; and HCO_3^-, 24 mmol/L. What is the single most appropriate next step in management?

   A Bilevel positive airway pressure
   B CPAP
   C Intravenous salbutamol
   D Intubation and invasive ventilation
   E Oropharyngeal airway adjunct

4. A 22-year-old woman falls off her bike on the way to work. When she gets to the office, she is not only shaken up but increasingly breathless. The breathlessness rapidly worsens, so she is taken to hospital. On arrival, her observations are temperature, 37.5°C; heart rate, 125 beats/min; respiratory rate, 30 breaths/min; blood pressure, 80/50 mmHg; and oxygen saturation, 90% on 6 L/min through a simple face mask. On examination, breath sounds are absent in the left hemithorax, and the trachea is deviated to the right. A tension pneumothorax is suspected.
   What is the single most appropriate location to insert a large-bore cannula?

   A Fourth intercostal space mid-axillary line
   B Fourth intercostal space mid-clavicular line
   C Second intercostal space anterior axillary line
   D Second intercostal space mid-axillary line
   E Second intercostal space mid-clavicular line

5. A 42-year-old woman has a postpartum haemorrhage. The bleeding is stopped in surgery and she is admitted to intensive care with the following results: T 37.3°C, BP 100/60mmHg, HR 130bpm, RR 22 breaths/min, Sats 98% intubated with Fi_{O_2} 0.4, Hb 5g/dL
   What is the single best intervention to give?

   A Fluid resuscitation using normal saline
   B Increase in Fi_{O_2} to 0.8
   C Increase in the PEEP delivered by the ventilator
   D Reduction of her heart rate using beta-blockers
   E Transfusion of packed red cells

6. A 60-year-old man has haemoptysis which he estimates at 250mL in the past 24 hours. He had TB in his 30s and received a full course of treatment. Otherwise he has had no respiratory problems and does not cough up sputum regularly. He has had 2 previous episodes of haemoptysis in the past year but these were smaller amounts. His weight is stable.
   What is the single most likely cause of his haemoptysis?

   A Aspergilloma
   B Arteriovenous malformation of the lung
   C Lung cancer
   D Pneumonia
   E Tuberculosis

SBA answers

Airway disease

1. B

The other answers are consistent with a life-threatening attack, but the inability to complete sentences is consistent with a severe but not life-threatening attack.

2. E

This patient has uncontrolled asthma. She is at step 1 in management. Therefore her treatment should be escalated to step 2: addition of regular preventer therapy in the form of an inhaled steroid.

Addition of an inhaled long-acting β_2 agonist would be step 3. Consideration of aminophylline would be step 4. Oral prednisolone would be step 5. Patients should be given home nebulisers for asthma only in highly selected cases.

3. D

This man has hypercapnoea. An increase in oxygen would further increase carbon dioxide retention. Evidence to support aminophylline as a treatment for a COPD exacerbation is lacking. Furthermore, aminophylline treatment would not address the hypercapnoea.

The patient needs non-invasive ventilation, because it delivers bilevel positive airway pressure. This aids the inspiratory phase and splints the airways open with a positive end-expiratory pressure to aid exhalation of carbon dioxide.

4. B

A patient with large airways obstruction would be expected to have reduced FEV_1 and reduced exercise tolerance. However, these are non-specific findings. Bronchiectasis can occur distal to the obstruction but again is non-specific. A wheeze is typical of small airways disease. In large airways obstruction, a monophonic stridor is typical.

A high Empey index score is characteristic of large airways obstruction. In this case, the cause may be a malignancy, as indicated by the haemoptysis. Urgent investigation is required.

5. B

The results of the pulmonary function tests confirm COPD. The history is consistent, and the spirometry results show an obstructive picture. This patient has a low symptom burden, a Medical Research Council breathlessness scale score of 2, and infrequent exacerbations. These features, in addition to the FEV_1 of 65%, mean that her condition is in the moderate severity category: group A (low risk and low symptom burden) on the GOLD classification. This knowledge will help guide treatment and predict prognosis.

6. A

There is little information available and a full history and examination would be required before any provisional diagnosis was given. However, the episodic pattern of breathlessness and her age makes asthma most likely. Ischaemic heart disease can cause intermittent short-lived dyspnoea but not cough and would be very unusual at this age. Cardiac failure and COPD are also very rare in the young and usually cause persisting dyspnoea. Pneumothorax is sudden onset and not episodic.

7. E

The history of dyspnoea is short and there are basal crepitations making COPD unlikely. Bronchiectasis is associated with a productive cough and the crepitations are usually coarse rather than fine. Pneumonia causes crepitations but there is usually a fever, the patient feels unwell and the crepitations are most often asymmetrical in their distribution. Pulmonary fibrosis and pulmonary oedema are both possible, but the more acute onset and the risk factors of smoking, diabetes and hypertension makes pulmonary oedema (due to ischaemic heart disease) more likely.

8. E

The superior thyroid vein drains the larynx and therefore metastatic spread would be most likely to occur via this vein. The bronchial veins drain the lungs, the pharyngeal venous plexus drains the pharynx and the pterygoid venous plexus drains the nose.

9. E

This man has COPD grade A. He does not require inhaled therapy unless he develops persistent symptoms or exacerbations. There is no suggestion that he has hypercapneoic respiratory failure so he does not need non-invasive ventilation. Oral prednisolone is used to treat exacerbations so is not required at present. Smoking cessation therapy will be the most effective treatment to prevent progression of COPD and improve symptoms of cough.

Interstitial lung disease

1. C

IPF is associated with finger clubbing in 15–25% of cases. Fine bibasal crepitations would be expected and the trachea would be central. Central cyanosis is usually seen in late stage disease rather than at diagnosis. IPF is a bilateral disease, so chest expansion is reduced bilaterally not unilaterally.

2. **B**

The characteristic findings are bibasal sub-pleural thickened intralobular septa, ground glass infiltration and honeycombing. Bilateral hilar lymphadenopathy is characteristic of sarcoidosis or tuberculosis. Patchy peripheral consolidation is seen in organising pneumonia. Nodular infiltrates with areas of coalescence and cavitation in an upper lobe distribution suggests pneumoconiosis. Upper lobe pre-dominant ground glass opacification with cysts is seen in hypersensitivity pneumonitis.

3. **B**

Episodic breathlessness, wheeze and cough that improve when not at work suggest exposure to an environmental agent, leading to hypersensitivity pneumonitis. Occupational asthma has a similar history but would not be associated with a restrictive pattern on spirometry or radiological abnormalities. Idiopathic pulmonary fibrosis and asbestosis would be more gradually progressive rather than episodic. Furthermore, neither occupa-tional asthma nor idiopathic pulmonary fibrosis would be expected in the patient's age group.

The antigen causing the patient's hyper-sensitivity pneumonitis needs to be identified so that he can take action to avoid it. Specific immunoglobulin G can then be tested.

4. **C**

Bilateral hilar lymphadenopathy is caused by tuberculosis, sarcoidosis or lymphoma. Sarcoidosis causes symmetrical hilar lymph-adenopathy; tuberculosis and lymphoma are usually asymmetrical. Sarcoidosis is more common in patients of African–Carribbean ethnicity. The lack of symptoms such as fever or weight loss makes tuberculosis less likely. The increased calcium concentration is also consistent with sarcoidosis. Further infor-mation, particularly to exclude lymphoma, would be obtained from a lymph node biopsy through endobronchial ultrasound.

5. **E**

The history of progressive dyspnoea and the examination findings of bibasal crepitations suggest IPF. IPF has a restrictive pattern on spirometry along with reduced lung volumes and a fall in transfer factor. Eosinophilia would indicate asthma, allergy, ABPA, vasculitis and pulmonary eosinophilia. Pleural effusions cause unilateral dull percussion note and decreased air entry rather than crepitations, and are only rarely associated with pulmonary fibrosis. A positive Mantoux test suggests previous exposure to tuberculosis.

6. **A**

Amiodarone is the only drug on the list that is known to cause pulmonary fibrosis. Azathio-prine is a possible treatment option for some forms of the disease.

7. **B**

Any patient under 65 years old with IPF who has failed pirfenidone should be considered for lung transplantation. This is independent of HRCT appearances and a fall in pulmonary function test values is an important trigger. Any patient with TLCO <40%, a fall of TLCO > 15% or FVC >10% in 6 months should be referred.

Sleep and ventilatory disorders

1. **A**

This patient has obesity hypoventilation syn-drome. As with other causes of hypoventilation it is rapidly identified by performing an arterial blood gas; this will show raised $PaCO_2$, a fall in PaO_2 and acidosis (i.e. a respiratory acidosis). CT scans of the brain and lungs will only show structural changes and although lung func-tion can show restrictive defects they cannot confirm physiological hypoventilation.

2. **E**

The patient has type 2 respiratory failure. Sev-eral neurological conditions affect the respira-tory muscles and put people at risk of this, including Guillain–Barré syndrome and motor neurone disease. In this case, the patient has a known chronic neurological condition. Therefore the answer must be motor neurone disease, because Guillain–Barré syndrome presents acutely.

3. **B**

This patient has severe obstructive sleep apnoea. This diagnosis is based on the results of the sleep study. He is a danger to himself and to others if he drives, because he could fall asleep at the wheel.

In the UK, those with a group 2 licence (to drive lorries, buses and other public vehicles) must inform the DVLA of their diagnosis and must not drive until successfully treated. This means they must have a sleep study on CPAP, be compliant with CPAP and be assessed by a physician who says they are now treated. They can then continue their job.

4. **A**

Polysomnography is the best investigation for OSA and an AHI of 18 indicates moder-ate severity. Patients may have ECG changes including right heart strain but this not diagnostic. Hyperexpanded lung fields and flattened diaphragms on chest X-ray indicate COPD which may co-exist with OSA but is a separate disease process. A high Mallampati score is 3 often seen in OSA but is not diagnostic. A sawtooth pattern on overnight oximetry is typical for OSA but is not as reliable as a polysomnography, and without an AHI index is not diagnostic.

Pleural disease

1. **D**

    The most likely diagnosis is primary spontaneous pneumothorax. Therefore a chest X-ray is needed to confirm this.

    There is no evidence of a tension pneumothorax, so insertion of a cannula would be premature. LMWH would be the treatment for pulmonary embolus, for which CTPA would be the investigation; however, this diagnosis is unlikely. Ibuprofen would be an appropriate treatment for costochondritis, which would cause pain but not decreased air entry.

2. **D**

    The patient's history suggests a number of possible causes for the pleural effusion. The pleural fluid results show that it is an exudate, which rules out heart failure, liver cirrhosis and nephrotic syndrome, all of which lead to transudates. There is no indication of tuberculosis from the history.

    The fact that the patient has had breast cancer makes malignancy (metastatic breast cancer) the most likely answer. The results of cytological investigations will be informative as it is very likely to show metastatic breast cancer cells in the pleural fluid.

3. **B**

    The loculations on ultrasound and the pleural fluid results, particularly the low pH, indicate that this is not a simple pleural effusion but an empyema. Several of the answers are reasonable in this situation. Advice from a microbiologist may help guide antibiotic choice, but most hospitals have standard guidance on empirical first-line choices. Computerised tomography of the chest may be helpful, but the findings would not change the immediate management plan. Diuretics are inappropriate in the context of sepsis; they would be useful only if the effusion were caused by cardiac failure. Referral to a cardiothoracic surgeon is premature.

    The most important action is to insert a chest drain to remove the infected fluid. Also, a prolonged course of an appropriate antibiotic (e.g. co-amoxiclav) should be started.

4. **B**

    This patient has a secondary spontaneous pneumothorax, because there is evidence of underlying lung disease (chronic obstructive pulmonary disease) from the pulmonary function tests. The pneumothorax is small, but nonetheless the patient is very breathless and hypoxaemic due to the severe underlying lung disease. Therefore intervention is required; in this case, a chest drain. Aspiration is appropriate only in primary and not in secondary spontaneous pneumothorax.

5. **A**

    The cause of the effusion is most likely to be heart failure. Therefore the aspirated pleural fluid should be a transudate (protein, < 25 g/L), with normal glucose (> 3.3 mmol/L), normal pH (> 7.2) and normal LDH pleura:serum ratio (< 0.6).

6. **C**

    Large bullae or a pneumothorax would lead to increased resonance. Obesity would not be expected to cause unilateral signs. Pneumonectomy and pleural effusion would both be possible, but in the absence of a scar pleural effusion is the most likely.

7. **A**

    Pleural plaques are caused by asbestos and identify patients who have had significant asbestos exposure in the past, usually during their occupation. Mesothelioma is a possible cause of pleural thickening but is more often associated with an effusion. Lung adenocarcinoma can also cause malignant effusions and pleural thickening, but adenocarcinoma and mesothelioma are progressive and usually cause significant chest wall pain and/or dyspnoea. Chronic aspergillosis and non-tuberculous mycobacteria infections are rare causes of pleural thickening and usually affect the lung apices.

8. **B**

    The pleural fluid results show a transudate. Hypothyroidism is a possibility but nothing from the history suggests this as a cause. Cardiac failure is a common cause of pleural effusions and can cause unilateral as well as bilateral effusions. Her history of hypertension is important and the fact that she is on 3 agents suggests it has been difficult to control. She is also a smoker so heart disease is the most likely.

9. **C**

    There is a change in pressure within the pleural cavity with inspiration and expiration, and therefore movement of the column of fluid in the drain, suggesting it is correctly sited in the pleural space. Since it is in the correct place, the lack of bubbling suggests that the pneumothorax has resolved.

10. D

Following the first aspiration he still has a large pneumothorax and is still symptomatic so any options that do not involve an additional intervention are incorrect. Repeating the aspiration could be considered but is unlikely to be successful and a chest drain is more appropriate. The size of the cannula used is not important; 16 or 18 gauge will be fine and the fact that 2.4L was aspirated shows the first attempt was successful to some degree.

Malignancy

1. E

This man's symptoms result from hypercalcaemia caused by parathyroid hormone-like protein released from a lung cancer. This is a paraneoplastic syndrome. The other options may explain some but not all of the symptoms.

2. C

Patients with COPD are at increased risk of lung cancer. Any patient's concerns should be taken seriously. A cough lasting 2 weeks would not be unusual in a patient with COPD, but a new cough lasting > 3 weeks should prompt consideration of referral in any patient. Bilateral end expiratory wheeze is a typical finding in COPD, and two exacerbations in a month is not necessarily concerning. An infection that fails to resolve despite appropriate treatment sometimes indicates obstruction to a bronchus from a cancer. Nausea is a non-specific finding possibly caused by a gastrointestinal problem or anxiety.

The lack of weight loss is reassuring. However, a hoarse voice is a red flag symptom. It could indicate recurrent laryngeal nerve palsy caused by a left hilar cancer. Therefore this symptom should prompt a chest X-ray and urgent referral to a chest physician.

3. A

In non-smokers, especially women, adenocarcinoma is the most common type of cancer. Adenocarcinomas are usually peripheral and grow slowly.

Bronchoalveolar carcinoma would also be possible, but this is much rarer. Small-cell lung cancers are usually central and metastasise early, often to mediastinal lymph nodes. Squamous cell carcinomas are much more common in smokers. These cancers usually arise from the bronchi and are therefore central. Lymphoma may affect young non-smokers, but if present in the lung parenchyma would be a

metastasis. Lymph node involvement would usually be visible.

4. C

This is a tricky question, so do not worry if unsure of the answer! Cytological analysis of sputum and bronchoscopy with bronchoalveolar lavage could provide a diagnosis but only in a minority of cases. Bronchoscopy would not reach a peripheral tumour. Therefore endobronchial biopsy of the primary mass is not possible. Video-assisted thoracoscopic surgery is occasionally used to biopsy most lung masses but is an operation; the vast majority of potential lung cancers are confirmed by less invasive biopsy methods.

The best answer is endobronchial ultrasound sampling of the mediastinal nodes. The results of this procedure will both provide a pathological diagnosis and help stage the tumour. The primary mass is peripheral and therefore accessible by CT-guided biopsy. However, the procedure would not determine whether or not the enlarged nodes are infiltrated with cancer or are reactive.

5. A

The primary tumour is 2–3 cm, which makes it T1a. In this case, the lack of nodal involvement makes in N0. There are no metastases, so it is M0.

6. D

This tumour is potentially curable, because the patient has good lung function and a good performance status (PS 0). Surgical resection provides the best chance of a cure; lobectomy is sufficient to give the required resection margin to ensure a low chance of recurrence. Pneumonectomy would have no additional benefit. It is not the best option, because the patient would have much less residual lung capacity, leaving him more disabled. Chemotherapy and chemoradiotherapy are offered for later stage cancers.

7. C

This tumour is incurable. Any radical treatment would be ineffective, so none is offered. Furthermore, the patient's performance status is poor. He should be offered palliative radiotherapy to the tumour encasing his right main bronchus. This option could reduce or stop the haemoptysis as well as perhaps prevent total lung collapse caused by obstruction. The overall aim of management is to prevent unnecessary hospital admissions and improve the quality of the patient's remaining life.

8. C

Pleural fluid analysis shows that the effusion is an exudate. However, all the answers would cause an exudate, so this finding is not especially helpful. The smoking history suggests lung cancer, but no parenchymal mass is visible on chest X-ray. The absence of a mass does not rule out metastatic lung cancer, but it does make the diagnosis less likely.

The occupational history, particularly of working in the automobile industry and the construction industry, suggests the possibility of exposure to asbestos. Mesothelioma is also more likely because of the pain, the blood-stained nature of the pleura fluid and the high protein but normal LDH.

9. C

A hoarse voice is a result of recurrent laryngeal nerve palsy and therefore left-sided node involvement. Chest wall pain would result from chest wall involvement from a peripheral tumour. Dilated veins over the chest wall would be from superior vena cava obstruction. Stridor is caused by major airway obstruction. Weight loss is often associated with metastatic spread but does not provide clues as to where the metastases are located.

10. D

Squamous cell carcinoma accounts for 30% of lung cancers and is the most likely type to cavitate. Squamous cell carcinomas sometimes produce parathyroid hormone-like protein leading to hypercalcaemia and symptoms such as lethargy, polyuria and constipation. Small cell carcinomas are more likely to be associated with SIADH or Cushing's syndrome as a paraneoplastic syndrome.

11. B

This patient is no longer able to carry out all normal activities, but remains ambulatory and able to carry out non-strenuous activities. She is therefore WHO performance status 1.

Lung infections

1. E

This man has community-acquired pneumonia. All the bacteria listed are possible causes, but by far the most common is *Strept. pneumoniae*. *H. influenzae* is also a common cause of exacerbation of chronic obstructive pulmonary disease, but this would not cause new focal crepitations.

2. D

This patient is hypoxic because of community-acquired pneumonia. She needs oxygen therapy. There is no justification for withholding treatment while awaiting the results for arterial blood gases. She is not in extremis, so high-flow oxygen is unnecessary and may have adverse consequences (e.g. masking a

deterioration). Oxygen through nasal cannula at 6 L/min is likely to be uncomfortable and dry the nasal mucosa. At this point, there is no indication for non-invasive ventilation. A Venturi mask gives accurate delivery of a given FiO_2. Use of the mask is likely to bring her saturations into the target range of 94–98%. Regular review is, of course, necessary.

3. D

This patient has hospital-acquired pneumonia. Hospital-acquired pneumonia is caused by several bacteria, including *Staph. aureus*, which can also cause multifocal cavitation. Anyone with rib fractures is at high risk of pneumonia, because pain prevents coughing and clearance of sputum. Cavitation occurs in tuberculosis, but this presentation is too acute. Also, there are no reasons to suspect that she is at risk of tuberculosis. Influenza A, *L. pneumophila* and *Strept. pneumoniae* cause community-acquired pneumonia but are rarer causes of hospital-acquired pneumonia.

4. B

Most respiratory pathogens are gram positive cocci. E. coli is a gram negative bacillus which is an unusual cause of community acquired pneumonia but a much more common cause of ventilator associated pneumonia.

5. A

This man has an upper respiratory tract infection, probably a rhinovirus (the 'common cold') or influenza. No features on examination suggest pneumonia, which would require assessment in hospital and antibiotics. Taking a nasal pharyngeal aspirate and throat swabs may confirm a virus but would not change management and are therefore unnecessary. Therefore the most appropriate action is to advise fluid, rest and analgesia.

6. B

The history suggests an acute problem, complicating the patient's COPD. Malignancy is unlikely to present acutely. The mild fever makes infection likely.

The X-ray shows many features of COPD, but the relevant finding for the acute presentation is the loss of the right heart border. This localises the pathology to the right middle lobe and makes right middle lobe pneumonia the correct answer. The decreased lung markings are likely to be bullae. These can be confused for pneumothorax and in some cases CT chest is required to differentiate them.

7. B

This patient scores 1 for age > 65 and 1 for urea > 7 mmol/L, giving her a CURB-65 score of 2 and an estimated mortality of 13%. An abbreviated mental test of 9/10 is not low enough to suggest confusion. She should be admitted to hospital.

8. **C**

The diagnosis of HIV and non-concordance with antiretroviral therapy make it extremely likely that this patient is immunocompromised. Therefore he is at risk from infection with unusual organisms, including fungi and viruses. The characteristic findings of a progressive history of breathlessness over a few weeks and desaturation on exercise despite normal saturations at rest make *Pneumocystis* pneumonia (caused by *P. jirovecii*) the most likely cause. *Pneumocystis* pneumonia is an AIDS-defining illness. Therefore the patient will need care from the HIV specialist team as well as the respiratory team.

9. **D**

The subacute presentation of weight loss and night sweats, with patchy consolidation and cavitation on X ray in a patient from a high-risk demographic group is characteristic for tuberculosis. *Pseudomonas* and *Aspergillus* both cause subacute lung infection but are less likely, especially if the patient is not immuno-compromised.

10. **E**

This patient probably has tuberculosis. The sputum cultures are likely to eventually come back positive for M. tuberculosis, but this takes at least 3–4 weeks. Treatment should be started before the culture results. The patient is relatively well and is smear-negative (her sputum is negative for alcohol- and acid-fast bacilli). Therefore she is unlikely to infect others; there is no reason to admit her to hospital, even though she lives in shared accommodation. Her housemates need to be contacted to determine whether one of them is the source of her infection and identify any that have caught the disease from her.

In the UK, about 7% of isolates are isoniazid-resistant (mainly in London). However, a standard regimen should be used until sensitivities are known. The patient has risk factors for poor adherence, including homelessness. Therefore she requires treatment under a directly observed therapy regimen three times weekly. Part of her care should be to facilitate securing a fixed address and access to state benefits.

11. **C**

Without additional factors such as HIV or other forms of immunocompromise the average rate of reactivation is 5%.

Chronic suppurative lung disease

1. **D**

Primary ciliary dyskinesia and cystic fibrosis cause bilateral bronchiectasis with other associated features from childhood, and are unlikely to present in a 55-year-old. Common variable immunodeficiency would also cause bilateral disease and is often associated with other infections (e.g. sinusitis and upper respiratory tract infection). An HIV test should be done, but HIV is unlikely to be the cause of focal bronchiectasis.

Symptoms of bronchiectasis dating from an episode of pneumonia, but not before, combined with CT evidence of focal rather than diffuse disease, suggest that the bronchiectasis was caused by the pneumonia damaging the bronchi.

2. **C**

Cystic fibrosis is an autosomal recessive inherited disease. Both parents are carriers, and each has a 50% chance of passing the affected gene to a future child. Therefore each child has a 1 in 4 chance of being affected by the disease, and a 1 in 2 chance of being a carrier.

3. **B**

Sweat chloride concentration is a test for CF and is likely to be one of the first tests in the investigation of the condition but genetic testing for a CFTR mutation is essential to confirm the diagnosis. High resolution will show evidence of bronchiectasis but is not specific for CF. Sputum microscopy is likely to isolate typical organisms such as P. aeruginosa but is not specific. Arterial blood gas analysis will not confirm the diagnosis but may reveal respiratory failure in the later stages of disease.

4. **E**

The common infecting organisms in bronchiectasis in mild disease include H. influenza, S. pneumoniae and M. catarrhalis. P. aeruginosa is isolated in severe disease. Neither C. albicans or L. pneumophila are specifically associated with bronchiectasis.

Circulatory disorders

1. **B**

Pulmonary angiography is the gold standard for diagnosis of PE but is invasive and not routinely available at most hospitals. V/Q scan is an excellent test for PE and is a lower radiation dose, but may be indeterminate, particularly in those with underlying lung disease. In massive or submassive PE an echocardiogram will show RV strain, but it is not a routine diagnostic test for PE. HRCT does not involve contrast and will not reveal filling defects in the pulmonary arteries; it is a test for abnormalities of the lung parenchyma not the vasculature.

2. **C**

The most likely diagnosis is primary pulmonary hypertension. A right heart catheterisation is the only investigation that will conclusively confirm the diagnosis. A CTPA can exclude pulmonary emboli and show enlarged pulmonary vessels and right ventricle, and any evidence of a chronic lung disease. Spirometry including lung volumes will also determine whether there is an underlying obstructive or restrictive chronic lung disease. An echocardiogram is a screening test for pulmonary hypertension and can identify raised right-sided pressures, right ventricular hypertrophy and tricuspid regurgitation, but it is not as sensitive or specific a test as right heart catheterisation. A bubble echocardiogram is used to look for right to left shunts. A myocardial perfusion scan is a test for ischaemic heart disease.

3. **C**

This woman has a condition which mimics pneumonia but has not responded to antibiotics. Her urine dip shows a nephritic picture due to the presence of blood and protein. This suggests a form of vasculitis, the most likely of which is GPA. Anti-GBM is also possible but less likely than GPA. There is no eosinophilia and no wheezing so EPA is less likely; renal involvement also does not typically occur in EPA. MCTD would include joint involvement and would be unlikely to cause a nephritic picture.

4. **B**

The examination and imaging findings show pulmonary hypertension and right ventricular failure in association with COPD; this condition is known as cor pulmonale. Chronic thromboembolism can lead to pulmonary hypertension. However, in this case there is no evidence of pulmonary embolism on the CTPA.

5. **E**

The diagnosis is granulomatosis with polyangiitis (previously known as Wegener's syndrome). Antineutrophil cytoplasmic antibody is likely to be increased, but this finding is not specific for granulomatosis with polyangiitis, and a confirmed diagnosis needs histological investigation.

A biopsy is required. The kidneys are affected (indicated by the haematuria and proteinuria), so a renal biopsy is highly likely to be diag-

nostic. Eosinophilia is commonly found in a different vasculitis, eosinophilic granulomatosis with polyangiitis (previously known as Churg–Strauss syndrome).

Respiratory emergencies

1. **B**

The history is consistent with a postpartum pulmonary embolus, probably from the pelvic veins. All the answers would be expected in pulmonary embolism. However, hypotension is the only one that indicates that this is a massive pulmonary embolism and therefore an emergency.

2. **A**

This patient has type 2 respiratory failure precipitated by community-acquired pneumonia on a background of obesity hypoventilation syndrome. Doxapram should be used only rarely as a temporary measure when non-invasive ventilation is unavailable.

The patient needs bilevel positive airway pressure, not CPAP, to enhance oxygenation and remove carbon dioxide. He has only a small effusion, so drainage would not reverse the respiratory acidosis. Intubation and invasive ventilation are the next steps if non-invasive ventilation fails to improve his condition.

3. **D**

This patient has a life-threatening asthma attack, indicated by the bradycardia, feeble respiratory effort, low Glasgow Coma Scale score and slightly increased $Paco_2$. $Paco_2$ is usually decreased in less severe asthma caused by hyperventilation. The patient is at risk of death and needs urgent intubation and invasive ventilation on an intensive care unit to give time for treatment to reduce the severe bronchoconstriction.

Bilevel positive airway pressure and CPAP would only delay intubation in a patient whose condition is highly unstable and who needs invasive ventilation. These interventions are not used to treat asthma. An oropharyngeal airway adjunct should be considered when the airway is compromised. In this case, the problem is bronchoconstriction and fatigue. Intravenous salbutamol is rarely used in this situation but should be in addition to, not instead of, intubation.

4. **E**

The second intercostal space in the mid-clavicular line is the most effective and safest location to insert a cannula to decompress a tension pneumothorax. A portable chest X-ray should be done once the patient's condition has been stabilised. A chest drain should then be inserted.

5. E

In this case the major problem is a lack of oxygen binding sites due to a low Hb. The oxygen content of the blood has fallen despite the Po_2 and saturations being normal levels. Fluid resuscitation with normal saline is a good idea as it will increase cardiac output, but this is a holding mechanism only until packed red cells are transfused. Increasing the Fio_2 will increase the amount of oxygen dissolved in plasma but this will have a small effect on oxygen delivery.

Increase in PEEP and reduction of heart rate will not increase oxygen delivery to the tissues.

6. A

Pneumonia is unlikely to cause major haemoptysis (>200 mL in 24 hours). Chronic sputum production or previous infections would be expected in bronchiectasis. Lung cancer is possible but less likely in the absence of weight loss, and would usually have progressed and caused additional symptoms if it had been causing haemoptysis for a year. TB reactivation would cause weight loss and progress quicker than a year.

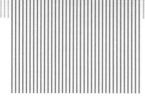

Index

Note: Page numbers in **bold** or *italic* refer to tables or figures, respectively.

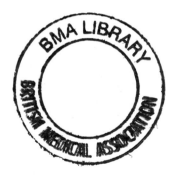